DIABETIC
COOKBOOK

800+ Days with Easy and Tasty Recipes Suitable for
Type 2 Diabetes and Prediabetes. 6-Week Healthy
Meal Plan Included to Help You Stay on Track!

OLIVIA PETERSON

TABLE OF CONTENTS

INTRODUCTION

Diabetes is a very serious disease that affects how your body converts food into energy. Most of the food you eat is used to produce glucose, which is then released into your bloodstream. Your pancreas is in charge of controlling your blood sugar. When blood sugar rises, it sends a signal to generate insulin. Insulin acts like a key that allows blood sugar to enter cells and be used as energy. Having diabetes can mean that you do not produce enough insulin, or the amount of insulin your body produces is not being used efficiently. When your body is not producing enough insulin or when your cells stop responding to insulin, a high amount of blood sugar remains in your bloodstream.

You must be aware of all the symptoms and early warning signs that come with this health condition if you have diabetes, or if you are at risk for developing diabetes. Living a healthy lifestyle can help avoid diabetes in the long run, especially if it runs in your family.

Simple lifestyle changes can also help you avoid or reverse prediabetes. Changes such as eating healthier food, exercising more frequently, and losing weight if you're overweight can make all the difference. Some programs can also assist you with making permanent healthy changes in your life, such as the CDC-led National Diabetes Prevention Program.

Diabetes does not have a cure. If you don't take care of yourself, you may develop more serious health problems such as heart disease, vision loss, or kidney disease. You must take your medication and attend all healthcare appointments to reduce the impact of diabetes on your life. You can also receive diabetes self-management education and support, which can help you take care of yourself better.

Knowing that you, your child, or someone you love has diabetes can be painful and shocking. However, you should know that there are several things you can do that can help manage the condition. Even with diabetes, you can live a normal life and go about your daily activities - as long as you know to be properly prepared for an insulin emergency.

Having diabetes does not mean that you can't still reach your highest life goals. There are many Olympic athletes, football players, actors, politicians, and others who have diabetes - and it never stopped them from achieving their goals. They live a healthy lifestyle that helps them manage diabetes and if you do the same, you can thrive. Bringing physical activity into your daily routine and eating healthier is the best way to manage this condition. This is why we created this book: to help you manage your diabetes and thrive in life.

Living With Diabetes

It can be very troubling to learn that you or a family member has diabetes. Not only might you become concerned, but your entire family might, too. You may have so many questions. How much are medical bills? What can happen when you're not at home? Where can you get appropriate medical care? You might find yourself suddenly feeling like you're carrying the weight of the entire world on your shoulders. Be careful not to overthink; don't believe for a second that your life is over or that you will only be remembered as "sickly." This is not the case. You are not alone. Many approaches exist that can help you and your family manage diabetes and help you live a happy, long, and healthy life.

VISIT A HEALTHCARE PROFESSIONAL

When you or a someone you love is diagnosed with diabetes, you may be at a loss wondering where to begin. Living with a medical condition can be extremely difficult, but you should know that many people can help you. Consult a doctor about what you can do to stay safe and healthy. Inquire about various diets and lifestyle changes you may need to make.

Make contact with any friends or family members who have been affected by this disease. Talk to people on the internet who are going through similar experiences. You are now officially a member of a worldwide community, and reaching out for help and support is the first step toward your new, healthy life.

Increase your Physical Activity

Physical activity is essential for diabetes management. You must try to be as active as possible. You don't have to spend two hours every day at the gym; simply engaging in 30 minutes or more of moderate physical activity for the majority of the week can make a big difference. Increased physical activity can help you drastically lower your blood glucose, cholesterol, and blood sugar levels. Exercise can also improve your mood, self-esteem, and sleep quality while reducing stress and anxiety. Increasing your physical activity can also help strengthen your muscles and bones.

If your doctor recommends that you lose weight, aim for at least an hour of physical activity most days of the week. It may seem to be a lot at first, but you can divide it over the course of the day in small segments of 10-15 minutes.

Improving your resistance is also strongly advised, particularly if you have diabetes. You can consult with an exercise physiologist who can help create a safe resistance exercise program for you. Make it a habit to engage in resistance training at least twice a week. Push-ups, squats, and lunges are examples of resistance exercises. If you want to exercise at home, you can also use dumbbells and resistance bands. Lifting, carrying, or digging during household chores can also boost your resistance. If you have the time and money, you can also join a gym and do weightlifting and other resistance exercises.

To increase your physical activity, you must also limit the amount of time you spend sitting at work or home. You can incorporate physical activity into the day by making simple changes such as taking the stairs instead of the elevator or parking further away from work so you can walk there. You can also take your dog, children, or grandchildren for a walk in the park. You can do your housework while watching television. You can also get off the bus one stop earlier and walk the rest of the way. There are numerous ways to incorporate physical activity into your daily routine. You don't need to join a gym; simply altering your activities will suffice.

Learn About Diabetes Support Programs

Diabetes is not something you can turn off when it is convenient for you. It must be managed 24 hours a day, seven days a week. If your child has diabetes, look into diabetes support programs that can assist your child in managing their diabetes throughout the day. Since you cannot always be with them while they are at school or participating in school activities such as field trips, summer camps, and recreational activities, they must learn how to act in case of an emergency.

Under federal law, students with diabetes have the same right as any other child to receive the care they need to stay safe and participate in school activities. With this, you should ensure that your child's school provides staff who have been trained in blood sugar (glucose) monitoring and insulin and glucagon administration, as well as staff who have been trained to provide diabetes care on field trips, at extracurricular events, and at all school-sponsored activities. In addition, your child must be able to manage their diabetes independently at any time and any location.

As a result, the schools where your children attend should be able to assist in managing your child's diabetes. You should not be required to go to the school in order to care for your child's diabetes. Along with that, your child should not be moved to a different school to receive necessary diabetes care, nor should they be barred from participating in school-sponsored activities.

Talk About It

It is perfectly normal to initially focus on the physical aspects of diabetes. However, you must manage the emotional aspects of it as well. Discussing your fears and frustrations, as well as your future goals, can be extremely beneficial. You should be aware that being open to discussing your health condition can help you manage it better.

If your child has diabetes, be aware that their emotions may shift as they grow. You should reassure your child that they have someone to talk to so that diabetes does not become a complete hindrance in their life. Share as much as you can with them, whether you talk about other family members or people you know who are going through the same thing as them. If you get stuck, you can seek the assistance of professionals who can assist you in identifying the emotions and fears that your child may be experiencing. This can also help the entire family express themselves more effectively.

Plan Ahead

Diabetes need not prevent you from living your life. It will go on regardless. Having said that, you must be prepared for any situation that may arise in the future. You can keep yourself prepared by doing the following:

- Before leaving the house to go on a trip, check with your doctor to ensure that your medications are up to date. In addition, you should obtain written prescriptions for insulin and other medications in case they are misplaced or you run out. A doctor's letter with treatment instructions should also be included.
- If you're looking for babysitters for your kids, consider hiring teenagers from diabetic families like yours. Since they are used to experiencing situations like yours, these teenagers will most likely know what to do in an emergency.
- When planning a party or holiday, contact the restaurant or location ahead of time to see what food is available. This is to ensure that you are still adhering to the meal plan prescribed by your dietitian. You can also notify party hosts ahead of time so that they are aware of what you or your child can and cannot eat.

Diabetes can have a significant impact on a person's life, but it is not always detrimental. While your options may be limited, diabetes allows you to be more conscious of what you put in your body and how you treat it. This book will go over the basics of diabetes, such as the different types, symptoms, risk factors, and ways to live with it.

CHAPTER 1: DIABETES AND ITS TYPES

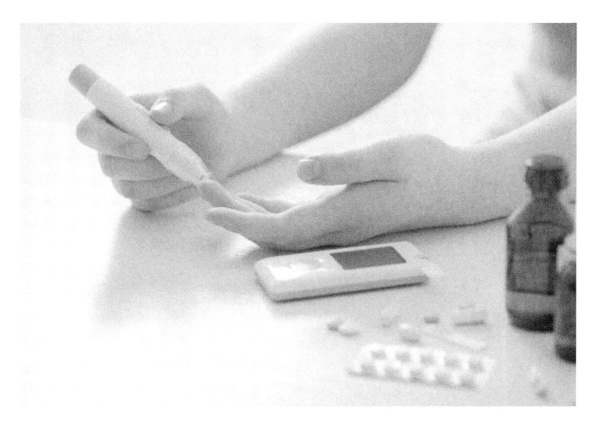

Diabetes is categorized into three types: type 1, type 2 , and gestational diabetes, which can develop in a mother during pregnancy. Aside from the three major types, some people may also develop prediabetes, a condition in which someone's blood sugar levels are greater than normal but not high enough to be diagnosed with type 2 diabetes.

TYPE 1 DIABETES

Experts believe that type 1 diabetes occurs when the body mistakenly attacks itself, preventing the body from producing the insulin that is needed to lower blood sugar levels. Type 1 diabetes affects approximately 5-10% of people with diabetes.

Increased thirst, increased urination, extreme hunger, fatigue, and blurred vision are some of the common symptoms of untreated type 1 diabetes. Type 1 diabetes symptoms may appear gradually or relatively suddenly.

To live with type 1 diabetes, a person must take insulin on a daily basis. It is unknown how to prevent type 1 diabetes, and the risk factors are not as clear as they are for type 2 diabetes and prediabetes. However, some known risk factors for type 1 diabetes are as follows:

- If you have a family member with type 1 diabetes
- Being at the age when type 1 diabetes most commonly occurs (anyone can develop type 1 diabetes regardless of age, but it is most common in children, teenagers, or young adults)

TYPE 2 DIABETES

Type 2 diabetes is not the same as type 1. When you have type 2 diabetes, your body does not use the insulin it produces efficiently, meaning that it cannot maintain normal blood sugar levels. Type 2 diabetes affects approximately 90-95% of people who have diabetes. It usually takes many years to develop and is most common in adults, but it is becoming more visible in children, teenagers, and young adults nowadays.

Type 2 diabetes may not reveal symptoms at first, which is why it is critical to have your blood sugar tested if you are at risk. It can be avoided or delayed by making healthy lifestyle changes such as increasing physical activity and eating healthier foods. The following are known type 2 diabetes risk factors:

- Presence of prediabetes
- Being overweight
- Age 45 years old or older
- Someone with type 2 diabetes is in your family
- Not being physically active
- You had gestational diabetes or given birth to a baby weighing over 9 pounds
- Being diagnosed with non-alcoholic fatty liver disease

GESTATIONAL DIABETES

Gestational Diabetes can develop in pregnant women even if the woman has no history of diabetes or prediabetes. The baby may be more vulnerable to developing the condition if the mother had gestational diabetes.

It usually resolves itself after your baby is born, but it does increase your chances of developing type 2 diabetes later in life. Your baby may also develop health problems such as obesity as a child or adolescent, and they are more likely to develop type 2 diabetes later in life. You may be at risk of developing gestational diabetes while pregnant if you have any of the following characteristics:

- Gestational diabetes was present in a previous pregnancy
- Had a baby weighing more than 9 pounds
- Are overweight
- Are over the age of 25
- Have a family member with type 2 diabetes
- Have been diagnosed with polycystic ovary syndrome (PCOS)
- Are of African American, Hispanic/Latino American, American Indian, Alaska Native, Native Hawaiian, or Pacific Islander descent

If you lose weight, eat healthier, and exercise regularly before becoming pregnant, you might be able to avoid gestational diabetes. While gestational diabetes is not permanent, the mother and baby may be at a high risk of developing type 2 diabetes later in life.

PREDIABETES

Prediabetes is very common, particularly in the United States. It affects about 88 million adults, or more than one-third of all adults. Most people are unaware that they have prediabetes.

Prediabetes is defined as having blood sugar levels that are greater than normal but not quite high enough to be classified as type 2 diabetes. If you have prediabetes, you are more likely to develop type 2 diabetes. The risks of other health issues like heart disease and stroke are also increased. The good news is that prediabetes can often be reversed if you make the necessary lifestyle changes. You may be at a high risk of developing prediabetes if any of the following applies:

- You are overweight
- You are over the age of 45 years
- A member of your family has type 2 diabetes
- You are not physically active
- You had gestational diabetes during a pregnancy
- You had a baby weighing more than 9 pounds
- You are of African American, Hispanic/Latino American, American Indian, Alaska Native, Asian American, or Pacific Islander descent

CHAPTER 2: CREATING A DIABETIC DIET

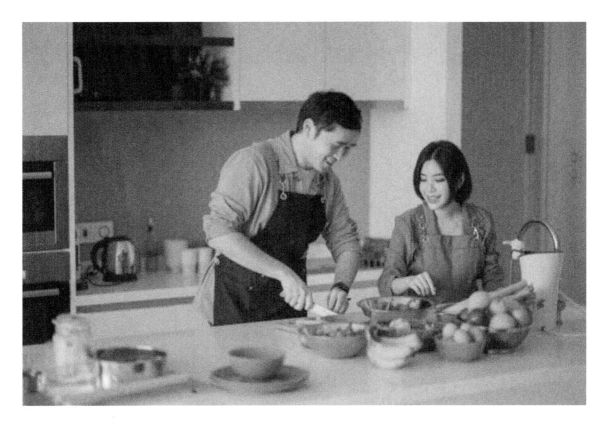

Your doctor may advise you to consult a registered dietitian if you are diagnosed with diabetes or prediabetes. Most dietitians will recommend that you go on a diabetic diet, and they can also help you develop a healthy eating plan that is perfect for you and your needs. A personalized eating plan can help you control your blood sugar levels, manage your weight, and reduce risk factors for heart disease.

A diabetic diet consists of three regular meals per day. This allows you to make better use of the insulin your body produces or that you obtain through medication. A registered dietitian can create eating plans that are designed for your specific health goals, preferences, and lifestyle. They can also give you advice on how to improve your eating habits, such as how to control your portions to ensure they are appropriate for your weight and activity level.

Eating too many calories and fat can lead to a rise in blood sugar. If this is not controlled, you may develop serious health issues such as diabetic retinopathy, nephropathy, macrovascular problems, and more. Additional long-term complications such as nerve, kidney, and heart damage may also occur. It's critical that you are aware of what you are putting into your body. Make healthy food choices and keep track of your eating habits to keep your blood sugar levels within a safe range.

BASIC GUIDELINES FOR A DIABETIC DIET

A healthy eating plan can be very beneficial if you have diabetes. If you choose to follow one, consider the following:

- Throughout the day, eat at regular intervals.
- Include vegetables in every meal. Do your best to fill half of your plate with vegetables that are not starchy.
- Make the size of your meals and snacks smaller.
- Include a small serving of carbohydrates that are high in fiber with every meal. Examples include brown rice, potatoes, whole grain bread, and whole grain pasta.
- Choose low-fat dairy products. Try to look for some that do not have a lot of added sugar.
- Consider different lean meats and alternatives such as skinless chicken and turkey, fish, eggs, and tofu.

- Decrease the amount of saturated fats in your food by limiting things like butter, processed meats, and fried foods. You can replace these with healthier options such as olive, canola, or sunflower oil, avocados, and unprocessed lean meats.
- Be sure to include oily fish in your diet such as salmon, sardines, and tuna at least two or three times per week.
- Only eat sweets on rare occasions.
- Avoid candies and sweet drinks.
- Limit your intake of salt and any foods that are overly salty.
- Consider using different herbs and spices to ensure your food does not taste bland.
- Limit alcohol consumption.

RECOMMENDED FOODS

If you have diabetes, you must learn to be more conscious of the foods you eat. It may seem difficult at first; however, you'll discover that living a healthy lifestyle is far more rewarding in the long run. Going on a diabetic diet does not mean you have to eat bland and tasteless food. There are many delicious recipes that are ideal for diabetics. We've provided a list of recommended foods to include in your eating plan, as well as some foods to avoid, in this chapter.

"Good" Carbohydrates

Carbohydrates are divided into two categories. Simple carbohydrates (sugar) and complex carbohydrates (starch). Simple carbohydrates can either be natural sugar that is usually found in fruits and milk or processed sugar that is found in soda and candies. Complex carbohydrates, on the other hand, refer to whole grains, legumes, and vegetables. Sugar and starch are the two ingredients that are broken down into glucose. If you have diabetes, it is important that you concentrate on good carbohydrates such as:

- Fruits
- Vegetables
- Whole grain cereals
- Legumes like beans and peas
- Low-fat dairy products like milk and cheese

Fibrous Foods

Eating food that is high in fiber can reduce the risk of different health conditions such as heart disease, constipation, and of course, diabetes. Fiber is used to control blood sugar levels by slowing down digestion. Fiber-rich foods include:

- Vegetables
- Fruits
- Nuts
- Legumes (such as beans and peas)
- Whole grains

Oily Fish

A diet that includes oily fish has been associated with a reduced risk of heart disease. Certain fish provide omega-3 fatty acids and include fish such as tuna, sardines, salmon, and mackerel. If you have diabetes, you should consume oily fish at least twice a week. It is also beneficial for pregnant or breastfeeding women to do so because it boosts the baby's immune system.

"Good" Fats

Fats are typically avoided in many diets, but there are some fats that are beneficial when eaten sparingly, even for people with diabetes. Monounsaturated and polyunsaturated fats are abundant in foods such as avocados, nuts, canola, olive, and peanut oils. These types of fats help lower cholesterol. However, it is still important to remember that fatty foods are high in calories and should be eaten in moderation.

FOODS TO AVOID

When you have diabetes, your chances of developing other health conditions such as heart disease or stroke are increased. The following are some food groups that you should avoid if you want to reduce the risk of other conditions and complications associated with type 2 diabetes:

- Saturated Fats: Products that are high in fat and proteins such as butter, bacon, sausages, hot dogs etc. should be avoided. You should also limit your use of coconut and palm oil.
- Sodium: Your doctor will most likely advise you to have less than 2,300 mg per day if you have high blood pressure.
- Trans Fat: Trans fat that is found in processed snacks, baked goods, and margarine should be avoided.
- Cholesterol: Dairy products and proteins that are high in fat, as well as organ meats like egg yolks and liver are high in cholesterol. In order to live a healthy lifestyle, you must limit your daily cholesterol intake to no more than 200 mg.

Our food choices have a huge impact on our wellbeing. As we live life, we must be aware of what is healthy and what is not. By being more conscious, we can reduce the risk of developing illnesses or health conditions later on in life.

Processed Carbohydrates

Carbohydrates that have been processed have been stripped of their beneficial bran and fiber, as well as vitamins and minerals. White flour, sugar, and white rice are examples of processed "enriched" carbohydrates. Consuming too many processed carbohydrates can cause blood sugar and insulin spikes. As you become older, you are considerably more likely to acquire type 2 diabetes. White bread, sugary baked desserts, and white pasta should also be limited because they can cause an increase in blood sugar if consumed in excess. Be wary of products that are marketed as being "enriched" for the same reason.

Sugary Drinks

A 2010 study published in *Diabetes Care* found that drinking more than one sugary drink per day has been found to increase the risk of type 2 diabetes by 26%[1]. Even if you don't think you're at risk of developing diabetes, it is critical that you limit your intake of sugary drinks. To stay hydrated, drink more water. In addition, you should avoid adding sugar and cream to your coffee or tea.

Saturated and Trans Fat

Although not all fats are bad for you, saturated and trans fats should be avoided. These fats are harmful and can raise cholesterol levels in the blood. Saturated fats are commonly found in fatty meats, cheese, butter, and milk, whereas trans fats are found both in packaged foods and fried foods. Because having high cholesterol is a risk factor for type 2 diabetes, these fats should be avoided.

Red and Processed Meat

It's been established that excessive consumption of red and processed meat is associated with type 2 diabetes. For instance, bacon, hot dogs, sausages, and other processed meats are examples of processed meats to avoid. These are especially bad for you because they contain a lot of sodium and nitrites.

CREATING A DIABETIC DIET PLAN

A diabetic diet plan can assist you in maintaining normal blood sugar levels. You can hire a professional dietitian to design a personalized meal plan for you based on your preferences and lifestyle. There are numerous types of meal plans available.

The Plate Method

This meal planning method was developed by the American Diabetes Association. This method encourages people to eat more vegetables by arranging your plate in the following ways:

- Half of your plate should be made up of non-starchy vegetables. Tomatoes, carrots, and other vegetables fall into this category.
- Protein should account for around one-quarter of your plate. This could be an oily fish, lean meat, or skinless meat.
- Whole grains should make up around one-quarter of your plate. These can include brown rice or a starchy vegetable.
- Remember, eating in moderation is key when it comes to healthy fats.
- Include some fruit or dairy products, as well as a glass of water, tea, or coffee.

Counting Carbohydrates

Carbohydrates are known to have the greatest impact on your blood sugar level because they are the food group that is broken down into glucose. It is essential that you learn how to count your carbohydrates in order to properly control your blood sugar. This can also help you adjust your insulin dose accordingly. You can learn to measure food portions and read food labels with the help of a professional dietitian. You should also consider learning about serving size and carbohydrate content.

Choose Your Foods

A professional dietitian may recommend specific foods that can assist you in meal and snack planning. With this method, you can choose foods from a variety of categories such as fats, carbohydrates, and proteins. Your "choice" is a single serving within a category. It must have roughly the same amount of carbohydrates, protein, fat, and calories as every other food in the same category. It must also have the same impact on your blood glucose levels.

---

[1] https://doi.org/10.2337/dc10-1079

Glycemic Index

The glycemic index is commonly used by a lot of people with diabetes for choosing food, particularly carbohydrates. This method ranks the effect of foods that contain carbohydrates on your blood glucose levels. It is best to consult a professional dietitian before trying this method to determine if it is right for you.

BENEFITS OF A DIABETIC DIET

The absolute best way to control your blood glucose levels is by sticking to your healthy eating plan. By doing so, you can reduce your risk of developing further complications that diabetes may bring. You can also tailor your meal plan according to your needs, so it would be really helpful if you're planning to lose weight or if you have a specific health goal you want to achieve.

A diabetic diet is not only helpful for managing diabetes, but it also comes with many benefits as well. Eating a diet abundant in vegetables, fruits, and fiber can reduce your risk of heart disease and certain types of cancer. Eating or drinking dairy products that are low in fat can reduce your chances of developing low bone mass in the future. Here is a list of great benefits that comes with eating a diabetic diet:

- Maintain general health
- Improve blood glucose control
- Obtain the desired blood lipid (fat) levels
- Maintain a normal blood pressure
- Keep a healthy body weight
- Stop or slow the progression of complications from diabetes

POSSIBLE RISKS

If you have diabetes, you must collaborate with your doctor and dietitian to develop a healthy eating plan that is perfect for you. Make sure to stick to your diet so that you don't risk having fluctuating blood sugar levels or other serious complications. You can manage your diabetes as long as you control your blood glucose levels by eating healthy foods, watching your portion sizes, and planning ahead of time.

SAMPLE MEAL PLAN

When creating a meal plan, it's important to select foods that you will enjoy that will also fill you up. You don't want your diet to be a hindrance to you; instead, you want it to perfectly fit your preferences. You can control your blood glucose levels by including a small amount of carbohydrates in each meal or snack. Your main course can be served at either lunch or dinner.

Breakfast

Here are a few meals you can eat in the morning:

- ¾ –1 cup of high-fiber cereal, low-fat milk, and a fruit of your choice
- ½ cup of muesli or oats with low-fat milk or low-fat yogurt
- 2 slices of whole grain toasted bread with peanut butter and a side of baked beans, boiled or poached eggs, or sardines
- Water, tea, or coffee

Light Meal

Some tasty light meals you can eat are:

- 1 sandwich made with slices of whole grain bread, or 6 small, high-fiber crackers and an avocado
- Salad
- 65–80g of lean meat or skinless poultry
- 100g of fish or other type of seafood
- 2 eggs or 1 cup of cooked legumes like beans or lentils
- Water, tea, or coffee

Main Meal

For your main meal you can have:

- ½ –1 cup cooked whole grain rice or pasta, or 1-2 small potatoes
- Other types of low-starch vegetables
- 65–80g of lean meat or skinless poultry
- 100g fish or other type of seafood
- 1 cup of cooked legumes like beans or lentils
- Water, tea, or coffee

Between-Meal Snacks

Snacks are tasty! Choosing ones that are healthy for persons with diabetes is crucial. If you don't know whether or not a certain snack food is appropriate for your way of eating, you can consult your diabetes educator or a dietitian. Here are several healthy snacks you might like:

- Fresh fruits
- A bit of reduced-fat natural yogurt
- A glass of skim milk
- 1 piece of whole grain bread with peanut butter, ricotta or cottage cheese, and tomato
- 1 slice of fruit bread
- High-fiber crackers with the same toppings as the bread above

You should consult a dietitian about your eating habits so that appropriate dietary recommendations can be developed for your specific needs. You should also talk with your doctor to ensure that the diet plan you choose is the best for your body and your condition.

This book will undoubtedly assist you on your journey. While you may believe that being diabetic limits your food options to bland, healthy foods, we are here to prove you wrong. This book contains a variety of recipes that are not only delicious but also nutritious. It's ideal for those who are new to a diabetic diet, and we've included a healthy meal plan to help you stay on track. It's a great resource not only for those with diabetes or prediabetes but also for those who want to try living a healthier lifestyle.

BREAKFAST

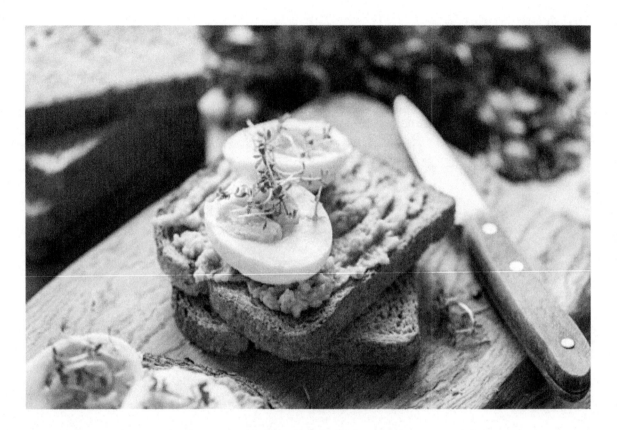

1. BREAKFAST QUESADILLA

Preparation Time: 13 minutes
Cooking Time: 16 minutes
Servings: 4
Ingredients:
- cooking spray
- ¼ cup of canned green chiles
- 4 beaten eggs
- ¼ teaspoon of black pepper
- Two 10-inch whole wheat tortillas
- 1½ cup of cheddar cheese (reduced fat)
- 4 slices turkey bacon (crumbled and cooked crisp)

Directions:
1. Lightly coat a small skillet with cooking spray.
2. Sauté the green chilies over medium-low heat for 1-2 minutes. Add beaten eggs and cook until scrambled and set aside. Season with some pepper.
3. Lightly coat a second large skillet with cooking spray. Place one tortilla in the skillet and cook over medium heat for about 1 minute, until the air bubbles begin to form. Cook for 1 minute more after flipping the tortilla (don't let the tortilla get crispy).
4. Layer half of the cheese thinly over the tortilla.
5. Reduce heat to low. Arrange half of the fried bacon and half of the egg mixture over the cheese. Now cook for about 1 minute, or until the cheese begins to melt.
6. To make a half-moon shape, fold the tortilla in half. Flip the folded tortilla over and cook for 1-2minutes until lightly toasted and the cheese filling is fully melted.

Nutrition:
Calories: 160
Fat: 19g
Carbohydrates: 8g
Sodium: 432

2. REDUCED CARB BERRY PARFAITS

Preparation Time: 7 minutes
Cooking Time: 23 minutes
Servings: 4
Ingredients:
For the Nut Granola:
- 2 cups of mixed nuts
- 1 tablespoon of flax seeds
- 1 tablespoon of sesame seeds
- 1 tablespoon of chia seeds
- 2 tablespoons of pumpkin seeds
- 2 tablespoons of coconut oil, melted
- 2 tablespoons of honey or low-carb sweetener to taste (optional)

- Pinch of salt

For the Blueberry Sauce:
- 2 cups of frozen blueberries
- 3 tablespoons of Xylitol (sugar alternative)
- 1 tablespoon of water

For the Parfait:
- Plain Greek yogurt
- Raspberries, fresh or any other fruit of your choice

Directions:
1. To prepare the granola, heat the oven to about 350°F and cover a baking tray with baking parchment paper.
2. Mix all the granola ingredients and put them in the oven, then drop them onto the baking tray.
3. Bake until the nuts are golden brown for 5-10 minutes. Regularly inspect the granola since it will quickly melt.
4. Allow to cool after you have removed from the oven.
5. Combine all the ingredients in a shallow saucepan to make the blueberry sauce and bring it to a boil. Allow the berries to cook for 5-10 minutes until their juice is released. Remove from the oven and allow a few minutes to cool.
6. Add the yogurt with granola, fresh fruit, and sauce to your bowl to make the parfaits. If the parfait is made in a pot, close the lid and place it overnight in the fridge before serving.

Nutrition:
Calories: 612.65
Protein: 17.79g
Fat: 48g
Carbs: 36g
Sodium: 290.83 mg
Sugars: 11.7g

3. HEALTHY AVOCADO TOAST

Preparation Time: 5 minutes
Cooking Time: 13 minutes
Servings: 4
Ingredients:
- 1 avocado peeled and seeded
- 2 tablespoons chopped cilantro
- Juice of half of a lime
- ½ tablespoon of red pepper flakes, optional
- Salt & pepper to taste
- 2 slices whole grain bread
- 2 eggs fried, scrambled, optional

Directions:
1. Toast 2 slices of whole grain bread in an oven until they are crispy and golden.
2. Mix and crush the avocado, lime, cilantro, salt, and pepper in a shallow bowl.
3. Spread on the toasted bread slices.
4. Top with fried, poached, or scrambled egg, if desired.

Nutrition:
Calories: 80.54
Fat: 4.6g
Protein: 2.34g
Carbs:8.5g
Sodium: 245mg

4. ZUCCHINI BREAD PANCAKES

Preparation Time: 5 minutes
Cooking Time: 20 minutes
Servings: 5
Ingredients:
- 2 cups spelt or kamut flour
- 2 tablespoon date sugar
- ¼ cup mashed burro banana
- 1 cup finely shredded zucchini
- 2 cups homemade walnut milk
- ½ cup chopped walnuts
- 1 tablespoon grapeseed oil

Directions:
1. Whisk flour in a large bowl with date sugar. Mix in walnut milk and mashed banana burro. Stir until just blended, make sure the bowl's bottom is scraped so there are no dry mix pockets. Stir in shredded walnuts and zucchini. Heat the grapeseed oil over medium-high heat in a griddle or skillet.
2. To make your pancakes, add batter onto the griddle. Cook on each side for 4-5 minutes. Serve with a syrup of agave and enjoy!

Nutrition:
Calories: 101
Protein :27g
Fiber: 14g
Carbs: 44g
Sodium: 13mg

5. RED PEPPER, GOAT CHEESE, AND ARUGULA OPEN-FACED GRILLED SANDWICH

Preparation Time: 5 minutes
Cooking Time: 15 minutes

Servings: 2
Ingredients:
- 1 red bell pepper, seeded
- Non-stick cooking spray
- 2 slice whole wheat thin-sliced bread
- 4 tablespoons crumbled goat cheese
- Pinch dried thyme
- 1 cup arugula

Directions:
1. Preheat the broiler to high heat. Line a baking sheet with parchment paper.
2. Cut the ½ bell pepper lengthwise into 2 pieces and arrange on the prepared baking sheet with the skin facing up.
3. Broil until the skin is blackened for about 5 to 10 minutes. Transfer to a covered container to steam for 5 minutes, then remove the skin from the pepper using your fingers. Cut the pepper into strips.
4. Heat a small skillet over medium-high heat. Spray it with nonstick cooking spray and place the bread in the skillet. Top with the goat cheese and sprinkle with the thyme. Pile the arugula on top, followed by the roasted red pepper strips. Press down with a spatula to hold in place.
5. Cook for 2 to 3 minutes until the bread is crisp and browned and the cheese is warmed through.

Nutrition:
Calories: 195
Fat: 10.45g
Protein: 9.7g
Carbs: 16.44g
Sodium: 210.35mg

6. WHOLE EGG BAKED SWEET POTATOES

Preparation Time: 30 minutes
Cooking Time: 60 minutes
Servings: 4
Ingredients:
For the Potatoes:
- 4 medium sweet potatoes
- 2 heads of garlic
- 2 teaspoons of extra virgin olive oil
- ½ tablespoon of taco seasoning
- ¼ cup of fresh cilantro, plus additional for garnish
- Salt and pepper

- 4 eggs

For the Sauce:
- ½ cup avocado, about 1 medium avocado
- 1 tablespoon of fresh lime juice
- 1 teaspoon of lime zest
- Salt and pepper
- 2 tablespoons of water

Directions:
1. Preheat the oven to 395°F, cover a baking sheet with tin foil then place the potatoes on it.
2. Rip off the garlic tips, keep the head intact, and softly rub them in the olive oil. Use 2 layers of tinfoil to make a small packet and wrap the garlic in it, then put it in the pan.
3. Bake the garlic for about 40 minutes, until it is tender. Remove from the pan and proceed to cook the potatoes for an additional 25-35 minutes, until fork-tender and soft.
4. When the potatoes are tender, set them aside for about 10 minutes until they're cool enough to eat. In addition, decrease the temperature of the oven to 375°F.
5. Break the potatoes down the middle and softly peel the skin back, leaving the skin intact on the sides. Carefully scoop out the skin, leaving a little amount on the sides of the potato to help maintain its form.
6. Mash the flesh of the sweet potato and then cut half of it from the bowl (you will not use this flesh, so use it at a later date in another meal). Add in the taco seasoning, cilantro and season with salt and pepper to taste. Finally, squeeze in all the fluffy oven-baked garlic. Blend well.
7. Divide the flesh between the 4 sweet potatoes, spreading it softly to fill each, leaving a large hole in the middle of each potato.
8. Place the sweet potatoes back on the baking sheet and crack an egg into each hole. Add pepper and salt. Bake until the egg is well-done (for a good runny yolk, it normally takes about 10-15 minutes). Blend until smooth.
9. Blend the mashed avocado, lime juice, and lime zest in a small food processor until smooth while the sweet potatoes are cooking. Then, while the food processor is on, slowly drizzle in the water until well blended—season with salt and pepper to taste.
10. When the potatoes are done, spread the avocado sauce among them and sprinkle it on top.
11. Garnish with sliced tomatoes and cilantro and enjoy!

Nutrition:
Calories: 298.8
Fat: 9.48g
Protein: 9.85g
Carbs: 44.94
Sodium: 441.64

7. BERRY AVOCADO SMOOTHIE

Preparation Time: 7 minutes
Cooking Time: 0 minutes
Servings: 2
Ingredients:
- ½ of an avocado
- 1 cup of strawberries
- ¼ cup of blueberries
- ½ cup of low-fat milk
- ½ cup of 2% Greek yogurt
- 1 teaspoon of raw honey, optional

Directions:
1. Fill the blender with avocado, strawberries, blueberries, and milk.
2. Blend until perfectly smooth.
3. Taste, then, if using honey, you can add.
4. Serve or put in a refrigerator for up to 2 days.

Nutrition:
Calories: 158.39
Fat: 6.79g
Protein: 9.33g
Carbs: 16.57g
Sodium: 49.21mg

8. BAGEL HUMMUS TOAST

Preparation Time: 30 minutes
Cooking Time: 4 hours
Servings: 2
Ingredients:
- 1 soft boiled egg, halved
- 6 tablespoons of plain hummus
- 2 pieces gluten-free bread, toasted
- Pinch of paprika
- 2 teaspoons of everything bagel spice
- Drizzle of olive oil

Directions:
1. Spread each bread piece with 3 tablespoons of hummus.
2. Add a slice of halved egg and finish with 1 teaspoon of bagel spice each.
3. Sprinkle a small amount of paprika, drizzle with olive oil, and serve at once.

Nutrition:
Calories: 213
Fat: 11.6g
Protein: 6.5g
Carbs: 19.23g
Sodium: 590mg

9. BLACK BEAN TACOS BREAKFAST

Preparation Time: 9 minutes
Cooking Time: 13 minutes
Servings: 4
Ingredients:
- ½ cup of red onion, diced
- 8 6-inch soft white corn tortillas, warmed
- 1 clove of garlic, minced
- 1 teaspoon avocado oil
- ¼ cup of chopped fresh cilantro
- 4 eggs
- 1 15-ounce can of black beans, rinsed and drained
- 1 small avocado, diced
- ¼ teaspoon of ground chipotle powder
- ½ cup fresh or your favorite jarred salsa

Directions:
1. Scramble Eggs.
2. Sauté the beans. Heat the avocado oil over moderate heat in a large skillet. Sauté the onion for about 3 minutes until tender.
3. Add the garlic and beans and heat until fully cooked, about 2-5 minutes.
4. Blister the tortillas or heat them in a dry skillet over an open fire on the range. Put aside, wrapped to keep them warm, in a cloth napkin.
5. Layer the beans, then top each tortilla with the eggs. Maintain only ¼ cup of beans per taco. You may be tempted but try not to overstuff the tortillas. Top up as needed with salsa, avocado, and cilantro.

Nutrition:
Calories: 299.37
Protein: 13.5g
Fat: 10.8g
Carbs: 35.55g
Sodium: 530.61mg

10. STRAWBERRY COCONUT BAKE

Preparation Time: 11 minutes
Cooking Time: 41 minutes
Servings: 2
Ingredients:

- ½ cup of chopped walnuts
- 2 cups of unsweetened coconut flakes
- 1 teaspoon cinnamon
- ¼ cup of chia seeds
- 2 cups of diced strawberries
- 1 ripe banana, mashed
- 1 teaspoon baking soda
- 4 large eggs
- ¼ teaspoon of salt
- 1 cup of unsweetened nut milk
- 2 tablespoons of coconut oil, melted

Directions:

1. Preheat oven to 375°F. Grease a square 8-inch pan and set it aside.
2. Combine the dry ingredients in a big bowl: walnuts, chia seeds, cinnamon, salt, and baking soda.
3. Whisk the milk and eggs in a smaller dish. Now, add mashed banana and coconut oil to the mixture. Add all ingredients, and thoroughly mix. Fold the strawberries in.
4. Bake for about 40 minutes, or until the top is golden and solid.
5. Serve hot!

Nutrition:
Calories: 395
Fat: 40g
Protein 7.5g
Carbs: 55g
Sodium: 457mg

11. PALEO BREAKFAST HASH

Preparation Time: 7 minutes
Cooking Time: 33 minutes
Servings: 5
Ingredients:

- 8 oz. white mushrooms, quartered
- 1 lb brussels sprouts, quartered
- Everything bagel seasoning
- 1 tablespoon olive oil or avocado oil
- 3 cloves of garlic, minced
- 1 small onion diced
- Crushed red pepper, optional
- 8 slices of nitrate-free bacon cut into pieces
- Sea salt and pepper to taste
- 6 large eggs

Directions:

1. Preheat oven to 425° F. Arrange the mushrooms and Brussels sprouts in a single layer on a sheet tray, drizzle with the olive oil and add pepper and salt. Sprinkle the onions and place the strips of bacon equally over the vegetables.
2. Roast for 15 mins in the preheated oven, then sprinkle with the garlic and stir gently. Again, roast for 10 minutes more or until the bacon and vegetables are crisp and fluffy, then remove from the oven.
3. For each egg, make tiny gaps in the hash, gently smash one at a time into a space, careful not to split the yolk. Sprinkle all the bagel seasoning and crushed red pepper over the bacon, eggs, and vegetables.
4. Put the baking tray in the oven and bake for another 5-10 minutes or until the eggs are ideally fried. Remove from the oven and quickly serve. Enjoy!

Nutrition:
Calories: 250
Protein: 14g
Fat: 18g
Carbs: 11.94g
Sodium: 558.44mg

12. OMELET WITH CHICKPEA FLOUR

Preparation Time: 10 minutes
Cooking Time: 20 minutes
Servings: 1
Ingredients:

- ½ teaspoon onion powder
- ¼ teaspoon black pepper
- 1 cup chickpea flour
- ½ teaspoon garlic powder
- ½ teaspoon baking soda
- ¼ teaspoon white pepper
- ⅓ cup nutritional yeast
- 3 finely chopped green onions
- 4 ounces sautéed mushrooms

Directions:

1. Combine the onion powder, white pepper, chickpea flour, garlic powder, black and white pepper, baking soda, and nutritional yeast.
2. Add 1 cup of water and create a smooth batter. On medium heat, put a frying pan and add the batter just like the way you would cook pancakes.
3. On the batter, sprinkle some green onion and mushrooms. Flip the omelet and cook evenly on both sides. Once both sides are cooked, serve the omelet with spinach, tomatoes, hot sauce, and salsa.

Nutrition:
Calories: 150
Fat: 1.9g
Carbohydrates: 24.4g
Protein: 10.2g
Sodium: 39mg

13. TOAST WITH EGG AND AVOCADO

Preparation Time: 17 minutes
Cooking Time: 0 minutes
Servings: 4
Ingredients:

- 4 eggs
- 4 slices of hearty whole grain bread
- 1 avocado (mashed)
- ½ teaspoon of salt (optional)
- ¼ teaspoon of black pepper
- ¼ cup of Greek yogurt (non-fat)

Directions:

1. To poach each egg, fill a microwaveable bowl or cup with ½ cup of water. Crack an egg into the water and make sure it's fully submerged. Cover with a saucer and microwave on high for 1 mninute, or before the white is set and the yolk starts to set, but still fluffy (not runny).
2. Toast the bread and use ¼ of the mashed avocado to cover each slice.
3. Sprinkle the avocado with salt (optional) and pepper. Top with a poached egg on each piece. Top the egg with 1 tablespoon of Greek yogurt.

Nutrition:
Calories: 188.7
Fat: 9.9g
Carbohydrates: 14.54g
Sodium: 167.88mg

14. HUEVOS RANCHEROS

Preparation Time: 12 minutes
Cooking Time: 33 minutes
Servings: 2
Ingredients:

- 4 corn tortillas
- 1 can of tomatoes (14.5-ounce, no-salt-added, diced, drained)
- 1 teaspoon of ground cumin
- ⅛ teaspoon of cayenne pepper (optional)
- ½ teaspoon of salt
- 4 large eggs

- 1 oz. part-skim mozzarella cheese or reduced-fat feta (shredded)
- ¼ cup of cilantro (chopped)

Directions:
1. Preheat the oven to 425°F.
2. Position the tortillas on the baking sheet and bake them on each side for 3 minutes.
3. Meanwhile, in a medium nonstick skillet, place the tomatoes, cumin, cayenne, and salt, and bring to a boil over medium-high heat. Now lower the heat to medium-low and cook, covered, until lightly thickened, or 3 minutes. Split one egg into a cup. Slide the egg gently over the tomato mixture. Repeat for the eggs that remain. Simmer gently, covered, over medium heat, 2 ½ to 3 minutes or until the whites are fully set and the yolks start to thicken slightly.
4. Put a tortilla on each of the 4 plates. Cover with the eggs and the tomato mixture. Sprinkle cheese and cilantro on top.

Nutrition:
Calories: 162
Fat: 8g
Carbohydrates: 14.6g
Sodium: 546mg

15. APPLE WALNUT FRENCH TOAST

Preparation Time: 12 minutes
Cooking Time: 14 minutes
Servings: 4
Ingredients:
- 4 slices of multi-grain Italian bread
- 1 cup of egg substitute
- 4 teaspoons of pure maple syrup
- 1 cup of diced apple
- Walnuts (chopped)

Directions:
1. Preheat your oven to 450°F. Meanwhile, put the bread in a 13"x9" baking pan, pour over all the egg substitutes, and turn several times until the bread slices are thoroughly coated and the egg mixture is used. Put bread slices coated with cooking spray on the baking sheet.
2. Bake for 6 minutes, turn, and bake for 5 minutes or until the bottom is golden. Serve with similar proportions of syrup, apples, and nuts in the mixture.

Nutrition:
Calories: 179.74
Fat: 7.8g
Carbohydrates: 22.26g
Sodium: 217.13mg

16. TOAST WITH CREAMY AVOCADO AND SPROUTS

Preparation Time: 10 minutes
Cooking Time: 15 minutes
Servings: 3
Ingredients:
- 2 slices of bread (Toasted)
- 1 cup of finely cut tomatoes
- 2 moderate size avocados
- 1 small cup of alfalfa
- Pure sea salt and bell pepper

Directions:
1. Add the avocado, alfalfa, and tomatoes to the toast and season to taste with pure sea salt and pepper. Have a sumptuous breakfast with any freshly extracted juice of your choice.

Nutrition:
Calories:194
Fiber:12g
Protein:4.9g
Sugar: 7g
Carbs: 20.35g
Sodium: 104mg

17. SCRAMBLED TURMERIC TOFU

Preparation Time: 5 minutes
Cooking Time: 15 minutes
Servings: 4
Ingredients:
- 1 crumbled serving of tofu
- 1 small cup of finely chopped onions
- 1 teaspoon of fresh parsley
- 1 teaspoon of coconut oil
- 1 cup of soft spinach
- 1 small teaspoon of turmeric
- 2 avocado slices
- 1 medium tomato, diced
- 1 small spoon of roasted paprika

Directions:
1. Make tofu crumbs with your hands and keep them separately. Sauté diced onions in oil until soft.
2. Combine tofu, tomatoes, and other seasonings and stir well. Add veggies and stir. Serve in a bowl alongside some avocado.

Nutrition:
Calories: 91

Fiber: 12g
Protein: 30g
Carbs: 6.91g
Sodium: 11.36mg
Sugar: 8g

18. BREAKFAST SALAD

Preparation Time: 5 minutes
Cooking Time: 15 minutes
Servings: 3
Ingredients:
- 1 cup of finely diced kale
- 1 cup of cabbage, red and Chinese
- 2 tablespoons of coconut oil
- 1 cup of spinach
- 2 medium avocados
- 8 c. of chickpeas
- 2 tablespoons of sunflower seed sprouts
- Pure sea salt (seasoning)
- Bell pepper (seasoning)
- Lemon juice (seasoning)

Directions:
1. Add spinach, Chinese and red cabbage, kale, coconut oil, to a container. Add seasoning to taste and mix adequately. Add other ingredients and mix.

Nutrition:
Calories: 112
Protein: 28g
Fiber: 10g
Carbs: 35g
Sodium: 269mg
Sugar: 1g

19. GREEN GODDESS BOWL WITH AVOCADO CUMIN DRESSING

Preparation Time: 10 minutes
Cooking Time: 20 minutes
Servings: 4
Ingredients:
- 3 heaping cups of finely sliced kale
- 1 small cup of diced broccoli florets
- ½ cup of zucchini spiral noodles
- ½ cup of soaked kelp noodles
- 3 cups of tomatoes
- 2 tablespoons of hemp seeds

For the Tahini Dressing:
- 1 small cup of sesame butter
- 1 cup of alkaline water
- 1 cup of freshly extracted lemon
- 1 garlic clove, finely chopped
- ¾ tablespoon of pure sea salt
- 1 tablespoon of olive oil

- 1 bell pepper

For the Avocado Dressing:
- 1 large avocado
- Juice of 2 freshly extracted limes
- 1 cup of alkaline water
- 1 tablespoon of olive oil
- 1 tablespoon of powdered cumin

Directions:
1. Simmer veggies (kale and broccoli) for about 4 minutes. Combine noodles and add avocado cumin dressing. Toss for a while. Add tomatoes and combine well. Put the cooked kale and broccoli on a plate, add Tahini dressing, add noodles and tomatoes. Add a couple of hemp seeds to the whole dish and enjoy it.

Nutrition:
Calories: 109
Protein: 25g
Fiber: 17g
Carbs: 22.99g
Sodium: 457mg
Sugar: 8g

20. QUINOA BURRITO

Preparation Time: 15 minutes
Cooking Time: 10 minutes
Servings: 8

Ingredients:
- 1 cup of quinoa
- 2 cups of black beans
- 4 finely chopped green onions
- 4 finely chopped garlic cloves
- 2 freshly cut limes
- 1 tablespoon of cumin
- 2 beautifully diced avocado
- 1 small cup of diced cilantro

Directions:
1. Boil quinoa. During this process, put the beans on low heat. Add other ingredients to the bean pot and let it cook for about 15 minutes. Serve quinoa and add the prepared beans.

Nutrition:
Calories: 300
Protein: 14.54g
Fiber: 11.6g
Carbs: 49.19g
Sodium: 9.37mg

21. BAKED BANANA NUT OATMEAL CUPS

Preparation Time: 17 minutes
Cooking Time: 40 minutes
Servings: 4

Ingredients:
- 3 cups of rolled oats.
- 1½ cups of low-fat milk
- 2 ripe bananas
- ¼ cup of packed brown sugar
- 2 large lightly beaten eggs
- 1 teaspoon of baking powder
- 1 teaspoon of ground cinnamon
- 1 teaspoon of vanilla extract
- ½ teaspoon of salt
- ½ cup of toasted chopped pecans

Directions:
1. Preheat oven to 375°F. Coat a pan with a cooking spray.
2. Combine oats, milk, bananas, refined sugar, eggs, cinnamon, vanilla, and salt in a giant bowl. Fold in pecans. Divide the mixture among baking cups (about ⅓ cup each). Bake till a pick inserted into the center comes out clean, within twenty-five minutes.
3. Cool in the pan for ten minutes, then move to a wire rack.
4. Serve hot or at room temperature.

Nutrition:
Calories: 178
Protein: 5.3g
Carbs: 42g
Sodium: 246mg
Fat: 6.3g

22. VEGGIE BREAKFAST WRAP

Preparation Time: 12 minutes
Cooking Time: 13 minutes
Servings: 2

Ingredients:
- 2 teaspoon of olive oil
- 1 cup of sliced mushrooms
- 2 eggs
- ½ cup of egg white or egg substitute
- 1 cup of firmly packed spinach or other greens
- 2 tablespoons of sliced scallions
- Non-stick cooking spray
- 2 whole wheat low-carb flour tortillas
- 2 tablespoons of salsa

Directions:
1. Add oil to the frying pan over medium heat. Add mushrooms and sauté till nicely brown at edges (about 3 minutes), set aside.
2. Beat eggs with egg substitute or egg whites in a medium-sized bowl, using a mixer or by hand, till emulsified. Stir in cut spinach and scallions. Use dried herbs like basil or parsley for more flavor.
3. Begin heating medium/large frying pan over medium-low heat. Coat pan with cooking spray. Pour in egg mixture and scramble it. Once eggs are done to your liking, stir in mushrooms.
4. Spread ½ the egg mixture down the middle of every tortilla shell and top with 1 tablespoon sauce of your choice. Garnish with additional toppings like avocado slices, bell pepper, or tomato if desired, then roll it up to form a wrap.

Nutrition:
Calories: 220
Fat: 11g
Carbs: 23g
Sodium: 490mg
Protein: 19g

23. BREAKFAST EGG AND HAM BURRITO

Preparation Time: 21 minutes
Cooking Time: 13 minutes
Servings: 3

Ingredients:
- 4 eggs
- Egg whites
- 1 dash hot pepper sauce
- ¼ teaspoon of black pepper
- 2 tablespoons of cheddar cheese
- 2 tablespoons of margarine
- 4 slices of deli ham
- ¼ cup of sliced onion
- ¼ cup of diced green pepper
- 4 heated corn tortillas
- Salsa

Directions:
1. Using a medium bowl, whisk together the eggs, egg whites, hot pepper sauce, black pepper, and cheese.
2. In a medium nonstick pan, heat the spread over medium heat. Sauté the ham for around 2-3 minutes. Remove the ham from the pan.
3. Add the onions and fresh peppers to the pan and cook for five minutes. Add the ham back to the pan.
4. Now reduce the heat to low and add the eggs to the pan. Gently mix the eggs with a spoon or spatula and continue to cook

gently over low heat until the eggs are broiled and set.

5. Equally divide the egg mixture into 4 servings. Spoon every portion of the egg mixture into a tortilla and top with 1 teaspoon salsa.

Nutrition:
Calories: 210
Fat: 9g
Carbohydrates: 16g
Sodium: 768mg

24. BREAKFAST CUPS FOR MEAT LOVERS

Preparation Time: 12 minutes
Cooking Time: 13 minutes
Servings: 4
Ingredients:
- 1 tablespoon of light sour cream
- 2 pre-cooked diced turkey breakfast sausage patties
- 1 clove of minced garlic
- 2 tablespoons of thinly sliced onion
- 1½ cup of frozen hash browns
- 1 teaspoon of canola oil
- ¼ teaspoon of salt
- A pinch of black pepper
- 1 cup of egg substitute
- 2 tablespoons of turkey bacon
- 2 tablespoons of Monterey jack cheese

Directions:
1. Heat oven to 400°F. Coat a six-cup muffin tin with cooking spray. Equally divide the hash browns among the cups and press firmly into the bottom and up the sides of every cup.
2. In a very large frying pan, heat the oil over medium heat. Sauté the onion till tender. Add the garlic and sausage; cook for one minute additional. Take away the frying pan from the heat; stir in the soured cream.
3. In a medium bowl, beat the egg substitute with the salt and black pepper, then pour it equally into the potato-lined cups. Top every cup with a bit of the sausage mixture, bacon, and cheese.
4. Bake fifteen to eighteen minutes, or till the eggs are set. Serve instantly or freeze for later.

Nutrition:
Calories: 193
Fat: 7.8g
Sodium: 529mg
Carbohydrates: 19.05g

25. SUMMER SMOOTHIE FRUIT

Preparation Time: 12 minutes
Cooking Time: 0 minutes
Servings: 4
Ingredients:
- 1 cup of fresh blueberries
- 1 cup of fresh strawberries (chopped)
- 2 peaches (peeled, seeded, and chopped)
- Peach flavored Greek-style yogurt (non-fat)
- 1 cup of unsweetened almond milk
- 2 tablespoons of ground flax seed
- ½ cup of ice

Directions:
1. Combine in a blender and puree all ingredients until creamy.

Nutrition:
Calories: 87.26
Fat: 2.38g
Carbohydrates: 16.19g
Sodium: 51.8mg

26. CHICKEN AND EGG SALAD

Preparation Time: 5 minutes
Cooking Time: 25 minutes
Servings: 2
Ingredients:
- 2 cooked chicken breasts
- 3 hard-boiled eggs
- 2 tablespoons of fat-free mayo
- 1 tablespoon of curry powder
- Chives or basil (optional)
- Salt (optional)

Directions:
1. Bake the chicken for 15 minutes in the oven at 360°F (confirm with just a meat thermometer that meat is cooked through).
2. For 8 minutes, cook the eggs. Cut the eggs and chicken into small-sized pieces.
3. Combine the cream cheese with curry powder
4. In a large bowl, combine everything and mix.
5. Allow a minimum of 10 minutes to chill in the refrigerator (it gets even better if you leave it overnight in the refrigerator).
6. Serve with chives on toast or muffins and a bit of salt on top.

Nutrition:
Calories: 504
Fat: 27.9g
Carbohydrates: 4.16g

Sodium: 358mg

27. NIÇOISE SALAD TUNA

Preparation Time: 12 minutes
Cooking Time: 5 minutes
Servings: 1
Ingredients:
- 4 oz. Ahi tuna steak
- 1 whole egg
- 2 cups of baby spinach (3oz)
- 2 oz. green beans
- 1½ oz. broccoli
- ½ red bell peppers
- 3 1/2 oz. cucumber
- 1 radish
- 3 large black olives
- Handful of parsley
- 1 teaspoon of olive oil
- 1 teaspoon of balsamic vinegar
- ½ teaspoon of Dijon mustard
- ½ teaspoon of pepper

Directions:
1. Cook the egg and place it aside to cool.
2. Steam beans and broccoli then set aside. 2-3 mins of a little water in the microwave or 3 minutes in a kettle of hot water does the trick.
3. In a pan, heat a bit of oil over high heat.
4. On all sides, season the seafood using pepper, then place it in the pan and cook on each edge for about 2 minutes.
5. To the salad bowl or pan, add the spinach.
6. Chop the red pepper, cucumber, and egg into pieces that are bite-sized. Add the spinach on top.
7. Cut the radish into slices and mix the broccoli, beans, and olives together. Add the spinach salad on top.
8. Break the tuna into strips and add it to the salad.
9. Toss the olive oil, balsamic vinegar, mustard, salt, and pepper together.
10. The parsley is chopped and added to the vinaigrette.
11. For drizzling the vinaigrette over a salad, use a spoon

Nutrition:
Calories: 346.36
Fat: 13.28g
Carbohydrates: 18.89g
Sodium: 366.11mg

28. ROLLS WITH SPINACH

Preparation Time: 15 minutes
Cooking Time: 40 minutes
Servings: 4
Ingredients:

- 16 ounces of frozen spinach leaves
- 3 eggs
- 2 ½ ounces of onion
- 2 ounces of carrots
- 1 ounce of low-fat mozzarella cheese
- 4 ounces of fat-free cottage cheese
- ½ cup of parsley
- 1 clove of garlic
- 1 teaspoon of curry powder
- ¼ teaspoon of chili flakes
- 1 teaspoon of salt
- 1 teaspoon of pepper
- Cooking spray

Directions:

1. Preheat the oven to 400°F.
2. Thaw the spinach if frozen and squeeze the water out (you can use a strainer). In order to accelerate the thawing process, you can microwave the spinach for a few minutes.
3. Mix the spinach, 2 eggs, mozzarella, ginger, half the salt, and pepper together in a baking bowl.
4. Coat a baking sheet with parchment paper and cooking spray. Move the spinach mixture, about half an inch thick and about 10 to 12 inches in length, to the sheet and press it down.
5. Bake for 15 minutes and then set aside to cool on a rack. Don't turn the oven off.
6. Finely chop the onion and parsley. Grate the carrots.
7. In a pan with a bit of cooking oil, fry the onions for about a minute. Cook for about 2 minutes after adding the carrots and parsley to the pan.
8. Add cottage cheese, curry, chili, salt, and pepper to the other half. Briefly mix.
9. Remove the pan from heat and add an egg, and mix it all together.
10. Spread the filling over the spinach that has been cooled. Do not stretch it all the way to the corners or as you fold it out, it will fall out.
11. Roll the spinach mat carefully and fill it, then bake for 25 minutes.
12. Take out the roll once the time is up, and let it cool for 5-10 minutes before cutting it into slices and serving.

Nutrition:
Calories: 149
Fat: 6.14g
Carbohydrates: 11.44g
Sodium: 844mg

29. KETO SALAD

Preparation Time: 11 minutes
Cooking Time: 0 minutes
Servings: 2
Ingredients:

- 4 cherry tomatoes
- ½ avocado
- 1 hardboiled egg
- 2 cups of mixed green salad
- 2 ounces of chicken breast, shredded
- 1 ounce of feta cheese (crumbled)
- ¼ cup of cooked bacon (crumbled)

Directions:

1. Slice the avocado and tomatoes. Slice the egg that is hard-boiled.
2. On a large plate, put the mixed greens.
3. Add the chicken breast, bacon, and feta cheese.
4. Position the tomatoes, egg, chicken, avocado, feta, and bacon on top of the greens in horizontal rows.

Nutrition:
Calories: 237
Fat: 18.51g
Carbohydrates: 5.7g
Sodium: 341mg

30. INSTANT POT CHICKEN CHILI

Preparation Time: 6 minutes
Cooking Time: 21 minutes
Servings: 2
Ingredients:

- 1 tablespoon of vegetable oil
- 1 yellow diced onion
- 4 minced garlic cloves
- 1 teaspoon of ground cumin
- 1 teaspoon of oregano
- 2½ lbs. chicken breasts, boneless & skinless
- 16 ounces of salsa verde

For Toppings:

- 2 packages of queso fresco (crumbled) or sour cream
- 2 diced avocados
- Finely chopped radishes
- 8 springs cilantro (optional)

Directions:

1. Set the Instant Pot to a medium sauté setting.
2. Add the oil to the vegetables.
3. Add the onion and simmer for 3 mins till the onion starts to soften, stirring regularly.
4. Apply the garlic, then stir for a minute.
5. Add the oregano and cumin and simmer for the one minute.
6. To the pot, add ½ of the salsa verde. Top chicken breasts and with salsa verde.
7. Position the cover on the Instant Pot, switch the nozzle to "seal," and choose "manual." set the timer to 10 minutes.
8. When the timer goes off, let the pressure naturally dissipate.
9. Lift the cover, move the chicken to a small bowl just after pressure has dropped, and slice it with a fork.
10. Mix with remaining ingredients, transfer the meat to the pot and stir.

Nutrition:
Calories: 144
Fat: 7g
Carbohydrates: 20g
Sodium: 575.65mg

31. SMOKED CHEESE WRAPS WITH SALMON AND CREAM

Preparation Time: 12 minutes
Cooking Time: 15 minutes
Servings: 2
Ingredients:

- 1 8-inch low carb flour tortilla
- 2 ounces of smoked salmon
- 2 teaspoons of low-fat cream cheese
- 1½ ounce of red onion
- Handful of arugula
- ½ teaspoon of fresh or dried basil
- A pinch of pepper

Directions:

1. In the oven or microwave, warm the tortilla (pro tip: to prevent it from drying out, warm it between 2 pieces of moist paper towel).
2. The cream cheese, basil, and pepper are mixed together and then spread over the tortilla.
3. With the salmon, arugula, and finely sliced onion, finish it off. Roll it up and enjoy the wrap!

Nutrition:
Calories: 84
Fat: 3.23g

Carbohydrates: 9g
Sodium: 329.19mg

32. CHEESE YOGURT

Preparation Time: 12 minutes
Cooking Time: 15 minutes
Servings: 2
Ingredients:
- 1 cup yogurt
- ½ teaspoon of kosher salt

Directions:
1. Line a strainer with twice the thickness of a normal or plastic cheesecloth.
2. Place the strainer on top of a bowl and add the yogurt.
3. Cover and refrigerate for 2 hours. Stir in the salt and continue to chill for another 22 hours until the yogurt cheese is ready to spread.

Nutrition:
Calories: 74.7
Protein: 4.25g
Fat: 3.98g
Carbs: 5.71g
Sodium: 521.46mg

33. SAVORY EGG MUFFINS

Preparation Time: 12 minutes
Cooking Time: 33 minutes
Servings: 6
Ingredients:
- 1½ cups of water
- 2 tablespoons of unsalted butter
- 1 (6-ounce) package Stove Top lower-sodium Stuffing Mix for chicken
- 3 ounces of bulk pork sausage
- Cooking spray
- 6 eggs, beaten
- ½ cup of (1.5 ounces) Monterey Jack cheese, shredded
- ½ cup of finely chopped red bell pepper
- ¼ cup of sliced green onions

Directions:
1. Preheat oven to 400°F.
2. In a medium saucepan, put 1 ½ cups of water and butter to a boil. Stir in the blend of stuffing. Cover, detach from heat and let stand for 5 minutes; use a fork to fluff. Let stand 10 minutes or before cool enough to hold, uncovered.
3. Cook the sausage in a small skillet over medium-high heat until browned while the stuffing is cooling; stir to crumble.
4. Coat a muffin pan with cooking spray.
5. Press approximately ¼ cup of stuffing into the bottom and sides of each of the 12 coated muffin cups with cooking oil. Pour the egg uniformly into the cups of stuffing. Layer cheese, ham, bell pepper, and green onions equally over the egg.
6. Bake for 18 to 20 minutes at 400°F or until the centers are cooked. Let it stand before serving for 5 minutes. Run a thin, sharp knife along the edges to loosen the muffin cups. Immediately serve.

Nutrition:
Calories: 292
Fat: 16.7g
Protein: 14.6g
Carbs: 23.19g
Sodium: 623.72mg

34. YOGURT AND WALNUT PARFAITS

Preparation Time: 5 minutes
Cooking Time: 5 minutes
Servings: 2
Ingredients:
- 1 ½ tablespoons maple syrup
- ½ cup walnuts, chopped
- ½ teaspoon ground cinnamon
- ¾ cup oats (Gluten-Free)

For Serving:
- 2 tablespoons pomegranate seeds
- 1 ½ cups plain yogurt (or vegan yogurt)
- Sprigs of mint
- 2 teaspoons maple syrup

Directions:
1. Heat the walnuts and oats in a dry frying pan over medium heat. Toast for 5 minutes, often stirring, until brown and aromatic, then whisk in the maple syrup and cinnamon. Cool for a few minutes.
2. Stir the maple syrup into the yogurt and stack the yogurt, granola, and pomegranate seeds in two glasses to serve. Garnish with a sprig of mint. Enjoy right now.
3. To make ahead, make the yogurt and set it in the fridge, and make the granola and store it in a container in a cold, dry location. Just before serving, layer the ingredients.

Nutrition:
Calories:495
Fat:24g
Protein:18g
Sugar: 29g
Carbs: 56g
Sodium: 3.95mg

35. GREEK-STYLE YOGURT

Preparation Time: 10 minutes
Cooking Time: 0
Servings: 4
Ingredients:
- 4 tbsp live yogurt
- 800 mL whole milk

Directions:
1. Heat the milk to 185 °F, then remove from the heat and set aside to cool to 110 °F.
2. Take a spoon of the yogurt into a clean jug and whisk in a few tablespoons of the warm milk, followed by the remainder of the milk and stirring well.
3. Pour into a big jar with a lid, cover with a cloth, and set aside in a warm location for 24 hours.
4. Refrigerate this yogurt overnight after straining it through a plastic strainer over a bowl.

Nutrition:
Calories: 134
Protein: 7g
Fat: 7g
Carbs:11g
Sugar: 11g
Sodium: 87.36mg

36. CAJUN-STYLE SHRIMP AND GRITS

Preparation Time: 12 minutes
Cooking Time: 20 minutes
Servings: 6
Ingredients:
- 1 tablespoon of olive oil
- ½ cups (2 ounces) of Tasso ham, minced
- 1 cup of chopped onion
- One garlic clove, minced
- 36 medium shrimp, peeled (about 1 ¼ pound)
- 1 teaspoon of Cajun seasoning
- 2½ cups of water, divided
- 1 tablespoon of unsalted butter
- 1 cup of fat-free milk
- ¼ teaspoon of salt
- 1 cup of uncooked quick-cooking grits
- 1 cup (4 ounces) of sharp cheddar cheese, shredded

- ½ cup of sliced green onions

Directions:
1. Heat the olive oil over medium-high heat in a large skillet.
2. Add Tasso; sauté for 2 minutes or until golden on the edges. Stir in the onion; sauté for 2 minutes. Stir in garlic; sauté for 1 minute.
3. Sprinkle with Cajun seasoning, add the shrimp to the pan, and cook for 3 minutes, rotating once. Add ¼ cup water to loosen the browned pieces. Remove from heat; mix with butter, stirring until melted. Cover.
4. On medium-high heat, put milk, salt, and 2 cups of water to a boil.. Add the grits steadily and cook until thick (about 5 minutes), stirring continuously with a whisk. Remove the grits from the heat; add the cheese and stir until the cheese melts, with a whisk.
5. On 6 plates, spoon grates evenly. Using the seafood and ham combination, add green onions to finish uniformly.

Nutrition:
Calories: 346
Fat:14g
Carbs: 20.44g
Protein:24g
Sodium: 1144mg

37. LOX, EGGS AND ONION SCRAMBLE

Preparation Time: 12 minutes
Cooking Time: 15 minutes
Servings: 4
Ingredients:
- Six eggs
- 4 egg whites
- 1 teaspoon of canola oil
- ⅓ cup of sliced green onions
- 4 ounces of smoked salmon, cut into ½-inch pieces
- ¼ cup of reduced-fat cream
- Cheese, cut into 12 pieces
- ¼ teaspoon of freshly ground black pepper
- 4 slices pumpernickel bread, toasted

Directions:
1. Place the eggs and egg whites in a bowl; stir until mixed with a whisk.
2. Over medium-high, heat a medium nonstick skillet. In a pan, add oil, swirl to coat. In the pan, add the green onions;

sauté for 2 minutes or until tender. Add the egg mixture. Until the mixture settles on the rim, cook without stirring.
3. Use a spatula to form curds over the bottom of the pan. Add the cream cheese and salmon. Continue to draw the spatula across the bottom of the pan until the egg mixture is somewhat thick but still moist; do not continuously stir.
4. Remove directly from the pan. Sprinkle the pepper with the egg mixture. Serve the toast of pumpernickel.

Nutrition:
Calories: 204.66
Fat: 9.99g
Protein: 14.26g
Carbs: 14.18g
Sodium: 465.87mg

38. PEACH AND BLUEBERRY PANCAKES

Preparation Time: 12 minutes
Cooking Time: 16 minutes
Servings: 6
Ingredients:
- 1½ cups of almond flour
- 2 tablespoons sugar
- 2 tablespoons of flaxseed (optional)
- 1 tablespoon of baking powder
- ½ teaspoon of kosher salt
- 1½ cups of nonfat buttermilk
- 1 teaspoon of grated lemon rind
- 2 eggs
- 1 cup of fresh or frozen blueberries, thawed
- 1 cup of chopped fresh or frozen peaches, thawed
- 2 tablespoons of unsalted butter
- Fresh blueberries (optional)

Directions:
1. Spoon the flour gently into dry measuring cups; level it with a knife. In a large cup, mix the flour, sugar, flaxseed, baking powder, and salt if necessary, and stir with a fork.
2. In a medium cup, mix the buttermilk, lemon rind, and eggs and stir with a fork. To the flour mixture, apply the buttermilk mixture, stirring only so it is moist. Fold in the blueberries and peaches.
3. Heat a nonstick griddle or nonstick skillet over medium heat. Pour ⅓ of a cup of flour into the pan per pancake. Cook

for 2 to 3 minutes over medium heat or until bubbles cover the tops and the edges appear fried. Flip the cakes over gently; cook for 2 - 3 mins or until the bottoms become golden brown.

Nutrition:
Calories: 255
Fat: 17g
Protein: 9.34g
Carbs:18.46g
Sodium: 482.88mg

39. OMELET WITH TURMERIC, TOMATO, AND ONIONS

Preparation Time: 8 minutes
Cooking Time: 15 minutes
Servings: 2
Ingredients:
- 4 large eggs
- Kosher salt
- 1 tablespoon of olive oil
- ¼ teaspoon of brown mustard seeds Turmeric powder
- 2 green onions, finely chopped
- ¼ cup of diced plum tomato
- Dash of black pepper

Directions:
1. Whisk the eggs and salt together.
2. Heat oil over medium-high heat in a large cast-iron skillet. Apply the mustard and turmeric seeds; simmer for 30 seconds or until the seeds pop up, stirring regularly. Add onions; simmer for 30 seconds or until tender, stirring regularly. Add the tomato; simmer for 1 minute or until very tender, stirring regularly.
3. Pour the plate with the egg mixture, scatter uniformly. Cook until the edges are set (about 2 minutes). Slide the spatula's front edge between the omelet edge and the plate. Raise the omelet edge softly, tilting the pan to allow the pan to come into contact with any uncooked egg mixture.
4. Repeat on the opposite edge. Continue to cook till the center is really just set (about 2 minutes). Loosen the omelet and fold it in half with a spatula. Slide the omelet carefully onto a platter. Halve the omelet and dust it with black pepper.

Nutrition:
Calories: 216
Fat: 16.9g
Protein: 13.3g

Carbs: 3.49g
Sodium: 533.49mg

40. BREAKFAST BOWL OF YOGURT

Preparation Time: 8 minutes
Cooking Time: 15 minutes
Servings: 4
Ingredients:
- 1 teaspoon of tandoori spice or curry powder
- ¼ cup of honey
- 2 cups of 2% plain Greek yogurt
- ½ cup of all-natural granola
- 1 cup of fresh berries
- 1 cup of freeze-dried mango, pineapple, and/or berries
- Small sprigs of fresh cilantro

Directions:
1. Toast the spices on low in a small skillet, stirring, until very fragrant, for about 2 minutes. Remove from heat, add honey, and stir.
2. Divide the yogurt into 4 cups. Drizzle with spiced honey; finish with cilantro, granola, and mango.

Nutrition:
Calories: 176
Fat : 3.23g
Protein: 7.26g
Carbs: 47g
Sodium: 132.61mg

41. TEX-MEX MIGAS

Preparation Time: 9 minutes
Cooking Time: 15 minutes
Servings: 4
Ingredients:
- 3 large eggs
- 3 egg whites
- 1 tablespoon of canola oil
- 4 corn tortillas, cut into ½-inch-wide strips
- ½ cup of chopped onion
- 2 large, seeded jalapeño peppers
- ⅔ cup of lower-sodium salsa
- ½ cup of Monterey Jack cheese, shredded
- ½ cup of sliced green onions
- Hot sauce (optional)
- Lower-sodium red salsa (optional)
- Lower-sodium green salsa (optional)

Directions:
1. Place the eggs and egg whites in a bowl; stir until mixed with a whisk.

2. Over medium-high, heat a medium nonstick skillet. In a pan, apply oil, swirl to coat. Apply tortilla strips to the skillet and cook, stirring constantly, for 3 minutes or until brown.
3. In a saucepan, add the onion and jalapeño peppers; sauté for 2 minutes or until tender. Stir in ⅔ of a cup of salsa, and simmer for 1 minute, stirring continuously.
4. Add the mixture of eggs; simmer for 2 minutes or until the eggs are tender, stirring periodically. Sprinkle the cheese with the egg mixture. Cook for thirty seconds or until the cheese is melted.
5. Cover with the green onions, then serve right away. If preferred, serve with hot sauce, red salsa, or green salsa.

Nutrition:
Calories: 193
Fat: 10.4g
Carbs: 17.45g
Protein: 10.2g
Sodium: 477mg

42. BARLEY BREAKFAST WITH BANANA & SUNFLOWER SEEDS

Preparation Time: 5 minutes
Cooking Time: 11 minutes
Servings: 1
Ingredients:
- ⅔ cup of water
- ⅓ cup of uncooked quick-Cooking pearl barley
- 1 banana, sliced
- 1 teaspoon of honey
- 1 tablespoon of unsalted sunflower seeds

Directions:
1. In a shallow microwave-safe cup, mix water and barley on high for 6 minutes in the microwave.
2. Remove and let stand for 2 minutes.
3. Cover with slices of banana, sunflower seeds, and honey.

Nutrition:
Calories: 410
Fat: 6g
Protein:10g
Carbs: 86g
Sodium: 10.9mg

43. BANANA SMOOTHIE FOR BREAKFAST

Preparation Time: 12 minutes
Cooking Time: 0 minute
Servings: 2
Ingredients:
- ½ cup of 1% low-fat milk
- ½ cup of crushed ice
- 1 tablespoon of honey
- ½ teaspoon ground nutmeg
- 1 frozen sliced ripe large banana
- 1 cup of plain 2% reduced-fat Greek yogurt

Directions:
1. In a blender, combine the first 5 ingredients; mix for 2 minutes or until smooth. Add the yogurt; just process until it's blended. Immediately serve.

Nutrition:
Calories: 112
Fat: 2.09g
Protein: 7.63g
Carbs: 32g
Sodium: 99.59mg

44. BLACKBERRY MANGO SHAKE

Preparation Time: 12 minutes
Cooking Time: 0 minutes
Servings: 4
Ingredients:
- 1 cup of orange juice
- 1 cup of refrigerated bottled mango slices
- ¼ cup of light firm silken tofu
- 3 tablespoons of honey
- 1½ cups of frozen blackberries

Directions:
1. In a blender, place all ingredients in the order given, process until smooth.

Nutrition:
Calories: 142
Fat: 0.7g
Protein: 1.86g
Carbs: 34.87g
Sodium: 2.62mg

45. BULGUR PORRIDGE BREAKFAST

Preparation Time: 5 minutes
Cooking Time: 15 minutes
Servings: 4
Ingredients:
- 4 cups of 1% low-fat milk
- 1 cup of bulgur
- ⅓ cup of dried cherries
- ¼ tablespoon of salt
- ⅓ cup of dried apricots, coarsely chopped
- ½ cup of sliced almonds

Directions:

1. Combine the milk, bulgur, dried cherries, and salt in a medium saucepan; bring it to a boil. Reduce heat to low and simmer, stirring regularly, until tender and the oatmeal consistency of the bulgur is tender (10-15 minutes).
2. Divide into 4 bowls of hot porridge: top with the apricots and almonds.

Nutrition:
Calories: 340
Fat: 6.7g
Protein: 15g
Carbs: 60.36g
Sodium: 552.32mg

46. TURKEY MEATBALLS

Preparation Time: 16 minutes
Cooking Time: 25 minutes
Servings: 5
Ingredients:

- 20 ounces of ground turkey
- 4 ounces of fresh or frozen spinach ¼ cup of oats
- 2 egg whites
- 2 celery sticks
- 3 cloves garlic
- ½ green bell peppers
- ½ red onion
- ½ cup of parsley
- ½ teaspoon of cumin
- 1 teaspoon of mustard powder
- 1 teaspoon of thyme
- ½ tablespoon of turmeric
- ½ teaspoon of chipotle pepper
- 1 teaspoon of salt
- Pinch of pepper

Directions:

1. Preheat the oven to 350°F.
2. Chop very finely (or use a food processor) the onion, garlic, and celery, and add to a large mixing cup.
3. In the dish, add the ham, egg whites, oats, and spices and combine well. Make sure the blend has no pockets of spices or oats.
4. Chop spinach, green peppers (stalked and seeded), and parsley. The bits need to be about a dime's size.
5. To the tpan, add the vegetables and mix them until well-combined.
6. Line the parchment paper with a baking sheet.
7. Roll the turkey mixture (about the size of golf balls) into 15

balls and put them on the baking sheet.
8. Bake for 25 minutes, until fully baked.

Nutrition:
Calories: 303
Fat: 7g
Carbs: 10.56g
Sodium: 600mg
Protein: 19g

47. BERRY OAT BREAKFAST BARS

Preparation Time: 10 minutes
Cooking Time: 25 minutes
Servings: 12
Ingredients:

- 2 cups fresh raspberries or blueberries
- 2 tablespoons sugar
- 2 tablespoons freshly squeezed lemon juice
- 1 tablespoon cornstarch
- 1½ cups rolled oats
- ½ cup whole wheat flour
- ½ cup walnuts
- ¼ cup chia seeds
- ¼ cup extra-virgin olive oil
- ¼ cup honey
- 1 large egg

Directions:

1. Preheat the oven to 350°F
2. In a small saucepan over medium heat, stir together the berries, sugar, lemon juice, and cornstarch. Bring to a simmer. Reduce the heat and simmer for 2 to 3 minutes, until the mixture thickens.
3. In a food processor or high-speed blender, combine the oats, flour, walnuts, and chia seeds. Process until powdered. Add the olive oil, honey, and egg. Pulse a few more times, until well combined. Press half of the mixture into a 9-inch square baking dish.
4. Spread the berry filling over the oat mixture. Add the remaining oat mixture on top of the berries. Bake for 25 minutes, until browned.
5. Let cool completely, cut into 12 pieces, and serve. Store in a covered container for up to 5 days.

Nutrition:
Calories: 219.96
Total Fat: 11.8g
Saturated Fat: 1g
Protein: 5g
Carbohydrates: 26g
Sugar: 9g

Fiber: 5g
Cholesterol: 16mg
Sodium: 8mg

48. WHOLE-GRAIN BREAKFAST COOKIES

Preparation Time: 20 minutes
Cooking Time: 10 minutes
Makes: 18 cookies
Ingredients:

- 2 cups rolled oats
- ½ cup whole-wheat flour
- ¼ cup ground flaxseed
- 1 teaspoon baking powder
- 1 cup unsweetened applesauce
- 2 large eggs
- 2 tablespoons vegetable oil
- 2 teaspoons vanilla extract
- 1 teaspoon ground cinnamon
- ½ cup dried cherries
- ¼ cup unsweetened shredded coconut
- 2 ounces dark chocolate, chopped

Directions:

1. Preheat the oven to 350°F.
2. In a large bowl, combine the oats, flour, flaxseed, and baking powder. Stir well to mix.
3. In a medium bowl, whisk the applesauce, eggs, vegetable oil, vanilla, and cinnamon. Pour the wet mixture into the dry mixture and stir until just combined.
4. Fold in cherries, coconut, and chocolate. Drop tablespoon-size balls of dough onto a baking sheet. Bake for 10 to 12 minutes, until browned and cooked through.
5. Let cool for about 3 minutes, remove from the baking sheet, and cool completely before serving. Store in an airtight container for up to 1 week.

Nutrition:
Calories: 136
Total Fat: 7g
Saturated Fat: 3g
Protein: 4g
Carbohydrates: 14g
Sugar: 4g
Fiber: 3g
Cholesterol: 21mg
Sodium: 11mg

49. BLUEBERRY BREAKFAST CAKE

Preparation Time: 15 minutes
Cooking Time: 45 minutes
Servings: 12
Ingredients:

For the Toppings:
- ¼ cup finely chopped walnuts
- ½ teaspoon ground cinnamon
- 2 tablespoons butter, chopped into small pieces
- 2 tablespoons sugar

For the Cake:
- Nonstick cooking spray
- 1 cup whole-wheat pastry flour
- 1 cup oat flour
- ¼ cup sugar
- 2 teaspoons baking powder
- 1 large egg, beaten
- ½ cup skim milk
- 2 tablespoons butter, melted
- 1 teaspoon grated lemon peel
- 2 cups fresh or frozen blueberries

Directions:

To Make the Topping:
1. In a small bowl, stir together the walnuts, cinnamon, butter, and sugar. Set aside.

To Make the Cake:
2. Preheat the oven to 350°F. Spray a 9-inch square pan with cooking spray. Set aside.
3. In a large bowl, stir together the pastry flour, oat flour, sugar, and baking powder.
4. Add the egg, milk, butter, and lemon peel, and stir until there are no dry spots.
5. Stir in the blueberries, and gently mix until incorporated. Press the batter into the prepared pan, using a spoon to flatten it into the dish.
6. Sprinkle the topping over the cake.
7. Bake for 40 to 45 minutes, until a toothpick inserted into the cake comes out clean and serve.

Nutrition:
Calories: 177
Total Fat: 7g
Saturated Fat: 3g
Protein: 4g
Carbohydrates: 26g
Sugar: 9g
Fiber: 3g
Cholesterol: 26mg
Sodium: 39mg

50. BUCKWHEAT GROUTS BREAKFAST BOWL

Preparation Time: 5 minutes, plus overnight to soak
Cooking Time: 10 to 12 minutes
Servings: 4
Ingredients:
- 3 cups skim milk

- 1 cup buckwheat grouts
- ¼ cup chia seeds
- 2 teaspoons vanilla extract
- ½ teaspoon ground cinnamon
- Pinch salt
- 1 cup water
- ½ cup unsalted pistachios
- 2 cups sliced fresh strawberries
- ¼ cup cacao nibs (optional)

Directions:
1. In a large bowl, stir the milk, groats, chia seeds, vanilla, cinnamon, and salt. Cover and refrigerate overnight.
2. The next morning, transfer the soaked mixture to a medium pot and add the water. Raise to a boil over medium-high heat, then lower to a simmer for 10 to 12 minutes, or until the buckwheat is soft and thickened.
3. Transfer to bowls and serve, topped with the pistachios, strawberries, and cacao nibs (if using).

Nutrition:
Calories: 340
Total Fat: 8g
Saturated Fat: 1g
Protein: 15g
Carbohydrates: 52g
Sugar: 14g
Fiber: 10g
Cholesterol: 4mg
Sodium: 140mg

51. WHOLE GRAIN DUTCH BABY PANCAKES

Preparation Time: 5 minutes
Cooking Time: 25 minutes
Servings: 4
Ingredients:
- 2 tablespoons coconut oil
- ½ cup whole-wheat flour
- ¼ cup skim milk
- 3 large eggs
- 1 teaspoon vanilla extract
- ½ teaspoon baking powder
- ¼ teaspoon salt
- ¼ teaspoon ground cinnamon
- Powdered sugar, for dusting

Directions:
1. Preheat the oven to 400°F.
2. Put the coconut oil in a medium oven-safe skillet and place the skillet in the oven to melt the oil while it preheats.
3. In a blender, milk, eggs, combine the flour, vanilla, baking powder, salt, and cinnamon. Process until smooth.

---

4. Then carefully remove the pan from the oven and tilt it to spread the oil around evenly.
5. Pour the batter into the pan and, then return it to the oven for 23 to 25 minutes, until the pancake puffs and lightly browns.
6. Remove, dust lightly with powdered sugar, cut into 4 wedges, and serve.

Nutrition:
Calories: 195
Total Fat: 11g
Saturated Fat: 7g
Protein: 8g
Carbohydrates: 16g
Sugar: 1g
Fiber: 2g
Cholesterol: 140mg
Sodium: 209mg

52. MUSHROOM, ZUCCHINI, AND ONION FRITTATA

Preparation Time: 10 minutes
Cooking Time: 20 minutes
Servings: 4
Ingredients:
- 1 tablespoon extra-virgin olive oil
- ½ onion, chopped
- 1 medium zucchini, chopped
- 1½ cups sliced mushrooms
- 6 large eggs, beaten
- 2 tablespoons skim milk
- Salt
- Freshly ground black pepper
- 1-ounce feta cheese, crumbled

Directions:
1. Preheat the oven to 400°F.
2. In a medium oven-safe skillet over medium-high heat, heat the olive oil.
3. Add the onion and sauté for 3 to 5 minutes, until translucent.
4. Add the zucchini and mushrooms, and cook for 3 to 5 more minutes, until the vegetables are tender.
5. Meantime, in a small bowl, whisk the eggs, milk, salt, and pepper. Pour the mixture into the skillet, stirring to combine, and transfer the skillet to the oven. Cook for 7-9 minutes, until set.
6. Sprinkle with the feta cheese, and cook for 1 to 2 minutes more, until heated through.
7. Remove, cut into 4 wedges, and serve.

Nutrition:
Calories: 178

Total Fat: 13g
Saturated Fat: 4g
Protein: 12g
Carbohydrates: 5g
Sugar: 3g
Fiber: 1g
Cholesterol: 285mg
Sodium: 234mg

53. SPINACH AND CHEESE QUICHE

Preparation Time: 10 minutes, plus 10 minutes to rest
Cooking Time: 50 minutes
Servings: 4 to 6
Ingredients:
- Nonstick cooking spray
- 8 ounces Yukon gold potatoes, shredded
- 1 tablespoon plus 2 teaspoons extra-virgin olive oil, divided
- 1 teaspoon salt, divided
- Freshly ground black pepper
- 1 onion, finely chopped
- 1 (10-ounce) bag fresh spinach
- 4 large eggs
- ½ cup skim milk
- 1-ounce Gruyère cheese, shredded

Directions:
1. Preheat the oven to 350°F. Spray a 9-inch pie dish with cooking spray. Set aside.
2. In a small bowl, toss the potatoes with 2 teaspoons of olive oil, ½ teaspoon of salt, and season with pepper. Press the potatoes into the sides and bottom of the pie dish to form a thin, even layer. Bake for 20 minutes, until golden brown. Now take from the oven and place on a cooling rack to cool.
3. In a large skillet over moderate-high flame, heat the remaining 1 tablespoon of olive oil.
4. Add the onion and sauté for 3 to 5 minutes, until softened.
5. By handfuls, add the spinach, stirring between each addition until it just starts to wilt before adding more. Cook for about 1 minute, until it cooks down.
6. In a medium bowl, whisk the milk and eggs. Add the gruyere, and season with the remaining ½ teaspoon of salt and some pepper. Fold the eggs into the spinach. Pour the mixture into the pie dish and bake for 25 minutes, until the eggs are set.
7. Let rest for 10 minutes before serving.

Nutrition:
Calories: 445
Total Fat: 14g
Saturated Fat: 4g
Protein: 19g
Carbohydrates: 68g
Sugar: 6g
Fiber: 7g
Cholesterol: 193mg
Sodium: 773mg

54. SPICY JALAPEÑO POPPER DEVILED EGGS

Preparation Time: 5 minutes
Cooking Time: 5 minutes
Servings: 4
Ingredients:
- 4 large whole eggs, hardboiled
- 2 tablespoons Keto-Friendly mayonnaise
- ¼ cup cheddar cheese, grated
- 2 slices bacon, cooked and crumbled
- 1 jalapeño, sliced

Directions:
1. Cut eggs in half, remove the yolk, and put them in a bowl
2. Lay egg whites on a platter
3. Mix in the remaining ingredients and mash them with the egg yolks
4. Transfer yolk mix back to the egg whites
5. Serve and enjoy!

Nutrition:
Calories: 176
Fat: 14g
Carbohydrates: 0.7g
Protein: 10g
Sodium: 233.14mg

55. LOVELY PORRIDGE

Preparation Time: 15 minutes
Cooking Time: Nil
Servings: 2
Ingredients:
- 2 tablespoons coconut flour
- 2 tablespoons vanilla protein powder
- 3 tablespoons golden flaxseed meal
- 1½ cups almond milk, unsweetened
- Powdered erythritol

Directions:
1. Take a bowl and mix in flaxseed meal, protein powder, coconut flour and mix well
2. Pour the mixture into the pot (placed over medium heat)

3. Stir in the almond milk and let aside to thicken.
4. Serve with your preferred quantity of sweetener.
5. Enjoy!

Nutrition:
Calories: 137
Carbohydrates: 17.5g
Fat: 7.79g
Protein: 7g
Sodium: 164.27mg

56. SALTY MACADAMIA CHOCOLATE SMOOTHIE

Preparation Time: 5 minutes
Cooking Time: Nil
Servings: 1
Ingredients:
- 2 tablespoons macadamia nuts, salted
- ⅓ cup chocolate whey protein powder, low carb
- 1 cup almond milk, unsweetened

Directions:
1. Add the listed ingredients to your blender and blend until you have a smooth mixture
2. Chill and enjoy it!

Nutrition:
Calories: 285
Fat: 17.67g
Carbohydrates: 7.46g
Protein: 26.62g
Sodium: 237mg

57. BASIL AND TOMATO BAKED EGGS

Preparation Time: 10 minutes
Cooking Time: 15 minutes
Servings: 4
Ingredients:
- 1 garlic clove, minced
- 1 cup canned tomatoes
- ¼ cup fresh basil leaves, roughly chopped
- ½ teaspoon chili powder
- 1 tablespoon olive oil
- 4 whole eggs
- Salt and pepper to taste

Directions:
1. Preheat your oven to 375°F
2. Take a small baking dish and grease it with olive oil
3. In a mixing bowl, combine the garlic, basil, tomatoes, chilli, and olive oil.
4. Crack eggs into a dish, keeping space between the 2
5. Sprinkle the whole dish with pepper and salt.

6. Cook for 12 minutes, or until the eggs are set and the tomatoes are boiling.
7. Serve with fresh basil on top.
8. Enjoy!

Nutrition:
Calories: 117.04
Fat: 7.99g
Carbohydrates: 5.39g
Protein: 6.7g
Sodium: 380mg

58. CINNAMON AND COCONUT PORRIDGE

Preparation Time: 5 minutes
Cooking Time: 5 minutes
Servings: 4
Ingredients:

- 2 cups of water
- 1 cup 36% heavy cream
- ½ cup unsweetened dried coconut, shredded
- 2 tablespoons flaxseed meal
- 1 tablespoon unsalted butter
- 1 and ½ teaspoon stevia
- 1 teaspoon cinnamon
- Salt to taste
- Toppings such as blueberries

Directions:
1. First add the above ingredients to a small pot, mix well
2. Place the saucepan on the stove over medium-low heat.
3. Bring to mix to a slow boil
4. Stir well and remove the heat
5. Divide the mix into equal servings and let them sit for 10 minutes
6. Top with your desired toppings and enjoy!

Nutrition:
Calories: 354
Fat: 35.45g
Carbohydrates: 8.22g
Protein: 3.4g
Sodium: 217.65mg

59. AN OMELET OF SWISS CHARD

Preparation Time: 5 minutes
Cooking Time: 5 minutes
Servings: 4
Ingredients:

- 4 eggs, lightly beaten
- 4 cups Swiss chard, sliced
- 2 tablespoons unsalted butter
- ½ teaspoon garlic salt
- Fresh pepper to taste

Directions:
1. Take a non-stick frying pan and place it over medium-low heat

2. Once the butter melts, add Swiss chard and stir cook for 2 minutes
3. Pour egg into the pan and gently stir them into Swiss chard
4. Season with garlic salt and pepper
5. Cook for 2 minutes
6. Serve and enjoy!

Nutrition:
Calories: 123.6
Fat: 9.8g
Carbohydrates: 2.4g
Protein: 6.44g
Sodium: 382mg

60. CHEESY LOW-CARB OMELET

Preparation Time: 5 minutes
Cooking Time: 5 minutes
Servings: 5
Ingredients:

- 2 whole eggs
- 1 tablespoon water
- 1 tablespoon unsalted butter
- 3 thin slices of salami
- 5 fresh basil leaves
- 5 thin slices, fresh ripe tomatoes
- 2 ounces fresh mozzarella cheese
- Salt and pepper as needed

Directions:
1. Take a small bowl and whisk in eggs and water
2. Take a non-stick Sauté pan and place it over medium heat, add butter and let it melt
3. Pour egg mixture and cook for 30 seconds
4. Spread salami slices on half of egg mix and top with cheese, tomatoes, basil slices
5. Season with pepper and salt according to your taste
6. Cook for 2 minutes and fold the egg with the empty half
7. Cover and cook on LOW for 1 minute
8. Serve and enjoy!

Nutrition:
Calories: 93.6
Fat: 7.42g
Carbohydrates: 1.13g
Protein: 5.57g
Sodium: 305mg

61. YOGURT AND KALE SMOOTHIE

Servings: 1
Preparation Time: 10 minutes
Ingredients:

- 1 cup whole milk yogurt

- 1 cup baby kale greens
- 1 pack Stevia
- 1 tablespoon MCT oil
- 1 tablespoon sunflower seeds
- 1 cup of water

Directions:
1. Add listed ingredients to the blender
2. Blend until you have a smooth and creamy texture
3. Serve chilled and enjoy!

Nutrition:
Calories: 321.45
Fat: 26g
Sodium: 119.89mg
Carbohydrates: 15g
Protein: 11g

62. CRISPY PITA WITH CANADIAN BACON

Preparation Time: 5 minutes
Cooking Time: 15 minutes
Servings: 2
Ingredients:

- 1 (6-inch) whole-grain pita bread
- 3 teaspoons extra-virgin olive oil, divided
- 2 eggs
- 2 Canadian bacon slices
- Juice of ½ lemon
- 1 cup microgreens
- 2 tablespoons crumbled goat cheese
- Freshly ground black pepper, to taste

Directions:
1. Heat a large skillet over medium heat. Cut the pita bread in half and brush each side of both halves with ¼ teaspoon of olive oil (using a total of 1 teaspoon oil). Cook for 2 to 3 minutes on each side, then remove from the skillet.
2. In the same skillet, heat 1 teaspoon of oil over medium heat. Crack the eggs into the skillet and cook until the eggs are set, 2 to 3 minutes. Remove from the skillet.
3. In the same skillet, cook the Canadian bacon for 3 to 5 minutes, flipping once.
4. In a large bowl, whisk together the remaining 1 teaspoon of oil and the lemon juice. Add the microgreens and toss to combine.
5. Top each pita half with half of the microgreens, 1 piece of bacon, 1 egg, and 1 tablespoon of goat cheese. Season with pepper and serve.

Nutrition:
Calories: 251
Fat: 13.9g
Protein: 13.1g
Carbohydrates: 20.1g
Fiber: 3.1g
Sugar: 0.9g
Sodium: 400mg

63. COCONUT AND CHIA PUDDING

Preparation Time: 5 minutes
Cooking Time: 0 minutes
Servings: 2
Ingredients:
- 7 ounces (198 g) light coconut milk
- ¼ cup chia seeds
- 3 to 4 drops liquid stevia
- 1 clementine
- 1 kiwi
- Shredded coconut (unsweetened)

Directions:
1. Start by taking a mixing bowl and adding in the light coconut milk. Add in the liquid Stevia to sweeten the milk. Mix well.
2. Add the chia seeds to the milk and whisk until well-combined. Set aside.
3. Peel the clementine and carefully remove the skin from the wedges. Set aside.
4. Also, peel the kiwi and dice it into small pieces.
5. Take a glass jar and assemble the pudding. For this, place the fruits at the bottom of the jar; then add a dollop of chia pudding. Now spread the fruits and then add another layer of chia pudding.
6. Finish by garnishing with the remaining fruits and shredded coconut.

Nutrition:
Calories: 486
Fat: 40.5g
Protein: 8.5g
Carbohydrates: 30.8g
Fiber: 15.6g
Sugar: 11.6g
Sodium: 24mg

64. COCONUT AND BERRY OATMEAL

Preparation Time: 10 minutes
Cooking Time: 35 minutes
Servings: 6
Ingredients:
- 2 cups rolled oats

- ¼ cup shredded unsweetened coconut
- 1 teaspoon baking powder
- ½ teaspoon ground cinnamon
- ¼ teaspoon sea salt
- 2 cups skim milk
- ¼ cup of melted coconut oil, plus extra for greasing the baking dish
- 1 egg
- 1 teaspoon pure vanilla extract
- 2 cups fresh blueberries
- ⅛ cup chopped pecans, for garnish
- 1 teaspoon of chopped fresh mint leaves, for garnish

Directions:
1. Preheat the oven to 350ºF (180ºC). Lightly oil a baking dish and set it aside.
2. In a medium bowl, stir together the oats, coconut, baking powder, cinnamon, and salt.
3. In a small bowl, whisk the milk, oil, egg, and vanilla until well blended.
4. Layer half the dry ingredients in the baking dish, top with half the berries, then spoon the remaining dry ingredients and the rest of the berries on top. Pour the wet ingredients evenly into the baking dish. Tap it lightly on the counter to disperse the wet ingredients throughout.
5. Bake the casserole, uncovered, until the oats are tender, about 35 minutes. Serve immediately, topped with pecans and mint.

Nutrition:
Calories: 296
Fat: 17.1g
Protein: 10.2g
Carbohydrates: 26.9g
Fiber: 4.1g
Sugar: 10.9g
Sodium: 154mg

65. GREEK YOGURT AND OAT PANCAKES

Preparation Time: 5 minutes
Cooking Time: 20 minutes
Servings: 4

Ingredients:
- 1 cup 2 percent plain Greek yogurt
- 3 eggs
- 1½ teaspoons pure vanilla extract
- 1 cup rolled oats

- 1 tablespoon granulated sweetener
- 1 teaspoon baking powder
- 1 teaspoon ground cinnamon
- Pinch ground cloves
- Nonstick cooking spray

Directions:
1. Place the yogurt, eggs, and vanilla in a blender and pulse to combine.
2. Add the oats, sweetener, baking powder, cinnamon, and cloves to the blender and blend until the batter is smooth.
3. Place a large nonstick skillet over medium heat and lightly coat it with cooking spray.
4. Spoon ¼ cup of batter per pancake, 4 at a time, into the skillet. Cook the pancakes until the bottoms are firm and golden, about 4 minutes.
5. Flip the pancakes over and cook the other side until they are cooked through about 3 minutes.
6. Remove the pancakes to a plate and repeat with the remaining batter.
7. Serve with fresh fruit.

Nutrition:
Calories: 244
Fat: 8.1g
Protein: 13.1g
Carbohydrates:28.1
Fiber: 4.0g
Sugar:3.0g
Sodium: 82mg

66. STYLISH CHICKEN-BACON WRAP

Preparation Time: 5 minutes
Cooking Time: 50 minutes
Servings: 3
Ingredients:
- 8 ounces lean chicken breast
- 6 bacon slices
- 3 ounces shredded cheese
- 4 slices ham

Directions:
1. Cut chicken breast into bite-sized portions
2. Transfer shredded cheese onto ham slices
3. Roll up chicken breast and ham slices in bacon slices
4. Take a pan and place it over moderate heat
5. Add olive oil and brown bacon
6. Remove rolls and transfer to your oven
7. Bake for 45 minutes at 325°F
8. Serve and enjoy!

Nutrition:

Calories: 420
Fat: 28g
Carbohydrates: 0.05g
Protein: 40g
Sodium: 1376mg

67. HEALTHY COTTAGE CHEESE PANCAKES

Preparation Time: 10 minutes
Cooking Time: 15
Servings: 1
Ingredients:
- ½ cup of Cottage cheese (low-fat)
- ⅓ cup (approx. 2 egg whites) Egg whites
- ¼ cup of oats
- 1 teaspoon of vanilla extract
- Olive oil cooking spray
- 1 tablespoon of Stevia (raw)
- Berries or sugar-free jam (optional)

Directions:
1. Begin by taking a food blender and adding in the egg whites and cottage cheese. Also add in the vanilla extract, a pinch of stevia, and oats. Blend until the consistency is smooth.
2. Get a nonstick pan and coat it nicely with the cooking spray. Put the pan on low heat.
3. After it has been heated, scoop out half of the batter and pour it into the pan. Cook for about 2½ minutes on each side.
4. Place the cooked pancakes on a serving plate and cover them with sugar-free jam or berries.

Nutrition:
Calories: 356
Fat: 11.98g
Protein: 29g
Carbohydrates: 40g
Sodium: 591mg

68. AVOCADO LEMON TOAST

Preparation Time: 10 minutes
Cooking Time: 13 minutes
Servings: 2
Ingredients:
- 2 slices whole-grain bread
- 2 tablespoons fresh cilantro (chopped)
- ¼ teaspoon lemon zest
- 1 pinch fine sea salt
- ½ Avocado
- 1 teaspoon fresh lemon juice
- 1 pinch cayenne pepper
- ¼ teaspoon chia seeds

Directions:

1. Begin by getting a medium-sized mixing bowl and adding in the avocado. Use a fork to crush it.
2. Then, add in the cilantro, lemon zest, lemon juice, sea salt, and cayenne pepper. Mix well until combined.
3. Toast the bread pieces till golden brown in a toaster. It should just take 3 minutes.
4. Drizzle the chia seeds over the toasted bread pieces and top with the avocado mixture.

Nutrition:
Calories: 116.81
Protein: 4.6g
Fat: 5.2g
Carbohydrates: 14.6g
Sodium: 153.65mg

69. HEALTHY BAKED EGGS

Preparation Time: 10 minutes
Cooking Time: 1 hour
Servings: 6
Ingredients:
- 1 tablespoon olive oil
- 2 cloves garlic
- 8 large eggs
- ½ teaspoon sea salt
- 3 cups shredded mozzarella cheese (medium fat)
- Olive oil spray
- 1 medium onion (chopped)
- 8 ounces spinach leaves
- 1 cup Half-and-Half
- 1 teaspoon black pepper
- ½ cup feta cheese

Directions:
1. Begin by heating the oven to 375°F.
2. Get a glass baking dish and grease it with olive oil spray. Set aside.
3. Now take a nonstick pan and pour in the olive oil. Place the pan on low heat.
4. Immediately toss in the garlic, spinach, and onion. Let it sit for about 5 minutes. Set aside.
5. In a large mixing bowl add in Half-and-Half, eggs, pepper, and salt. Whisk thoroughly to combine.
6. Put in the feta cheese and chopped mozzarella cheese (reserve ½ cup of mozzarella cheese for later).
7. Put the egg mixture and prepared spinach into the glass baking dish. Blend well to combine. Drizzle the reserved cheese over the top.

8. Bake the egg mix for about 45 minutes.
9. Remove the baking dish from the oven and allow it to stand for 10 minutes.
10. Dice and serve!

Nutrition:
Calories: 387
Fat: 28.78g
Protein: 24.7g
Carbohydrates: 7.9g
Sodium: 662mg

70. QUICK LOW-CARB OATMEAL

Preparation Time: 10 minutes
Cooking Time: 15 minutes
Servings: 2
Ingredients:
- ½ cup almond flour
- 2 tablespoons flax meal
- 1 teaspoon ground cinnamon (ground)
- 1½ cups almond milk (unsweetened)
- Salt, as per taste
- 2 tablespoons chia seeds
- 10 – 15 drops liquid Stevia
- 1 teaspoon vanilla extract

Directions:
1. Begin by taking a large mixing bowl and adding in the coconut flour, almond flour, ground cinnamon, flax seed powder, and chia seeds. Mix properly to combine.
2. Position a stockpot on low heat and add in the dry ingredients. Also add in the liquid Stevia, vanilla extract, and almond milk. Mix well to combine.
3. Prepare the flour and almond milk for about 4 minutes. Add salt if needed.
4. Move the oatmeal to a serving bowl and top with nuts, seeds, and pure and neat berries.

Nutrition:
Calories: 267.59
Protein: 9.71g
Fat: 20.3g
Carbohydrates: 14.22g
Sodium: 529mg

71. TOFU AND VEGETABLE SCRAMBLE

Preparation Time: 10 minutes
Cooking Time: 15 minutes
Servings: 2
Ingredients:
- 16 ounces firm tofu (drained)
- ½ teaspoon Sea salt
- 1 teaspoon garlic powder
- Fresh coriander, for garnishing

- ½ medium red onion
- 1 teaspoon cumin powder
- Lemon juice, for topping
- 1 medium green bell pepper
- 1 teaspoon garlic powder

Directions:

1. Begin by preparing the ingredients. Remove the seeds of the tomato and green bell pepper.
2. Shred the onion, bell pepper, and tomato into small cubes.
3. Get a small mixing bowl and put the fairly hard tofu inside it. Make use of your hands to break the fairly hard tofu. Set aside.
4. Get a nonstick pan and add in the onion, tomato, and bell pepper. Mix and cook for about 3 minutes.
5. Put the somewhat hard crumbled tofu into the pan and combine well.
6. Get a small bowl and put in the water, turmeric, garlic powder, cumin powder, and chili powder. Combine well and stream it over the tofu and vegetable mixture.
7. Allow the tofu and vegetable crumble to cook with seasoning for 5 minutes. Continuously stir so that ingredients do not stick to the pan.Drizzle the tofu scramble with chili flakes and salt. Combine well.
7. Transfer the prepared scramble to a serving bowl and give it a spray of lemon juice.
8. Finalize by garnishing with coriander. Serve while hot!

Nutrition:
Calories: 238
Carbohydrates: 8.6g
Fat: 9.89g
Sodium: 553.56mg

72. BREAKFAST SMOOTHIE BOWL WITH FRESH BERRIES

Preparation Time: 10 minutes
Cooking Time: 5 minutes
Servings: 2
Ingredients:

- ½ cup almond milk (unsweetened)
- ½ teaspoon psyllium husk powder
- 2 ounces strawberries (chopped)
- 1 tablespoon coconut oil
- 3 cups crushed ice

- 5 to 10 drops of liquid Stevia
- ⅓ cup pea protein powder

Directions:

1. Begin by taking a blender and adding in the mashed ice cubes. Allow them to rest for about 30 seconds.
2. Then put in the almond milk, strawberries, pea protein powder, psyllium husk powder, coconut oil, and liquid Stevia. Blend well until it turns into a smooth and creamy puree.
3. Pour the prepared smoothie into 2 glasses.
4. Cover with coconut flakes and strawberries.

Nutrition:
Calories: 150
Fat: 9.2g
Sodium: 224.57mg
Carbohydrates: 4.1g
Protein: 14.6g

73. CHIA AND COCONUT PUDDING

Preparation Time: 10 minutes
Cooking Time: 5 minutes
Servings: 2
Ingredients:

- 7 ounces light coconut milk
- 3 to 4 drops liquid Stevia
- 1 kiwi
- ¼ cup chia seeds
- 1 clementine
- shredded coconut (unsweetened)

Directions:

1. Begin by getting a mixing bowl and putting in the light coconut milk. Add the liquid Stevia to sweeten the milk. Combine well.
2. Put the chia seeds into the milk and whisk until well-combined. Set aside.
3. Peel the clementine and carefully extract the skin from the wedges. Leave aside.
4. Also, peel the kiwi and dice it into small pieces.
5. Get a glass bowl and add the pudding. For this, position the fruits at the bottom of the jar; then put a dollop of chia pudding. Then spread the fruits and then put another layer of chia pudding.
6. Finalize by garnishing with the rest of the fruits and chopped coconut.

Nutrition:
Calories: 244.8
Protein: 5.4g

Fat: 10g
Sodium: 13.19mg
Carbohydrates: 22.8g

74. BANANA BARLEY PORRIDGE

Preparation Time: 15 minutes
Cooking Time: 5 minutes
Servings: 2
Ingredients:

- 1 cup unsweetened coconut milk
- 1 small peeled and sliced banana
- ½ cup barley
- 3 drops liquid Stevia
- ¼ cup chopped coconuts

Directions:

1. In a bowl, mix barley with half the coconut milk and Stevia.
2. Cover the blending bowl, then refrigerate for about 6 hours.
3. In a saucepan, mix the barley mixture with coconut milk.
4. Cook for about 5 minutes on moderate heat.
5. Then top it with the chopped coconuts and, therefore, the banana slices.
6. Serve.

Nutrition:
Calories: 468
Fat: 24g
Carbohydrates: 54g
Protein: 4.6g
Sodium: 59.94mg

75. COCONUT AND BERRY SMOOTHIE

Preparation Time: 5 minutes
Cooking Time: 0 minutes
Servings: 2
Ingredients:

- ½ cup mixed berries (blueberries, strawberries, blackberries)
- 1 tablespoon ground flaxseed
- 2 tablespoons unsweetened coconut flakes
- ½ cup unsweetened plain coconut milk
- ½ cup leafy greens (kale, spinach)
- ¼ cup unsweetened vanilla nonfat yogurt
- ½ cup ice

Directions:

1. In a blender, combine the berries, flaxseed, coconut flakes, coconut milk, greens, yogurt, and ice.
2. Process until smooth. Serve.

Nutrition:
Calories: 182

Fat: 14.9g
Protein: 5.9g
Carbohydrates: 8.1g
Fiber: 4.1g
Sugar: 2.9g
Sodium: 25mg

76. APPLE AND PUMPKIN WAFFLES

Preparation Time: 10 minutes
Cooking Time: 20 minutes
Servings: 6
Ingredients:

- 2¼ cups whole wheat pastry flour
- 2 tablespoons granulated sweetener
- 1 tablespoon baking powder
- 1 teaspoon ground cinnamon
- 1 teaspoon ground nutmeg
- 4 eggs
- 1¼ cups pure pumpkin purée
- 1 apple, peeled, cored, and finely chopped
- Melted coconut oil, for cooking

Directions:

1. Combine the flour, sweetener, baking powder, cinnamon, and nutmeg in a large mixing basin. Whisk together the eggs and pumpkin in a small bowl. Whisk together the wet and dry ingredients until smooth.
2. Stir the apple into the batter.
3. Make the waffles according to the manufacturer's instructions, brushing your waffle iron with melted coconut oil, until all the batter is gone. Serve immediately.

Nutrition:
Calories: 232
Fat: 4.1g
Protein: 10.9g
Carbohydrates: 40.1g
Fiber: 7.1g
Sugar: 5.1g
Sodium: 52mg

77. BUCKWHEAT CRÊPES

Preparation Time: 20 minutes
Cooking Time: 20 minutes
Servings: 5
Ingredients:

- 1½ cups skim milk
- 3 eggs
- 1 teaspoon extra-virgin olive oil, plus more for the skillet
- 1 cup buckwheat flour
- ½ cup whole wheat flour
- ½ cup 2% plain Greek yogurt

- 1 cup sliced strawberries
- 1 cup blueberries

Directions:

1. In a large bowl, whisk together the milk, eggs, and 1 teaspoon of oil until well combined.
2. Into a medium bowl, sift together the buckwheat and whole wheat flours. Whisk together the wet and dry ingredients until thoroughly blended and extremely smooth.
3. Allow the batter to rest for at least 2 hours before cooking.
4. Place a large skillet or crêpe pan over medium-high heat and lightly coat the bottom with oil.
5. Pour about ¼ cup of batter into the skillet. Swirl the pan until the batter completely coats the bottom.
6. Cook the crêpe for about 1 minute, then flip it over. Cook the other side of the crêpe for another minute, until lightly browned. Transfer the cooked crêpe to a plate and cover with a clean dish towel to keep warm. Then repeat until the batter is used up; you should have about 10 crêpes.
7. Spoon 1 tablespoon of yogurt onto each crêpe and place 2 crêpes on each plate. Top with berries and serve.

Nutrition:
Calories: 330
Fat: 6.9g
Protein: 15.9g
Carbohydrates: 54
Sugar: 11.1g
Sodium: 100mg

78. MUSHROOM FRITTATA

Preparation Time: 10 minutes
Cooking Time: 15 minutes
Servings: 4
Ingredients:

- 8 large eggs
- ½ cup skim milk
- ¼ teaspoon ground nutmeg
- Freshly ground black pepper & Sea salt, to taste
- 2 teaspoons extra-virgin olive oil
- 2 cups sliced wild mushrooms (cremini, oyster, shiitake, portobello, etc.)
- ½ red onion, chopped
- 1 teaspoon minced garlic
- ½ cup goat cheese, crumbled

Directions:

1. Preheat the broiler. In a medium basin, mix together the milk, eggs, and nutmeg until well combined.
2. Season the egg mixture lightly with salt and pepper and set it aside.
3. Place an ovenproof pan over medium heat and add the oil, coating the bottom completely by tilting the pan.
4. Sauté the mushrooms, onion, and garlic until translucent, about 7 minutes. Pour the egg mixture into the skillet and cook until the bottom of the frittata is set, lifting the edges of the cooked egg to allow the uncooked egg to seep under.
5. Place the skillet under the broiler until the top is set for about 1 minute. Sprinkle the goat cheese on the frittata and broil until the cheese is melted, about 1 minute more.
6. Remove from the oven. Cut into 4 wedges to serve.

Nutrition:
Calories: 227
Fat: 15.1g
Protein: 17.1g
Carbohydrates: 5.1g
Fiber: 0.9g
Sugar: 4.1g
Sodium: 224mg

79. TROPICAL YOGURT KIWI BOWL

Preparation Time: 5 minutes
Cooking Time: 0 minutes
Servings: 2
Ingredients:

- 1½ cups plain low-fat Greek yogurt
- 2 kiwis, peeled and sliced
- 2 tablespoons shredded unsweetened coconut flakes
- 2 tablespoons halved walnuts
- 1 tablespoon chia seeds
- 2 teaspoons honey, divided (optional)

Directions:

1. Divide the yogurt between 2 small bowls.
2. Top each serving of yogurt with half of the kiwi slices, coconut flakes, walnuts, chia seeds, and honey (if using).

Nutrition:
Calories: 261
Fat: 9.1g
Protein: 21.1g
Carbohydrates: 23.1g
Fiber: 6.1g
Sugar: 14.1g

Sodium: 84mg

80. BANANA CRÊPE CAKES

Preparation Time: 5 minutes
Cooking Time: 20 minutes
Servings: 4
Ingredients:
- Avocado oil cooking spray
- 4 ounces (113g) reduced-fat plain cream cheese, softened
- 2 medium bananas
- 4 large eggs
- ½ teaspoon vanilla extract
- ⅛ teaspoon salt

Directions:
1. Heat a large skillet over low heat. Coat the cooking surface with cooking spray and allow the pan to heat for another 2 to 3 minutes.
2. Meanwhile, in a medium bowl, mash the cream cheese and bananas together with a fork until combined. The bananas can be a little chunky.
3. Add the vanilla, salt, and eggs, and mix well.
4. For each cake, drop 2 tablespoons of the batter onto the warmed skillet and use the bottom of a large spoon or ladle to spread it thin. Let it cook for 7 to 9 minutes.
5. Flip the cake over and cook briefly for about 1 minute.

Nutrition:
Calories: 176
Fat: 9.1g
Protein: 9.1g
Carbohydrates: 15.1g
Fiber: 2.1g
Sugar: 8.1g
Sodium: 214mg

81. TACOS WITH PICO DE GALLO

Preparation Time: 5 minutes
Cooking Time: 10 minutes
Servings: 4
Ingredients:
For the Taco Filling:
- Avocado oil cooking spray
- 1 medium green bell pepper, chopped
- 8 large eggs
- ¼ cup shredded sharp cheddar cheese
- 4 6-inch whole wheat tortillas
- 1 cup fresh spinach leaves
- ½ cup pico de gallo
- Scallions, chopped, for garnish (optional)
- Avocado slices, for garnish (optional)

For the Pico De Gallo:
- 1 tomato, diced
- ½ large white onion, diced
- 2 tablespoons chopped fresh cilantro
- ½ jalapeño pepper stemmed, seeded, and diced
- 1 tablespoon freshly squeezed lime juice
- ⅛ teaspoon salt

Directions:
To Make the Taco Filling:
1. Heat a medium skillet over medium-low heat. When hot, coat the cooking surface with cooking spray and put the pepper in the skillet. Cook for 4 minutes.
2. Meantime, mix the eggs in a medium bowl, then add the cheese and whisk to combine. Pour the eggs and cheese into the skillet with the green peppers and scramble until the eggs are fully cooked about 5 minutes.
3. Microwave the tortillas very briefly, about 8 seconds.
4. For each serving, top a tortilla with one-quarter of the spinach, eggs, and pico de gallo. Garnish with scallions and avocado slices (if using).

To Make the Pico de Gallo:
1. In a medium bowl, combine the cilantro, onion, tomato, pepper, lime juice, and salt. Mix well and serve.

Nutrition:
Calories: 277
Fat: 12.
Protein: 16.1g
Carbohydrates: 28.1g
Fiber: 2.9g
Sugar: 8.
Sodium: 563mg

82. TOMATO WAFFLES

Preparation Time: 15 minutes
Cooking Time: 40 minutes
Servings: 8
Ingredients:
- 2 cups low-fat buttermilk
- ½ cup crushed tomato
- 1 medium egg
- 2 medium egg whites
- 1 cup gluten-free all-purpose flour
- ½ cup almond flour
- ½ cup coconut flour
- 2 teaspoons baking powder
- ½ teaspoon baking soda
- ½ teaspoon dried chives
- Non-stick cooking spray

Directions:
1. Heat waffle iron.
2. In a medium bowl, whisk the buttermilk, tomato, egg, and egg whites together.
3. In another bowl, whisk the all-purpose flour, almond flour, coconut flour, baking powder, baking soda, and chives together.
4. To the dry ingredients, add the wet ingredients.
5. Lightly spray the waffle iron with cooking spray.
6. Gently pour ¼-½-cup portions of batter into the waffle iron. Cooking time for waffles will vary depending on the kind of waffle iron you use, but it is usually 5 minutes per waffle. (Note: Once the waffle iron is hot, the cooking process is a bit faster.) Repeat until no batter remains.
7. Enjoy the waffles warm with dandelion greens with sweet onion.

Nutrition:
Calories: 144
Fat: 4.1g
Protein: 7.1g
Carbohydrates: 21.2g
Fiber: 5.1g
Sugar: 2.9g
Sodium: 171mg

83. VEAL SCALOPPINI TOPPED WITH CAPERS

Preparation Time: 10 minutes
Cooking Time: 20 minutes
Servings: 4
Ingredients:
- 1 pound veal cutlets
- ½ teaspoon sea salt
- ¼ teaspoon black pepper
- 1 tablespoon olive oil
- 3 tablespoons butter
- 4 cloves garlic (minced)
- ½ cup white cooking wine
- ½ cup chicken bone broth
- ¼ cup lemon juice
- ¼ cup capers (drained)
- 2 tablespoons fresh parsley

Directions:
1. Place the veal cutlets onto a flat surface and use a meat tenderizer to pound the same. Make sure the thickness of the veal cutlets is about ⅛ inch.

Generously season both sides of the veal with pepper and salt.

2. Take a medium-sized cast-iron skillet and place it on a medium-high flame. Pour in the olive oil and let it heat through.

3. Once the oil is hot, place half of the veal cutlets into the skillet and cook for about 45 seconds on each side. Transfer the meat onto a plate and add in the remaining oil and veal cutlets. Cook for 45 seconds on each side. Transfer the meat onto the plate. Cover the plate with an aluminum foil sheet. Set aside.

4. Return the skillet to the flame and reduce the flame to medium. Add in 1 tablespoon of butter and let it melt.

5. Toss in the minced garlic and cook for about 1 minute. To prevent the garlic from burning, keep stirring.

6. Pour in the white wine, lemon juice, and chicken broth. Use the spatula to scrape the browned bits from the bottom of the pan.

7. Toss in the capers and increase the flame to medium-high. Cook until the sauce comes to a boil. Let the sauce simmer for about 8-10 minutes or until the sauce is reduced to half.

8. Add in the remaining butter and stir until it melts and incorporates into the sauce. This will take about 4-5 minutes.

9. Taste the sauce and add the pepper and salt as per your taste.

10. Return the seared veal cutlets to the prepared sauce and toss well. Put off the flame.

11. Garnish with fresh parsley and serve!

Nutrition:
Calories: 266
Fat: 15.8g
Protein: 25.5g
Carbohydrates: 4.45g
Sugar: 0.9g
Sodium: 659.86mg

84. BRUSSELS SPROUT HASH AND EGGS

Preparation Time: 15 minutes
Cooking Time: 15 minutes
Servings: 4
Ingredients:

- 3 teaspoons extra-virgin olive oil, divided
- 1 pound Brussels sprouts, sliced
- 2 garlic cloves, thinly sliced
- ¼ teaspoon salt
- Juice of 1 lemon
- 4 eggs

Directions:

1. In a large skillet, heat 1½ teaspoon of oil over medium heat. Add the Brussels sprouts and toss. Cook, stirring regularly, for 6 to 8 minutes until browned and softened. Add the garlic and continue to cook until fragrant, about 1 minute. Season with salt and lemon juice. Transfer to a serving dish.

2. In the same pan, heat the remaining 1½ teaspoons of oil over medium-high heat. Crack the eggs into the pan. Fry for 2 to 4 minutes, flip, and continue cooking to desired doneness. Serve over the bed of hash.

3. Make-ahead tip: Brussels sprouts, like other brassica vegetables, are easy to prep in advance and hold up well both raw and cooked. Prep the Brussels sprouts up to 5 days in advance by slicing them when you have a free moment. Refrigerate in an airtight container until ready for use.

Nutrition:
Calories: 158
Total Fat: 9g
Protein: 10g
Carbohydrates:12g
Sugar: 4g
Fiber: 4g
Sodium: 234mg

LUNCH

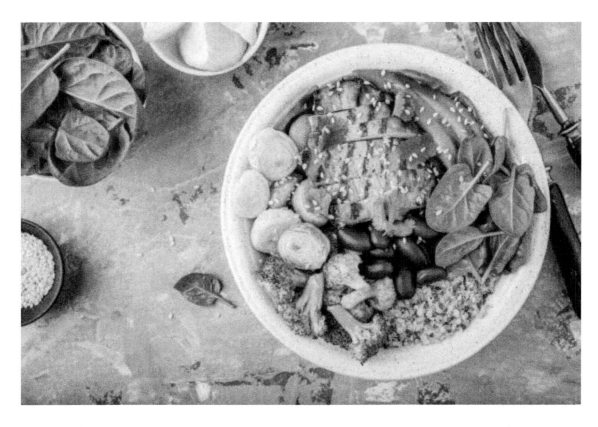

85. CHICKEN CHILI

Preparation Time: 6 minutes
Cooking Time: 1 hour
Servings: 4
Ingredients:

- 3 tablespoons vegetable oil
- 2 cloves garlic, minced
- 1 green bell pepper, chopped
- 1 onion, chopped
- 1 stalk celery, sliced
- ¼ pound mushrooms, chopped
- 1-pound chicken breast
- 1 tablespoon chili powder
- 1 teaspoon dried oregano
- 1 teaspoon ground cumin
- ½ teaspoon paprika
- ½ teaspoon cocoa powder
- ¼ teaspoon salt
- 1 14.5-oz can tomatoes with juice
- 1 pinch crushed red pepper flakes
- 1 pinch ground black pepper
- 1 19-oz can kidney beans

Directions:

1. Add 2 tablespoons of oil into a big skillet and heat it at moderate heat. Add mushrooms, celery, onion, bell pepper, and garlic, sautéing for 5 minutes. Put it to one side.
2. Insert the leftover 1 tablespoon of oil into the skillet. At high heat, cook the chicken until browned and its exterior turns firm. Transfer the vegetable mixture back into the skillet.
3. Stir in ground black pepper, hot pepper flakes, salt, cocoa powder, paprika, oregano, cumin, and chili powder. Continue stirring for several minutes to avoid burning. Pour in the beans and tomatoes and lead the entire mixture to boiling point then adjust the setting to low heat. Place a lid on the skillet and leave it simmering for 15 minutes. Uncover the skillet and leave it simmering for another 15 minutes.

Nutrition:
Calories: 401.26
Carbohydrates: 30g
Protein: 27g
Sodium: 677.28mg

86. CHICKEN VERA CRUZ

Preparation Time: 7 minutes
Cooking Time: 10 hours
Servings: 5
Ingredients:

- 1 medium onion, cut into wedges
- 1 pound yellow-skin potatoes
- 6 skinless, boneless chicken thighs
- 2 14.5-oz. cans of no-salt-added diced tomatoes
- 1 fresh jalapeño chili pepper

- 2 tablespoons Worcestershire sauce
- 1 tablespoon chopped garlic
- 1 teaspoon dried oregano, crushed
- ¼ teaspoon ground cinnamon
- ⅛ teaspoon ground cloves
- ½ cup snipped fresh parsley
- ¼ cup chopped pimiento-stuffed green olives

Directions:
1. Put the onion in a 3½- or 4-quart slow cooker. Place chicken thighs and potatoes on top. Drain and discard juices from a can of tomatoes. Stir undrained and drained tomatoes, cloves, cinnamon, oregano, garlic, Worcestershire sauce, and jalapeño pepper together in a bowl. Pour over all in the cooker.
2. Cook with a cover for 10 hours on a low heat setting.
3. To make the topping: Stir chopped pimiento-stuffed green olives and snipped fresh parsley together in a small bowl. Drizzle the topping over each serving of chicken.

Nutrition:
Calories: 275
Sugar: 6.37g
Carbohydrates: 24g
Sodium: 333.79mg

87. CHICKEN AND CORNMEAL DUMPLINGS

Preparation Time: 8 minutes
Cooking Time: 8 hours
Servings: 4
Ingredients:
For the Chicken and Vegetable Filling:
- 2 medium carrots, thinly sliced
- 1 stalk celery, thinly sliced
- ⅓ cup corn kernels
- ½ of a medium onion, thinly sliced
- 2 cloves garlic, minced
- 1 teaspoon snipped fresh rosemary
- ¼ teaspoon ground black pepper
- 2 chicken thighs, skinned
- 1 cup reduced-sodium chicken broth
- ½ cup fat-free milk
- 1 tablespoon almond flour
For the Cornmeal Dumplings:
- ¼ cup flour
- ¼ cup cornmeal

- ½ teaspoon baking powder
- 1 egg white
- 1 tablespoon fat-free milk
- 1 tablespoon canola oil

Directions:
1. Mix ¼ teaspoon pepper, carrots, garlic, celery, rosemary, corn, and onion in a 1½ or 2-quart slow cooker. Place chicken on top. Pour the broth atop the mixture in the cooker.
2. Close and cook on low heat for 7 to 8 hours.
3. If cooking with the low-heat setting, switch to a high-heat setting (or if the heat setting is not available, continue to cook). Place the chicken onto a cutting board and let cool slightly. Once cool enough to handle, chop off the chicken from bones and get rid of the bones. Cut the chicken and place it back into the mixture in the cooker. Mix flour and milk in a small bowl until smooth. Stir into the mixture in the cooker.
4. Drop the cornmeal dumplings dough into 4 mounds atop hot chicken mixture using 2 spoons. Cover and then cook for 20 to 25 minutes more or until a toothpick comes out clean when inserted into a dumpling. (Avoid lifting lid when cooking.) Sprinkle each of the servings with coarse pepper if desired.
5. Mix together ½ teaspoon baking powder, ¼ cup flour, a dash of salt, and ¼ cup cornmeal in a medium bowl. Mix 1 tablespoon canola oil, 1 egg white, and 1 tablespoon fat-free milk in a small bowl. Pour the egg mixture into the flour mixture. Mix just until moistened.

Nutrition:
Calories: 222.86
Sugar: 4.8g
Carbohydrates: 23.67g
Sodium: 311mg

88. CHICKEN AND PEPPERONI

Preparation Time: 4 minutes
Cooking Time: 4 hours
Servings: 5
Ingredients:
- 3½ to 4 pounds meaty chicken pieces
- ⅛ teaspoon salt

- ⅛ teaspoon black pepper
- 2 ounces sliced turkey pepperoni
- ¼ cup sliced pitted ripe olives
- ½ cup reduced-sodium chicken broth
- 1 tablespoon tomato paste
- 1 teaspoon dried Italian seasoning, crushed
- ½ cup shredded part-skim mozzarella cheese (2 ounces)

Directions:
1. Put the chicken into a 3½ to 5-qt. slow cooker. Sprinkle pepper and salt on the chicken. Slice pepperoni slices in half. Put olives and pepperoni into the slow cooker. In a small bowl, blend Italian seasoning, tomato paste, and chicken broth together. Transfer the mixture into the slow cooker.
2. Cook with a cover for 3-3½ hours on high.
3. Transfer the olives, pepperoni, and chicken onto a serving platter with a slotted spoon. Discard the cooking liquid. Sprinkle cheese over the chicken. Use foil to loosely cover and allow to sit for 5 minutes to melt the cheese.

Nutrition:
Calories: 513
Carbohydrates: 1.8g
Protein: 41g
Sodium: 643mg

89. CHICKEN AND SAUSAGE GUMBO

Preparation Time: 6 minutes
Cooking Time: 4 hours
Servings: 5
Ingredients:
- ⅓ cup almond flour
- 1 14-ounce can reduced-sodium chicken broth
- 2 cups cubed chicken breast
- 8 ounces smoked turkey sausage links
- 2 cups sliced fresh okra
- 1 cup water
- 1 cup coarsely chopped onion
- 1 cup sweet pepper
- ½ cup sliced celery
- 4 cloves garlic, minced
- 1 teaspoon dried thyme
- ½ teaspoon ground black pepper
- ¼ teaspoon cayenne pepper
- 3 cups hot cooked brown rice

Directions:
1. To make the roux: Cook the flour upon a medium heat in a

heavy medium-sized saucepan, stirring periodically, for roughly 6 minutes or until the flour browns. Take off the heat and slightly cool, then slowly stir in the broth. Cook the roux until it bubbles and thickens up.

2. Pour the roux in a 3½- or 4-quart slow cooker, then add in cayenne pepper, black pepper, thyme, garlic, celery, sweet pepper, onion, water, okra, sausage, and chicken.

3. Cook the soup covered on a high setting for 3-3½ hours. Take the fat off the top and serve atop hot cooked brown rice.

Nutrition:
Calories: 376
Sugar: 5.8g
Protein: 25g
Carbs: 38g
Sodium: 655mg

90. CHICKEN, BARLEY, AND LEEK STEW

Preparation Time: 10 minutes
Cooking Time: 3 hours
Servings: 6
Ingredients:
- 1 pound chicken thighs
- 1 tablespoon olive oil
- 1 49-ounce can reduced-sodium chicken broth
- 1 cup regular barley (not quick-cooking)
- 2 medium leeks, halved lengthwise and sliced
- 2 medium carrots, thinly sliced
- 1½ teaspoons dried basil or Italian seasoning, crushed
- ¼ teaspoon cracked black pepper

Directions:
1. In a large skillet, cook the chicken in hot oil until brown on all sides. In the 4-5-qt. slow cooker, whisk the pepper, dried basil, carrots, leeks, barley, chicken broth, and chicken.
2. Keep covered and cook over high heat setting for 2-2.5 hours or till the barley softens. Drizzle with the parsley or fresh basil prior to serving.

Nutrition:
Calories: 248
Fiber: 6g
Sodium: 587mg
Carbohydrates: 27g

91. CIDER PORK STEW

Preparation Time: 9 minutes
Cooking Time: 12 hours
Servings: 5
Ingredients:
- 2 pounds pork shoulder roast
- 3 medium cubed potatoes
- 3 medium carrots
- 2 medium onions, sliced
- 1 cup coarsely chopped apple
- ½ cup coarsely chopped celery
- 3 tablespoons quick-cooking tapioca
- 2 cups apple juice
- 1 teaspoon salt
- 1 teaspoon caraway seeds
- ¼ teaspoon black pepper

Directions:
1. Chop the meat into 1-in. cubes. In a 3.5- 5.5 qt. slow cooker, mix the tapioca, celery, apple, onions, carrots, potatoes, and meat. Whisk in pepper, caraway seeds, salt, and apple juice.
2. Keep covered and cook over low heat setting for 10-12 hours. If you want, use the celery leaves to decorate each of the servings.

Nutrition:
Calories: 494
Fiber: 4.6g
Carbohydrates: 44g
Sodium: 607.78mg

92. CREAMY CHICKEN NOODLE SOUP

Preparation Time: 7 minutes
Cooking Time: 8 hours
Servings: 4
Ingredients:
- 1 32-ounce container of low-sodium chicken broth
- 3 cups of water
- 2½ cups cooked chicken
- 3 medium carrots, sliced
- 3 stalks of celery
- 1½ cups sliced fresh mushrooms
- ¼ cup diced onion
- 1½ teaspoons thyme
- 2 cloves garlic
- 3 ounces reduced-fat cream cheese
- 2 cups of dry egg noodles

Directions:
1. Mix together the garlic-pepper seasoning, thyme, onion, mushrooms, celery, carrots, chicken, water, and broth in a 5- to 6-quart slow cooker.

2. Put the cover and let it cook for 6-8 hours on a low heat setting.
3. Increase to a high-heat setting if you are using a low-heat setting. Mix in the cream cheese until blended. Mix in uncooked noodles. Cover and let it cook for an additional 20-30 minutes or just until the noodles become tender.

Nutrition:
Calories: 394
Sugar: 5g
Fiber: 3.25g
Carbs: 31.8g
Sodium: 254.64mg

93. GAZPACHO

Preparation Time: 15 minutes
Cooking Time: 0 minutes
Servings: 4
Ingredients:
- 3 pounds ripe tomatoes
- 1 cup low-sodium tomato juice
- ½ red onion, chopped
- 1 cucumber
- 1 red bell pepper
- 2 celery stalks
- 2 tablespoons parsley
- 2 garlic cloves
- 2 tablespoons extra-virgin olive oil
- 2 tablespoons red wine vinegar
- 1 teaspoon honey
- ½ teaspoon salt
- ¼ teaspoon freshly ground black pepper

Directions:
1. In a blender, combine the tomatoes, tomato juice, onion, cucumber, bell pepper, celery, parsley, garlic, olive oil, vinegar, honey, salt, and pepper. Pulse until blended but still slightly chunky.
2. Adjust the seasonings as needed and serve.

Nutrition:
Calories: 170
Carbohydrates: 24g
Sodium: 362mg
Sugar: 16g

94. TOMATO AND KALE SOUP

Preparation Time: 10 minutes
Cooking Time: 15 minutes
Servings: 4
Ingredients:
- 1 tablespoon extra-virgin olive oil
- 1 medium onion

- 2 carrots
- 3 garlic cloves
- 4 cups low-sodium vegetable broth
- 1 28-ounce can crushed tomatoes
- ½ teaspoon dried oregano
- ¼ teaspoon dried basil
- 4 cups chopped baby kale leaves
- ¼ teaspoon salt

Directions:
1. In a large pot, heat oil over medium heat. Sauté the onion and carrots for about 3 to 5 minutes. Then add the garlic and sauté it for 30 seconds or so.
2. Add in the vegetable broth, along with the tomatoes, oregano, and basil and boil it all before decreasing the heat to low and simmering for 5 minutes.
3. Use a blender to purée the soup.
4. Add in the kale and let it simmer for 3 more minutes. Season with salt and then serve immediately.

Nutrition:
Calories: 254
Carbohydrates: 46.7g
Sugar: 18g
Sodium: 712mg

95. COMFORTING SUMMER SQUASH SOUP WITH CRISPY CHICKPEAS

Preparation Time: 10 minutes
Cooking Time: 20 minutes
Servings: 4
Ingredients:
- 1 15-ounce can low-sodium chickpeas
- 1 teaspoon extra-virgin olive oil
- ¼ teaspoon smoked paprika
- Pinch salt, plus ½ teaspoon
- 3 medium zucchinis
- 3 cups low-sodium vegetable broth
- ½ onion
- 3 garlic cloves
- 2 tablespoons plain low-fat Greek yogurt
- Freshly ground black pepper

Directions:
1. Preheat the oven to 425°F. Line a baking sheet with parchment paper.
2. In a medium mixing bowl, toss the chickpeas with 1 teaspoon of olive oil, the smoked paprika, and a pinch of salt. Place to the prepared baking sheet and roast until crispy, about 20 minutes, stirring once. Set aside.
3. Meanwhile, heat the remaining 1 tablespoon of oil in a separate saucepan over medium heat.
4. Add the zucchini, broth, onion, and garlic to the pot, and boil. Simmer, and cook for 20 minutes.
5. In a blender, purée the soup. Return to the pot.
6. Add the yogurt, remaining ½ teaspoon of salt, and pepper, and stir well. Serve topped with roasted chickpeas.

Nutrition:
Calories: 227.33
Carbohydrates: 39.7g
Sugar: 12g
Sodium: 310mg

96. CURRIED CARROT SOUP

Preparation Time: 10 minutes
Cooking Time: 5 minutes
Servings: 6
Ingredients:
- 1 tablespoon extra-virgin olive oil
- 1 small onion
- 2 celery stalks
- 1½ teaspoons curry powder
- 1 teaspoon ground cumin
- 1 teaspoon minced fresh ginger
- 6 medium carrots
- 4 cups low-sodium vegetable broth
- ¼ teaspoon salt
- 1 cup canned coconut milk
- ¼ teaspoon freshly ground black pepper
- 1 tablespoon chopped fresh cilantro

Directions:
1. Heat an Instant Pot to high and add the olive oil.
2. Sauté the onion and celery for 2 to 3 minutes. Add the curry powder, cumin, and ginger to the pot and cook until fragrant, about 30 seconds.
3. Add the carrots, vegetable broth, and salt to the pot. Close and seal and set for 5 minutes on high. Allow the pressure to release naturally.
4. In a blender jar, carefully purée the soup in batches and transfer it back to the pot.

5. Stir in the coconut milk and pepper, and heat through. Top with the cilantro and serve.

Nutrition:
Calories: 204
Carbohydrates: 24.59g
Sugar: 7.67g
Sodium: 255mg

97. THAI PEANUT, CARROT, AND SHRIMP SOUP

Preparation Time: 10 minutes
Cooking Time: 10 minutes
Servings: 4
Ingredients:
- 1 tablespoon coconut oil
- 1 tablespoon Thai red curry paste
- ½ onion
- 3 garlic cloves
- 2 cups chopped carrots
- ½ cup whole unsalted peanuts
- 4 cups low-sodium vegetable broth
- ½ cup unsweetened plain almond milk
- ½ pound shrimp
- Minced fresh cilantro, for garnish

Directions:
1. In a large pan, heat up oil over medium-high heat.
2. Cook curry paste, stirring continuously, for 1 minute. Add the onion, garlic, carrots, and peanuts to the pan, and continue to cook for 2 to 3 minutes.
3. Boil broth. Reduce the heat to low and simmer for 5 to 6 minutes.
4. Purée the soup until smooth and return it to the pot. Over low heat, pour almond milk and stir to combine. Cook shrimp in the pot for 2 to 3 minutes.
5. Garnish with cilantro and serve.

Nutrition:
Calories: 33%
Carbohydrates: 37.88g
Sugar: 11g
Sodium: 500mg

98. CHICKEN TORTILLA SOUP

Preparation Time: 10 minutes
Cooking Time: 35 minutes
Servings: 4
Ingredients:
- 1 tablespoon extra-virgin olive oil

- 1 onion, thinly sliced
- 1 garlic clove, minced
- 1 jalapeño pepper, diced
- 2 boneless, skinless chicken breasts
- 4 cups low-sodium chicken broth
- 1 Roma tomato, diced
- ½ teaspoon salt
- 2 6-inch corn tortillas
- Juice of 1 lime
- Minced fresh cilantro, for garnish
- ¼ cup shredded cheddar cheese, for garnish

Directions:
1. In a medium pot, cook oil over medium-high heat. Add the onion and cook for 3 to 5 minutes until it begins to soften. Add the garlic and jalapeño, and cook until fragrant, about 1 minute more.
2. Add the chicken, chicken broth, tomato, and salt to the pot and boil. Lower heat to medium and simmer mildly for 20 to 25 minutes. Remove the chicken from the pot and set it aside.
3. Preheat a broiler to high.
4. Spray the tortilla strips with non-stick cooking spray and toss to coat. Spread in a single layer on a baking sheet and broil for 3 to 5 minutes, flipping once, until crisp.
5. Once the chicken is cooked, shred it with 2 forks and return to the pot.
6. Season the soup with lime juice. Serve hot, garnished with cilantro, cheese, and tortilla strips.

Nutrition:
Calories: 268.62
Carbohydrates: 13.7g
Sugar: 2g
Sodium: 461mg

99. BEEF AND MUSHROOM BARLEY SOUP

Preparation Time: 10 minutes
Cooking Time: 80 minutes
Servings: 6
Ingredients:
- 1 pound beef stew meat, cubed
- ¼ teaspoon salt
- ¼ teaspoon freshly ground black pepper
- 1 tablespoon extra-virgin olive oil
- 8 ounces sliced mushrooms
- 1 onion, chopped
- 2 carrots, chopped

- 3 celery stalks, chopped
- 6 garlic cloves, minced
- ½ teaspoon dried thyme
- 4 cups low-sodium beef broth
- 1 cup water
- ½ cup pearl barley

Directions:
1. Season the meat well.
2. In an Instant Pot, heat the oil over high heat. Cook meat on all sides. Remove from the pot and set aside.
3. Add the mushrooms to the pot and cook for 1 to 2 minutes. Remove the mushrooms and set them aside with the meat.
4. Sauté onion, carrots, and celery for 3 to 4 minutes. Add the garlic and continue to cook until fragrant, about 30 seconds longer.
5. Return the meat and mushrooms to the pot, then add the thyme, beef broth, and water. Adjust the pressure on high and cook for 15 minutes. Let the pressure release naturally.
6. Open the Instant Pot and add the barley. Use the slow cooker function on the Instant Pot, affix the lid (vent open), and continue to cook for 1 hour. Serve.

Nutrition:
Calories: 215.3
Carbohydrates: 19.6g
Sugar: 3g
Sodium: 447.12mg

100. TOMATO AND GUACA SALAD

Preparation Time: 10 minutes
Cooking Time: 0 minutes
Servings: 4
Ingredients:
- 1 cup cherry tomatoes
- 1 large cucumber
- 1 small red onion
- 1 avocado
- 2 tablespoons chopped fresh dill
- 2 tablespoons extra-virgin olive oil
- Juice of 1 lemon
- ¼ teaspoon salt
- ¼ teaspoon freshly ground black pepper

Directions:
1. In a big mixing bowl, mix the tomatoes, cucumber, onion, avocado, and dill.

2. In a small bowl, combine the oil, lemon juice, salt, and pepper, and mix well.
3. Drizzle the dressing over the vegetables and toss to combine. Serve.

Nutrition:
Calories: 132
Carbohydrates: 7.89g
Sugar: 3g
Sodium: 151.44mg

101. COLESLAW

Preparation Time: 15 minutes
Cooking Time: 0 minutes
Servings: 4
Ingredients:
- 2 cups green cabbage
- 2 cups red cabbage
- 2 cups grated carrots
- 3 scallions
- 2 tablespoons extra-virgin olive oil
- 2 tablespoons rice vinegar
- 1 teaspoon honey
- 1 garlic clove
- ¼ teaspoon salt

Directions:
1. Throw together the green and red cabbage, carrots, and scallions.
2. In a small bowl, whisk together the oil, vinegar, honey, garlic, and salt.
3. Pour the dressing over the veggies and mix to thoroughly combine.
4. Serve immediately or cover and chill for several hours before serving.

Nutrition:
Calories: 120
Carbohydrates: 13.6g
Sugar: 7.4g
Sodium: 208mg

102. GREEN SALAD WITH BERRIES AND SWEET POTATOES

Preparation Time: 15 minutes
Cooking Time: 20 minutes
Servings: 4
Ingredients:
For the Vinaigrette:
- 1 pint blackberries
- 2 tablespoons red wine vinegar
- 1 tablespoon honey
- 3 tablespoons extra-virgin olive oil
- ¼ teaspoon salt
- Freshly ground black pepper
For the Salad:

- 1 sweet potato, cubed
- 1 teaspoon extra-virgin olive oil
- 8 cups salad greens (baby spinach, spicy greens, romaine)
- ½ red onion, sliced
- ¼ cup crumbled goat cheese

Directions:

For the Vinaigrette:

1. In a blender jar, combine the blackberries, vinegar, honey, oil, salt, and pepper, and process until smooth. Set aside.

For the Salad:

1. Preheat the oven to 425°F. Line a baking sheet with parchment paper.
2. Mix the sweet potato with olive oil. Transfer everything onto the baking sheet and then roast for 20 minutes, stirring once halfway through, until tender. Remove and cool for a few minutes.
3. In a large bowl, toss the greens with the red onion and cooled sweet potato, and drizzle with the vinaigrette. Serve topped with 1 tablespoon of goat cheese per serving.

Nutrition:
Calories: 253.56
Carbohydrates: 24.6g
Sugar: 11.49g
Sodium: 230.87mg

103. 3 BEAN AND SCALLION SALAD

Preparation Time: 10 minutes
Cooking Time: 0 minutes
Servings: 8
Ingredients:

- 1 15-ounce can low-sodium chickpeas
- 1 15-ounce can low-sodium kidney beans
- 1 15-ounce can low-sodium white beans
- 1 red bell pepper
- ¼ cup chopped scallions
- ¼ cup finely chopped fresh basil
- 3 garlic cloves, minced
- 2 tablespoons extra-virgin olive oil
- 1 tablespoon red wine vinegar
- 1 teaspoon Dijon mustard
- ¼ teaspoon freshly ground black pepper

Directions:

1. Toss chickpeas, kidney beans, white beans, bell pepper,

scallions, basil, and garlic gently.
2. Blend together olive oil, vinegar, mustard, and pepper. Toss with the salad.
3. Wrap and chill for 1 hour.

Nutrition:
Calories: 225.21
Carbohydrates: 29g
Sugar: 3g
Sodium: 226.25mg

104. RAINBOW BEAN SALAD

Preparation Time: 15 minutes
Cooking Time: 0 minutes
Servings: 5
Ingredients:

- 1 15-ounce can low-sodium black beans
- 1 avocado, diced
- 1 cup cherry
- 3 tomatoes, halved
- 1 cup chopped baby spinach
- ½ cup red bell pepper
- ¼ cup jicama
- ½ cup scallions
- ¼ cup fresh cilantro
- 2 tablespoons lime juice
- 1 tablespoon extra-virgin olive oil
- 2 garlic cloves, minced
- 1 teaspoon honey
- ¼ teaspoon salt
- ¼ teaspoon freshly ground black pepper

Directions:

1. Mix black beans, avocado, tomatoes, spinach, bell pepper, jicama, scallions, and cilantro.
2. Blend lime juice, oil, garlic, honey, salt, and pepper. Add to the salad and toss.
3. Chill for 1 hour before serving.

Nutrition:
Calories: 182.16
Carbohydrates: 26.34g
Sugar: 6.57g
Sodium: 247.38mg

105. WARM BARLEY AND SQUASH SALAD

Preparation Time: 20 minutes
Cooking Time: 40 minutes
Servings: 8
Ingredients:

- 1 small butternut squash
- 3 tablespoons extra-virgin olive oil
- 2 cups broccoli florets
- 1 cup pearl barley
- 1 cup toasted chopped walnuts
- 2 cups baby kale

- ½ red onion, sliced
- 2 tablespoons balsamic vinegar
- 2 garlic cloves, minced
- ½ teaspoon salt
- ¼ teaspoon black pepper

Directions:

1. Preheat the oven to 400°F. Line a baking sheet with parchment paper.
2. Peel the squash, and slice. In a large bowl, toss the squash with 2 teaspoons of olive oil. Transfer everything onto the baking sheet and then roast it for 20 minutes.
3. While the squash is roasting, toss the broccoli in the same bowl with 1 teaspoon of olive oil. After 20 minutes, flip the squash and push it to one side of the baking sheet. Add the broccoli to the other side and continue to roast for 20 more minutes until tender.
4. While the veggies are roasting, in a medium pot, cover the barley with several inches of water. Boil, then adjust heat, cover, and simmer for 30 minutes until tender. Drain and rinse.
5. Transfer the barley to a large bowl, and toss with the cooked squash and broccoli, walnuts, kale, and onion.
6. In a small bowl, mix the remaining 2 tablespoons of olive oil, balsamic vinegar, garlic, salt, and pepper. Drizzle dressing over the salad and toss.

Nutrition:
Calories: 271
Carbohydrates: 32g
Sugar: 3g
Sodium: 159.45mg

106. CITRUS AND CHICKEN SALAD

Preparation Time: 10 minutes
Cooking Time: 0 minutes
Servings: 4
Ingredients:

- 4 cups baby spinach
- 2 tablespoons extra-virgin olive oil
- 1 tablespoon lemon juice
- ⅛ teaspoon salt
- 2 cups chopped cooked chicken
- 2 mandarin oranges
- ½ peeled grapefruit, sectioned
- ¼ cup sliced almonds

Directions:

1. Toss spinach with olive oil, lemon juice, pepper, and salt.
2. Add the chicken, oranges, grapefruit, and almonds to the bowl. Toss gently.
3. Arrange on 4 plates and serve.

Nutrition:
Calories: 288.49
Carbohydrates: 9.39g
Sugar: 7g
Sodium: 140.97mg

107. BLUEBERRY AND CHICKEN SALAD

Preparation Time: 10 minutes
Cooking Time: 0 minutes
Servings: 4
Ingredients:
- 2 cups chopped cooked chicken
- 1 cup fresh blueberries
- ¼ cup almonds
- 1 celery stalk
- ¼ cup red onion
- 1 tablespoon fresh basil
- 1 tablespoon fresh cilantro
- ½ cup plain, vegan mayonnaise
- ¼ teaspoon salt
- ¼ teaspoon freshly ground black pepper
- 8 cups salad greens

Directions:
1. Toss chicken, blueberries, almonds, celery, onion, basil, and cilantro.
2. Blend yogurt, salt, and pepper. Stir chicken salad to combine.
3. Situate 2 cups of salad greens on each of 4 plates and divide the chicken salad among the plates to serve.

Nutrition:
Calories: 392
Carbohydrates: 10.61g
Sugar: 6g
Sodium: 368mg

108. CRUNCHY STRAWBERRY SALAD

Preparation Time: 10 minutes
Cooking Time: 0 minutes
Servings: 5
Ingredients:
- 0.6 lb. romaine lettuce leaves, roughly torn
- 0.6 lb. strawberries, sliced
- 0.2 lb. nuts of choice

Directions:
1. In a large mixing bowl add strawberry slices, lettuce, and nuts; toss to combine.
2. Add to a serving bowl.

Nutrition:

Calories: 136
Fat: 10.1g
Protein: 4.6g
Carbs: 9.55g
Sodium: 54.23mg

109. ZUCCHINI NOODLE SALAD WITH ALMONDS

Preparation Time: 35 minutes
Cooking Time: 10 minutes
Servings: 4
Ingredients:
- 2-3 zucchini, noodled
- 2 tablespoon olive oil
- 1 carrot, peeled, noodled
- 0.2 lb. red cabbage, thinly sliced
- 2 tablespoon lime juice
- Kosher salt and pepper, to taste
- 0.3 lb. toasted almonds, chopped
- 3-4 tablespoon cilantro leaves

Directions:
1. Combine zucchini, carrots, cabbage, and almonds. Season with salt, pepper, lemon juice, and olive oil then toss it well.
2. Add to a serving platter.

Nutrition:
Calories: 299
Fat: 26.77g
Protein: 8.81g
Carbs: 12.37g
Sodium: 332mg

110. CARROT AND SPINACH SALAD

Preparation Time: 60 minutes
Cooking Time: 0 minutes
Servings: 4
Ingredients:
- 0.8 lb. baby spinach leaves
- 2 carrots, peeled, grated
- 5 tablespoon olive oil
- 4 tablespoon lemon juice
- Salt and black pepper, to taste
- 1 teaspoon thyme
- 1-2 garlic cloves, minced
- ¼ teaspoon onion powder

Directions:
1. Stir in lemon juice, olive oil, salt, pepper, onion powder, and garlic. Mix well.
2. Add carrots and spinach leaves to the mixture. Toss to combine.
3. Cover the bowl with a plastic wrapper. Place it in the refrigerator for about 50 minutes before serving.

Nutrition:
Calories: 195

Fat: 18g
Protein: 3.04g
Carbs: 7.6g
Sodium: 285.91mg

111. RED CABBAGE SALAD

Preparation Time: 15 minutes
Cooking Time: 0 minutes
Servings: 4
Ingredients:
- 1 lb. red cabbage, thinly sliced
- 2 carrots, peeled, thinly sliced
- 2 tablespoon olive oil
- Salt and black pepper, to taste
- 2 tablespoon lemon juice
- 2 tablespoon coriander leaves, chopped
- 1 tablespoon mint leaves, chopped

Directions:
1. Combine cabbage, carrots, mint, and coriander. Mix in salt, pepper, lemon juice, and olive oil then toss it well. Transfer salad onto a serving platter.

Nutrition:
Calories: 105
Fat: 7.37g
Protein: 1.61g
Carbs: 9.97g
Sodium: 237.33mg

112. QUINOA FRUIT SALAD

Preparation Time: 15 minutes
Cooking Time: 0 minutes
Servings: 3
Ingredients:
- 1 lb. cooked quinoa
- 1 mango, peeled and diced
- ½ lb. strawberries, quartered
- ½ lb. blueberries
- 2 tablespoon pine nuts
- Chopped mint leaves, for garnish
- 4 tablespoon olive oil
- Zest of 1 lemon
- 3 tablespoons freshly squeezed lemon juice
- 1 tablespoon date sugar

Directions:
1. For the vinaigrette, beat the olive oil, lemon zest, juice, and sugar in a small bowl. Set aside.
2. Mix quinoa, mango, strawberries, blueberries, and pine nuts in a large bowl. Add the lemon vinaigrette.

Nutrition:
Calories: 518
Fat: 26g
Protein: 9.1g

Carbs: 66.89g
Sodium: 17.83mg

113. BEEF AND RED BEAN CHILI

Preparation Time: 10 minutes
Cooking Time: 6 hours
Servings: 8
Ingredients:

- 1 cup dry red beans
- 1 tablespoon olive oil
- 2 pounds boneless beef chuck
- 1 large onion, coarsely chopped
- 1 14-ounce can beef broth
- 2 chipotle chili peppers in adobo sauce
- 2 teaspoons dried oregano, crushed
- 1 teaspoon ground cumin
- ½ teaspoon salt
- 1 14.5-ounce can tomatoes with mild green chilis
- 1 15-ounce can tomato sauce
- ¼ cup snipped fresh cilantro
- 1 medium red sweet pepper

Directions:

1. Rinse out the beans and place them into a Dutch oven or big saucepan, then add in water enough to cover them. Allow the beans to boil then drop the heat down. Simmer the beans without a cover for 10 minutes. Take off the heat and keep covered for an hour.
2. In a big frying pan, heat the oil on medium-high heat, then cook onion and half the beef until they brown a bit over medium-high heat. Move into a 3½- or 4-quart crockery cooker. Do this again with what's left of the beef. Add in tomato sauce, tomatoes (not drained), salt, cumin, oregano, adobo sauce, chipotle peppers, and broth, stirring to blend. Strain out and rinse beans and stir in the cooker.
3. Cook while covered on a low setting for around 10-12 hours or on a high setting for 5-6 hours. Spoon the chili into bowls or mugs and top with sweet pepper and cilantro.

Nutrition:
Calories: 419
Carbohydrates: 24g
Sodium: 777.83mg
Sugar: 5g

114. BERRY APPLE CIDER

Preparation Time: 15 minutes
Cooking Time: 3 hours
Servings: 3
Ingredients:

- 4 cinnamon sticks, cut into 1-inch pieces
- 1½ teaspoons whole cloves
- 4 cups apple cider
- 4 cups low-calorie cranberry-raspberry juice drink
- 1 medium apple

Directions:

1. To make the spice bag, cut out a 6-inch square from double-thick, pure cotton cheesecloth. Put in the cloves and cinnamon, then bring the corners up, tie it closed using a clean kitchen string that is pure cotton.
2. In a 3½- 5-quart slow cooker, combine cranberry-raspberry juice, apple cider, and the spice bag.
3. Cook while covered over low heat setting for around 4-6 hours or on a high heat setting for 2-2 ½ hours.
4. Throw out the spice bag. Serve right away or keep it warm while covered on a warm or low heat setting up to 2 hours, occasionally stirring. Garnish each serving with apples (thinly sliced).

Nutrition:
Calories: 343
Carbohydrates: 84g
Sugar: 76g
Sodium: 84.72mg

115. BRUNSWICK STEW

Preparation Time: 10 minutes
Cooking Time: 45 minutes
Servings: 3
Ingredients:

- 4 ounces diced salt pork
- 2 pounds chicken parts
- 8 cups water
- 3 potatoes, cubed
- 3 onions, chopped
- 1 28-ounce can whole peeled tomatoes
- 2 cups canned whole kernel corn
- 1 10-ounce package frozen lima beans
- 1 tablespoon Worcestershire sauce
- ½ teaspoon salt
- ¼ teaspoon ground black pepper

Directions:

1. Mix and boil water, chicken, and salt pork in a big pot on high heat. Lower heat to low. Cover then simmer until chicken is tender for 45 minutes.
2. Take out chicken. Let cool until easily handled. Take the meat out. Throw out bones and skin. Chop meat into bite-sized pieces. Put back in the soup.
3. Add ground black pepper, salt, Worcestershire sauce, lima beans, corn, tomatoes, onions, and potatoes. Mix well. Stir well and simmer for 1 hour, uncovered.

Nutrition:
Calories: 368
Carbohydrates: 25.9g
Protein: 27.9g
Sodium: 867mg

116. BUFFALO CHICKEN SALAD

Preparation Time: 7 minutes
Cooking Time: 3 hours
Servings: 5
Ingredients:

- 1½ pounds chicken breast halves
- ½ cup Wing Time® buffalo chicken sauce
- 4 teaspoons cider vinegar
- 1 teaspoon Worcestershire sauce
- 1 teaspoon paprika
- ⅓ cup light mayonnaise
- 2 tablespoons fat-free milk
- 2 tablespoons crumbled blue cheese
- 2 romaine hearts, chopped
- 1 cup whole grain croutons
- ½ cup very thinly sliced red onion

Directions:

1. Place chicken in a 2-quart slow cooker. Mix together Worcestershire sauce, 2 teaspoons of vinegar, and Buffalo sauce in a small bowl; pour over chicken. Dust with paprika. Close and cook for 3 hours on a low heat setting.
2. Mix the leftover 2 teaspoons of vinegar with milk and light mayonnaise together in a small bowl at serving time; mix in blue cheese. While chicken is still in the slow cooker, pull meat into bite-sized pieces using 2 forks.

3. Split the romaine among 6 dishes. Spoon sauce and chicken over lettuce. Pour with blue cheese dressing then add red onion slices and croutons on top.

Nutrition:
Calories: 356.35
Carbohydrates: 14.28g
Fiber: 4.88g
Sodium: 931.38mg

117. CACCIATORE STYLE CHICKEN

Preparation Time: 10 minutes
Cooking Time: 4 hours
Servings: 6
Ingredients:
- 2 cups sliced fresh mushrooms
- 1 cup sliced celery
- 1 cup chopped carrot
- 2 medium onions, cut into wedges
- 1 green, yellow, or red sweet pepper
- 4 cloves garlic, minced
- 12 chicken drumsticks
- ½ cup chicken broth
- ¼ cup dry white wine
- 2 tablespoons quick-cooking tapioca
- 2 bay leaves
- 1 teaspoon dried oregano, crushed
- 1 teaspoon sugar
- ½ teaspoon salt
- ¼ teaspoon pepper
- 1 14.5-ounce can diced tomatoes
- ⅓ cup tomato paste
- Hot cooked pasta or rice

Directions:
1. Mix garlic, sweet pepper, onions, carrot, celery, and mushrooms in a 5- or 6-qt. slow cooker. Cover veggies with the chicken. Add pepper, salt, sugar, oregano, bay leaves, tapioca, wine, and broth.
2. Cover. Cook for 3-3½ hours in a high-heat setting.
3. Take chicken out; keep warm. Discard bay leaves. Turn to a high-heat setting if using a low-heat setting. Mix tomato paste and undrained tomatoes in. Cover. Cook on high heat setting for 15 more minutes. For serving, put the veggie mixture on top of pasta and chicken.

Nutrition:
Calories: 369.86
Sugar: 6.56g

Carbohydrates: 20.94g
Sodium: 567.91mg

118. CARNITAS TACOS

Preparation Time: 10 minutes
Cooking Time: 5 hours
Servings: 4
Ingredients:
- 3 to 3½-pound bone-in pork shoulder roast
- ½ cup chopped onion
- ⅓ cup orange juice
- 1 tablespoon ground cumin
- 1½ teaspoons kosher salt
- 1 teaspoon dried oregano, crushed
- ¼ teaspoon cayenne pepper
- 1 lime
- 2 5.3-ounce containers plain low-fat Greek yogurt
- 1 pinch kosher salt
- 16 6-inch soft yellow corn tortillas, such as Mission® brand
- 4 leaves green cabbage, quartered
- 1 cup very thinly sliced red onion
- 1 cup salsa (optional)

Directions:
1. Take off meat from the bone; throw away bone. Trim meat fat. Slice meat into 2 to 3-inch pieces; put in a slow cooker of 3 ½ or 4-quart in size. Mix in cayenne, oregano, salt, cumin, orange juice, and onion.
2. Cover and cook for 4 to 5 hours on high. Take out the meat from the cooker. Shred meat with 2 forks. Mix in enough cooking liquid to moisten.
3. Take out 1 teaspoon zest (put aside) for lime crema, then squeeze 2 tablespoons lime juice. Mix dash salt, yogurt, and lime juice in a small bowl.
4. Serve lime crema, salsa (if wished), red onion, and cabbage with meat in tortillas. Scatter with lime zest.

Nutrition:
Calories: 879.71
Carbohydrates: 67g
Sugar: 9.21g
Sodium: 1009.89mg

119. CUBAN PULLED PORK SANDWICH

Preparation Time: 6 minutes
Cooking Time: 5 hours
Servings: 5

Ingredients:
- 1 teaspoon dried oregano, crushed
- ¾ teaspoon ground cumin
- ½ teaspoon ground coriander
- ¼ teaspoon salt
- ¼ teaspoon black pepper
- ¼ teaspoon ground allspice
- 2 to 2½-pound boneless pork shoulder roast
- 1 tablespoon olive oil
- Non-stick cooking spray
- 2 cups sliced onions
- 2 green sweet peppers, cut into bite-size strips
- ½ to 1 fresh jalapeño pepper
- 4 cloves garlic, minced
- ¼ cup orange juice
- ¼ cup lime juice
- 6 heart-healthy wheat hamburger buns, toasted
- 2 tablespoons coarse grain mustard or Jalapeno mustard
- 1 slice Avocado slices

Directions:
1. Mix allspice, oregano, black pepper, cumin, salt, and coriander together in a small bowl. Press each side of the roast into the spice mixture. On medium-high heat, heat oil in a big non-stick pan; put in the roast. Cook for 5mins until both sides of the roast are light brown, turn the roast one time.
2. Using a cooking spray, grease a 3½ or 4qt slow cooker; arrange the garlic, onions, jalapeño, and green peppers in a layer. Pour in lime juice and orange juice. Slice the roast if needed to fit inside the cooker; put on top of the vegetables covered or 4½-5 hrs on high heat setting.
3. Move roast to a cutting board using a slotted spoon. Drain the cooking liquid and keep the jalapeño, green peppers, and onions. Shred the roast with 2 forks then place it back in the cooker. Remove fat from the liquid. Mix ½ cup of cooking liquid and reserved vegetables into the cooker. Pour in more cooking liquid if desired. Discard the remaining cooking liquid.
4. Slather mustard on rolls. Split the meat between the bottom roll halves. Add avocado on top if desired. Place the roll tops on sandwiches.

Nutrition:

Calories: 604
Carbohydrates: 44.3g
Fiber: 4g
Sodium: 592mg

120. LEMON TARRAGON SOUP

Preparation Time: 10 minutes
Cooking Time: 10 minutes
Servings: 2
Ingredients:
- 1 tablespoon avocado oil
- ½ cup diced onion
- 3 garlic cloves, crushed
- ¼ plus ⅛ teaspoon sea salt
- ¼ plus ⅛ teaspoon freshly ground black pepper
- 1 13.5-ounce can full-fat coconut milk
- 1 tablespoon freshly squeezed lemon juice
- ½ cup raw cashews
- 1 celery stalk
- 2 tablespoons chopped fresh tarragon

Directions:
1. In a medium skillet over medium-high heat, heat up avocado oil. Sauté onion, garlic, salt, and pepper for 4 minutes.
2. In a high-speed blender, blend together the coconut milk, lemon juice, cashews, celery, and tarragon with the onion mixture until smooth. Adjust seasonings, if necessary.
3. Pour into 2 small bowls or 1 large and enjoy immediately, or transfer to a medium saucepan and warm on low heat for 3 to 5 minutes before serving.

Nutrition:
Calories: 661
Fiber: 2.17g
Fat: 63.65g
Carbs: 22.88g
Sodium: 285.9mg

121. CHILLED CUCUMBER AND LIME SOUP

Preparation Time: 25 minutes
Cooking Time: 0 minute
Servings: 2
Ingredients:
- 1 cucumber, peeled
- ½ zucchini, peeled
- 1 tablespoon freshly squeezed lime juice
- 1 tablespoon fresh cilantro leaves
- 1 garlic clove, crushed
- ¼ teaspoon sea salt

Directions:
1. In a blender, blend together the cucumber, zucchini, lime juice, cilantro, garlic, and salt until well combined. Add more salt, if necessary.
2. Pour into 1 large or 2 small bowls and enjoy immediately or refrigerate for 15 to 20 minutes to chill before serving.

Nutrition:
Calories: 26.41
Protein: 1.32g
Fat: 0.27g
Carbs: 6g
Sodium: 243mg

122. COCONUT, CILANTRO, AND JALAPEÑO SOUP

Preparation Time: 5 minutes
Cooking Time: 5 minutes
Servings: 2
Ingredients:
- 2 tablespoons avocado oil
- ½ cup diced onions
- 3 garlic cloves, crushed
- ¼ teaspoon sea salt
- 1 13.5-ounce can full-fat coconut milk
- 1 tablespoon freshly squeezed lime juice
- ½ to 1 jalapeño
- 2 tablespoons fresh cilantro leaves

Directions:
1. Using a medium skillet over medium-high heat, heat up avocado oil. Sauté onion, garlic, and salt for 4 minutes.
2. In a blender, blend together the coconut milk, lime juice, jalapeño, and cilantro with the onion mixture until creamy.
3. Pour into 1 large or 2 small bowls and enjoy.

Nutrition:
Calories: 521.44
Fat: 54.52g
Protein: 4.6g
Carbs: 11g
Sodium: 264.38mg

123. SPICY WATERMELON GAZPACHO

Preparation Time: 5 minutes
Cooking Time: 0 minutes
Servings: 2
Ingredients:
- 2 cups cubed watermelon
- ¼ cup diced onion
- ¼ cup packed cilantro leaves
- ½ to 1 jalapeño
- 2 tablespoons freshly squeezed lime juice

Directions:
1. In a blender or food processor, pulse to combine the watermelon, onion, cilantro, jalapeño, and lime juice only long enough to break down the ingredients, leaving them very finely diced and taking care to not over process.
2. Pour into 1 large or 2 small bowls and enjoy.

Nutrition:
Calories: 58
Fat: 0.28g
Protein: 1.26g
Carbs: 14.7g
Sodium: 3.56mg

124. ROASTED CARROT AND LEEK SOUP

Preparation Time: 10 minutes
Cooking Time: 30 minutes
Servings: 2 to 4
Ingredients:
- 6 carrots
- 1 cup chopped onion
- 1 fennel bulb, cubed
- 2 garlic cloves, crushed
- 2 tablespoons avocado oil
- 1 teaspoon sea salt
- 1 teaspoon freshly ground black pepper
- 2 cups almond milk, plus more if desired

Directions:
1. Preheat the oven to 400°F. Line a baking sheet with parchment paper. Cut the carrots into thirds, and then cut each third in half. Transfer to a medium bowl.
2. Add the onion, fennel, garlic, and avocado oil, and toss to coat. Toss once more with salt and pepper.
3. Place the veggies on the baking sheet that has been prepared, and roast for 30 minutes. Allow the veggies to cool after they have been removed from the oven.
4. In a high-speed blender, blend together the almond milk and roasted vegetables until creamy and smooth. Adjust the seasonings, if necessary, and add additional milk if you prefer a thinner consistency.
5. Pour into 2 large or 4 small bowls and enjoy.

Nutrition:

Calories: 173
Fiber: 4.7g
Protein: 2.31g
Carbs: 23.3g
Sodium: 632mg

125. LEMON CAULIFLOWER & PINE NUTS

Preparation Time: 5 minutes
Cooking Time: 20 minutes
Servings: 4
Ingredients:

- 1 teaspoon lemon zest
- ¼ teaspoon sea salt
- 1 10-ounce package cauliflower florets
- 2 tablespoons extra-virgin olive oil
- 2 tablespoons pine nuts
- 1 tablespoon parsley, fresh flat-leaf
- 1 ½ teaspoon lemon juice
- ¼ teaspoon fresh ground black pepper

Directions:

1. Preheat your oven to 400°F.
2. In a large bowl, combine all of your ingredients. Then set onto a baking sheet.
3. Bake for 20 minutes, serve and enjoy!

Nutrition:
Calories: 108
Protein: 1.9g
Fat: 9.9g
Carbs: 4.51g
Sodium: 139mg

126. BEEF TENDERLOIN & AVOCADO CREAM

Preparation Time: 10 minutes
Cooking Time: 8 minutes
Servings: 2
Ingredients:

- 1 teaspoon mustard
- 2 6-ounce beef steaks
- ¼ cup sour cream
- 2 teaspoons lemon juice, fresh
- ⅓ avocado
- 1 tablespoon olive oil-slicked
- Sea salt along with fresh ground black pepper as needed

Directions:

1. Preheat your oven to 450° Fahrenheit.
2. Sprinkle the beef steaks with some salt and pepper.
3. Mix the mustard and oil and spread the mixture over the meat.

4. Place the steaks into a skillet over medium-high heat for 3 minutes.
5. Transfer the steaks to a baking sheet and place in the oven, then bake for 6 minutes.
6. Blend the avocado with lemon juice and sour cream.
7. Serve steaks with avocado cream and enjoy!

Nutrition:
Calories: 305
Protein: 24g
Fat: 22.4g
Carbs: 3.5g
Sodium: 468.71mg

127. SALMON & CITRUS SAUCE

Preparation Time: 10 minutes
Cooking Time: 15 minutes
Servings: 2
Ingredients:

- ¾ lb. salmon fillets
- ⅓ cup fresh orange juice
- 1 tablespoon fresh lime juice
- 1 tablespoon fresh lemon juice
- 1 tablespoon honey
- 1 tablespoon olive oil
- 1½ tablespoons mustard
- Sea salt along with fresh ground black pepper as needed
- ¼ teaspoon smoked paprika

Directions:

1. Sprinkle fillets with paprika, salt, and pepper. Then, cook in a skillet over medium-high heat for 5 minutes per side.
2. While fillets are cooking, mix the lemon, orange, lime juices, and honey, then add to a small saucepan. Add the mustard and stir to combine. Cook over low heat for 10 minutes.
3. Add the salmon fillets to serving dishes, then pour the sauce over the fillets. Serve and enjoy!

Nutrition:
Calories: 443.68
Protein: 35g
Fat: 27.6g
Carbs: 15g
Sodium: 549.96mg

128. ORANGE-AVOCADO SALAD

Preparation Time: 10 minutes
Cooking Time: 0 minutes
Servings: 2
Ingredients:

- ½ teaspoon arugula
- 1 avocado
- 1 navel orange

- 1 tablespoon fresh lime juice
- 1 tablespoon extra-virgin olive oil

Directions:

1. Mix your lime juice, arugula, and oil in a bowl.
2. Add the peeled and sectioned pieces of orange, then toss.
3. Add the diced avocado just before serving, then enjoy!

Nutrition:
Calories: 177.72
Protein: 1.59g
Fat: 15.34g
Carbs: 11.52g
Sodium: 4.7mg

129. AVOCADOS WITH WALNUT-HERB

Preparation Time: 7 minutes
Cooking Time: 5 minutes
Servings: 2
Ingredients:

- 1 avocado
- ¼ cup walnuts
- 1½ teaspoons virgin olive oil
- 1½ teaspoons lemon juice (fresh)
- 1 tablespoon fresh basil
- Sea salt and black pepper to taste

Directions:

1. Fry the chopped nuts for about 5 minutes over medium-low heat in a pan.
2. In a small bowl, mix the chopped basil, lemon juice, oil, sea salt, and pepper.
3. Slice avocado in half, then top slices with the walnut mixture, serve, and enjoy!

Nutrition:
Calories: 253.68
Protein: 4.9g
Fat: 24.7g
Carbs: 8.11g
Sodium: 343mg

130. BARBECUE BRISKET

Preparation Time: 15 minutes
Cooking Time: 5 hours
Servings: 4
Ingredients:

- 1 cup beef broth
- 2 lb. beef brisket
- 1 sweet onion, diced
- ½ cup barbecue sauce
- ½ tablespoon steak seasoning

Directions:

1. Add the prepared onion to your slow cooker. Rub the trimmed brisket with seasoning.

2. Cut the brisket into pieces and add to your slow cooker.
3. Pour the beef broth and barbecue sauce over the brisket.
4. Cook on low for 5 hours, slice brisket. Serve and enjoy!

Nutrition:
Calories: 562
Protein: 36.7g
Fat: 37g
Carbs: 18g
Sodium: 796mg

131. BROCCOLI & HOT SAUCE

Preparation Time: 5 minutes
Cooking Time: 5 minutes
Servings: 4
Ingredients:
- 4 cups broccoli florets
- 1 tablespoon extra-virgin olive oil
- ½ teaspoon hot sauce
- Sea salt along with black ground pepper as needed

Directions:
1. Arrange your broccoli in a steamer basket. Steam your broccoli for about 5 minutes or until tender.
2. Drizzle with the oil and sprinkle with hot sauce, sea salt, and black pepper. Serve and enjoy!

Nutrition:
Calories: 55.71
Protein: 2g
Fat: 1.8g
Carbs: 4.7g
Sodium: 208mg

132. CHICKEN THIGHS

Preparation Time: 10 minutes
Cooking Time: 40 minutes
Servings: 4
Ingredients:
- 4 bone-in skinless chicken thighs
- ½ teaspoon ginger
- 1 tablespoon olive oil
- 2 tablespoons soy sauce
- ¼ teaspoon dry mustard
- 1 garlic clove
- ¼ teaspoon red pepper
- ¼ teaspoon all-spice

Directions:
1. Preheat the oven to 400°F and sauté the minced garlic, ground allspice, ground ginger, crushed red pepper, and mustard in hot oil for 5 minutes. Remove from heat.

2. Whisk in soy sauce, then place the chicken thighs on a baking sheet. Add the garlic mixture over the chicken, and toss.

Nutrition:
Calories: 169.23
Protein: 21.89g
Fat: 8.08g
Carbs: 1g
Sodium: 551.17mg

133. CREAMY BELL PEPPER-CORN SALAD & SEARED ZUCCHINI

Preparation Time: 10 minutes
Cooking Time: 20 minutes
Servings: 5
Ingredients:
- 2 zucchinis
- ½ cup celery
- 1 green bell pepper, sliced and seeded
- 1 dozen cherry tomatoes
- 2 cups kernel corn
- 4 tablespoons sour cream
- ½ cup mayonnaise
- 2 teaspoons sweetener
- Sea salt along with ground black pepper as needed

Directions:
1. Cook corn by following package instructions.
2. Mix the chopped celery, sliced bell pepper, whole cherry tomatoes, mayonnaise, sour cream, sweetener, salt, and pepper in a large salad bowl.
3. Heat a skillet over medium-high heat. Cook the zucchini sliced lengthwise for about 10 minutes. Turn occasionally, then add salt to zucchini.
4. Once zucchini is cooked, add it to the corn mixture.
5. You can serve this dish alongside your favorite meat dish!

Nutrition:
Calories: 249.54
Protein: 3.61g
Fat: 20g
Carbs: 17.81g
Sodium: 269.46mg

134. CORN TORTILLAS & SPINACH SALAD

Preparation Time: 3 minutes
Cooking Time: 5 minutes
Servings: 4
Ingredients:
- 2 cups baby spinach, chopped
- 4 corn tortillas

- 2 tablespoons red onion, chopped
- 4 cherry tomatoes, whole
- 2 teaspoons balsamic vinegar
- 8 olives, ripe and pitted
- 1 tablespoon extra-virgin olive oil
- Salt and pepper to taste

Directions:
1. Heat your tortillas according to their package instructions.
2. Mix the remaining ingredients in a bowl.
3. Serve the tortillas along with your salad and enjoy!

Nutrition:
Calories: 103.54
Protein: 2.12g
Fat: 5.16g
Carbs: 13.25g
Sodium: 274mg

135. SMOKY CARROT & BLACK BEAN STEW

Preparation Time: 15 minutes
Cooking Time: 25 minutes
Servings: 2
Ingredients:
- 1 15-ounce can of salt-free black beans
- 1 cup carrots, chopped
- 1 15-ounce can diced tomatoes
- 1 carton chicken broth
- 2 teaspoons smoked paprika
- ¾ cup onion, chopped
- 1 ½ teaspoon extra virgin olive oil
- 2 garlic cloves, minced
- 1 avocado, pitted and chopped

Directions:
1. Add extra-virgin olive oil to a pan over medium-high heat.
2. Add onion and carrots, then fry for 5 minutes.
3. Stir in the minced garlic, paprika, and cook for one minute.
4. Add the beans, broth, and diced tomatoes, then bring to a boil.
5. Reduce the pan heat, simmer until carrots are tender.
6. Top each serving with chopped avocado, then serve and enjoy!

Nutrition:
Calories: 425.48
Protein: 18.9g
Fat: 14.23g
Sodium: 2006mg
Carbs: 60.47g

136. OVEN-BAKED POTATOES & GREEN BEANS

Preparation Time: 10 minutes
Cooking Time: 30 minutes
Servings: 4
Ingredients:

- ½ lb. green beans
- ½ lb. potatoes, peeled and sliced into chunks
- 2 teaspoons extra virgin olive oil
- ½ teaspoon garlic powder
- 2 teaspoons Dijon mustard
- Sea salt along with fresh ground black pepper as needed

Directions:

1. Preheat oven to 375°F.
2. Mix chunks of potatoes with oil and mustard. Spread prepared potato chunks over a baking sheet. Bake for 15 minutes to make the first layer.
3. Add green beans, garlic powder, sea salt, and black pepper to your potatoes and toss. Bake for an additional 15 minutes. Serve and enjoy!

Nutrition:
Calories: 80
Protein: 2.27g
Fat: 2.8g
Carbs: 12.55g
Sodium: 182mg

137. HUMMUS & SALAD PITA FLATS

Preparation Time: 15 minutes
Cooking Time: 0 minutes
Servings: 2
Ingredients:

- 2 ounces whole wheat pitas
- 8 black olives, pitted
- ¼ cup sweet roasted red pepper hummus
- 2 large eggs
- 2 teaspoons spring mix
- 1 teaspoon dried oregano
- 2 teaspoons extra-virgin olive oil

Directions:

1. Heat pitas according to the package instructions.
2. Spread the hummus over the pitas.
3. Top pitas with hard-boiled eggs, dried oregano, and olives.
4. Add the spring mix and extra-virgin olive oil. Serve and enjoy!

Nutrition:
Calories: 299.51
Protein: 11.57g
Fat: 19.21g

Carbs: 20.28g
Sodium: 395.95mg

138. LETTUCE SALAD WITH LEMON

Preparation Time: 5 minutes
Cooking Time: 5 minutes
Servings: 2
Ingredients:

- 2 ounces arugula
- ½ head Romaine lettuce, chopped
- 1 avocado, pitted and sliced
- 2 teaspoons extra-virgin olive oil
- 1 tablespoon lemon juice
- ¼ teaspoon mustard
- Sea salt along with fresh ground black pepper as needed

Directions:

1. Whisk your torn arugula, lemon juice, chopped avocado, olive oil, sea salt, and pepper.
2. Add the chopped lettuce and toss to coat. Serve and enjoy!

Nutrition:
Calories: 166.76
Protein: 3.79g
Fat: 13.58g
Carbs: 11.6g
Sodium: 369mg

139. PORK CHOPS & BUTTERNUT SQUASH SALAD

Preparation Time: 20 minutes
Cooking Time: 25 minutes
Servings: 4
Ingredients:

- 4 boneless pork chops
- 1½ tablespoon fresh lemon juice
- 1 pkg. pomegranate seeds
- 1 pkg. baby arugula
- 3 cups butternut squash, peeled and cubed
- ½ cup pine nuts
- 2 tablespoons extra-virgin olive oil (divided)
- 2 garlic cloves, minced
- 6 tablespoons balsamic vinaigrette
- Sea salt along with fresh ground black pepper as needed

Directions:

1. Preheat oven to 475°F.
2. Combine a tablespoon of olive oil, minced garlic, and lemon juice.
3. Mix your pork chops with oil mixture, sprinkle the top of the chops with sea salt and pepper.

4. Mix squash and 1 tablespoon of oil, sprinkle with salt and pepper.
5. Place your pork chops onto a baking sheet, add place cubed squash around the chops. Bake for 25 minutes, then turn chops.
6. Toast your pine nuts for about 5 minutes in a small pan over medium-high heat.
7. Combine your squash, nuts, arugula, and pomegranate seeds. Drizzle with balsamic vinaigrette and toss. Serve and enjoy!

Nutrition:
Calories: 575.74
Protein: 35.45g
Fat: 38.35g
Carbs: 24.9g
Sodium: 495.86mg

140. LOW CARB STUFFED PEPPERS

Preparation Time: 15 minutes
Cooking Time: 30 minutes
Servings: 4
Ingredients:

- 1 onion, diced
- 2 lb. ground steak
- 4 green bell peppers, seeds removed and cut in half
- Sea salt along with black ground pepper
- 1 tablespoon Worcestershire sauce
- Thin slices of mozzarella cheese
- 2 teaspoons garlic, minced

Directions:

1. Heat your oil, add diced onions and minced garlic along with some salt and pepper in the pan over medium-high heat.
2. Add diced steak pieces into the pan along with Worcestershire sauce and cook for 5 minutes.
3. Add cooked steak and other ingredients into a bowl and combine (except cheese slices and pepper halves).
4. Fill the pepper halves with steak mixture and top with a thin piece of mozzarella cheese on top of each half pepper.
5. Place the peppers into a baking pan and bake for 30 minutes. Serve and enjoy!

Nutrition:
Calories: 350.81
Protein: 53.68g
Fat: 11.87g
Carbs: 8.26g
Sodium: 383.93mg

141. CHICKEN CORDON BLEU

Preparation Time: 20 minutes
Cooking Time: 23 minutes
Servings: 8
Ingredients:

- 8 chicken breasts, boneless and skinless
- ½ cup fat-free sour cream
- ⅔ cup skim milk
- 1½ cups mozzarella cheese, grated
- 8 slices ham
- 1 cup corn flakes, crushed
- 1 can low-fat condensed cream of chicken soup
- 1 teaspoon lemon juice
- 1 teaspoon paprika
- ½ teaspoon garlic powder
- ½ teaspoon black pepper
- ¼ teaspoon sea salt
- Non-stick cooking spray as needed

Directions:

1. Heat oven to 350°F. Spray a 13×9 baking dish lightly with cooking spray.
2. Flatten the chicken breasts to ¼-inch thick. Sprinkle with pepper and top with a slice of ham and 3 tablespoons of cheese down the middle. Roll up, and tuck ends under and secure with toothpicks.
3. Pour the milk into a shallow bowl. In another bowl, combine corn flakes and seasoning. Dip the chicken into milk, roll in the cornflake mixture, and then place on a prepared baking dish.
4. Bake for 30 minutes or until chicken is cooked through.
5. In a small pan, whisk the soup, lemon juice, and sour cream until well-combined. Cook over medium heat until hot.
6. Remove the toothpicks from your chicken and place onto serving plates. Top with sauce, serve and enjoy!

Nutrition:
Calories: 443.95
Fat: 13g
Protein: 58.56g
Carbs: 20.64g
Sodium: 1006mg

142. BEEF GOULASH

Preparation Time: 15 minutes
Cooking Time: 60 minutes
Servings: 6
Ingredients:

- 2 lb. chuck steak, trim the fat, and cut into bite-sized pieces
- 1 orange pepper, chopped
- 1 red pepper, chopped
- 1 green pepper, chopped
- 3 onions, quartered
- 3 garlic cloves, diced fine
- 1 cup low-sodium beef broth
- 1 can tomatoes, chopped
- 2 tablespoons tomato paste
- 3 cups water
- 2 bay leaves
- 1 tablespoon paprika
- 1 tablespoon olive oil
- 2 teaspoons hot smoked paprika
- Sea salt and black pepper to taste

Directions:

1. Heat oil in a soup pot over medium-high heat. Add the steak and cook until browned, stirring often.
2. Add onions and continue to cook for another 5 minutes or until soft. Add the garlic and cook for another minute, stirring often.
3. Add remaining ingredients, then bring to a boil. Reduce the heat to a low simmer for 50 minutes, stirring occasionally. The Goulash is done when the steak is tender. Stir well, then add to serving bowls and enjoy!

Nutrition:
Calories: 321.54
Fat: 15.7g
Protein: 34.8g
Carbs: 12.39g
Sodium: 376.5mg

143. CAJUN BEEF & RICE SKILLET

Preparation Time: 10 minutes
Cooking Time: 25 minutes
Servings: 4
Ingredients:

- 2 cups cauliflower rice, cooked
- ¾ lb. lean ground beef
- 1 red bell pepper, sliced thin
- 1 jalapeño pepper, with seeds removed and diced fine
- 1 celery stalk, sliced thin
- ½ yellow onion, diced
- ¼ cup parsley, fresh diced
- 4 teaspoons cajun seasoning
- ½ cup low-sodium beef broth

Directions:

1. Place the beef along with 1½ teaspoon of Cajun seasoning into a large skillet over medium-high heat.
2. Add the vegetables, except cauliflower and remaining cajun seasoning. Cook, occasionally stirring, for about 8 minutes or until vegetables are tender.
3. Add the broth and stir. Cook for 3 minutes or until the mixture has thickened. Stir in your cauliflower rice and cook until heated through. Remove from heat and add to serving bowls, then top with parsley, serve and enjoy!

Nutrition:
Calories: 198
Fat: 6g
Protein: 28g
Carbs: 6.29g
Sodium: 666mg

144. CHEESY BEEF & NOODLES

Preparation Time: 10 minutes
Cooking Time: 15 minutes
Servings: 4
Ingredients:

- 1 lb. lean ground beef
- 2 cups mozzarella cheese, grated
- 1 onion, diced
- ½ cup + 2 tablespoons fresh parsley, diced
- 1 package fettuccine noodles
- 2 tablespoons tomato paste
- 1 tablespoon Worcestershire sauce
- 1 tablespoon extra-virgin olive oil
- 3 garlic cloves, minced
- 1 teaspoon red pepper flakes
- Sea salt and black pepper to taste

Directions:

1. Heat oil in a large skillet placed over medium-high heat. Add the beef and cook while breaking up with the spatula for about 2 minutes.
2. Cook the noodles according to package instructions.
3. Lower the heat of skillet to medium, then season with salt and pepper. Stir in your garlic, pepper flakes, onion, tomato paste, ½ cup parsley, Worcestershire sauce, and ½ cup of water. Bring to a simmer while occasionally stirring for about 8 minutes.
4. Stir in the cooked noodles and continue to cook for another 2

minutes. Stir in 1 cup of cheese over the top and cover with a lid until cheese melts. Serve with remaining parsley as garnish and enjoy!

Nutrition:
Calories: 712
Fat: 26g
Protein: 46g
Carbs: 70.78g
Sodium: 596mg

145. BISTRO STEAK SALAD WITH HORSERADISH DRESSING

Preparation Time: 8 minutes
Cooking Time: 30 minutes
Servings: 2
Ingredients:
- 1 12-oz. rib-eye steak
- ¼ teaspoon of each:
- Pepper
- Salt
- 1 2.1-oz. small red onion
- 1 7-oz. bag romaine salad greens
- 4 slices uncured bacon
- ½ cup sliced radishes
- 4.2 oz. cherry tomatoes

For the Dressing:
- 2 tablespoon prepared horseradish
- ¼ cup mayonnaise
- Pepper and salt

Directions:
1. Thinly slice the onion and radishes.
2. Place parchment paper on a baking tin. Set the oven temperature to 350ºF. Arrange the bacon in a single layer in the pan. Bake for 15 minutes. Drain and break into small pieces.
3. Pat the steak with paper towels. Season with pepper and salt. Grill for 4 minutes and flip. Continue cooking for another 12-15 minutes (medium is approximately 12 minutes or an internal temperature of 155ºF).
4. Let it cool down for five minutes, and slice against the grain into small slices.
5. Prepare the dressing and enjoy it.

Nutrition:
Calories: 889.66
Protein: 46.52g
Fat: 73.7g
Carbs: 10.92g
Sodium: 1804mg

146. CAPRESE SALAD WITH HORSERADISH DRESSING

Preparation Time: 10 minutes
Cooking Time: 19 minutes
Servings: 4
Ingredients:
- 3 cups grape tomatoes
- 4 peeled garlic cloves
- 2 tablespoon avocado oil
- 10 pearl-sized mozzarella balls
- 4 cups baby spinach leaves
- ¼ cup fresh basil leaves
- 1 tablespoon Brine reserved from the cheese
- 1 tablespoon pesto

For the Dressing:
- 1 egg yolk
- 1-2 tsp. white vinegar/lemon juice
- 1 tablespoon Dijon mustard
- 1 cup light olive oil

Directions:
1. Use aluminum foil to cover a baking tray. Set the oven to 400ºF. Put the cloves and tomatoes on the baking pan and cover with the oil.
2. Bake 20-30 minutes until the tops are slightly browned.
3. Drain the liquid (saving one tablespoon) from the mozzarella. Mix the pesto in with the brine.
4. Arrange the spinach in a large bowl, then move it and the tomatoes to the dish along with the roasted garlic. Drizzle with the pesto sauce.
5. Garnish with the balls of mozzarella and the basil leaves.

For the Dressing:
6. Ahead of time, take out the egg and mustard to become room temperature.
7. Mix the mustard and egg. Slowly, pour the oil until the mixture thickens.
8. Pour in the lemon juice/vinegar. Stir well. Add a pinch of salt and pepper for additional flavoring.

Nutrition:
Calories: 736
Protein: 41.4g
Carbs: 21.6g
Sodium: 976mg
Fat: 59.4g

147. EGG SALAD STUFFED AVOCADO

Preparation Time: 10 minutes
Cooking Time: 28 minutes
Servings: 6

Ingredients:
- 6 large hard-boiled eggs
- 3 celery ribs
- ⅓ med. red onion
- 4 tablespoon mayonnaise
- 2 tablespoon fresh lime juice
- 2 tsp brown mustard
- Pepper & salt to taste
- ½ teaspoon cumin
- 1 teaspoon hot sauce
- 3 med. avocados

Directions:
1. Begin by chopping the onions, celery, and eggs. Discard the pit and slice the avocado in half.
2. Combine with all of the other fixings except for the avocado.
3. Scoop the salad into the avocado and serve!

Nutrition:
Calories: 230.57
Fat: 20.83g
Protein: 7.32g
Carbs: 6.69g
Sodium: 305mg

148. THAI PORK SALAD

Preparation Time: 9 minutes
Cooking Time: 30 minutes
Servings: 2
Ingredients:
For the Salad:
- 2 cups romaine lettuce
- 10 oz. pulled pork
- ¼ medium chopped red bell pepper
- ¼ cup chopped cilantro

For the Sauce:
- 2 tablespoons of each: Tomato paste & Chopped cilantro
- Juice & zest of 1 lime
- 2 tablespoon + 2 tsp. soy sauce
- 1 teaspoon of each: Red curry paste, Five Spice & Fish sauce
- ¼ teaspoon red pepper flakes
- 1 tablespoon (+) 1 teaspoon rice wine vinegar
- ½ teaspoon mango extract
- 10 drops liquid Stevia

Directions:
1. Zest half of the lime and chop the cilantro.
2. Mix all of the sauce fixings.
3. Blend the barbecue sauce components and set them aside.
4. Pull the pork apart and make the salad. Pour a glaze over the pork with a bit of the sauce.

Nutrition:
Calories: 440
Fat: 28.6g
Protein: 34.2g
Carbs: 11.98g

Sodium: 3343mg

149. VEGETARIAN CLUB SALAD

Preparation Time: 10 minutes
Cooking Time: 22 minutes
Servings: 3
Ingredients:

- 2 tablespoons of each: Mayonnaise & Sour cream
- ½ teaspoon of each: Onion powder & Garlic powder
- 1 tablespoon milk
- 1 teaspoon dried parsley
- 3 large hard-boiled eggs
- 4 oz. cheddar cheese
- ½ cup cherry tomatoes
- 1 c. diced cucumber
- 3 cups torn romaine lettuce
- 1 tablespoon Dijon mustard

Directions:

1. Slice the hard-boiled eggs and cube the cheese. Cut the tomatoes into halves and dice the cucumber.
2. Prepare the dressing (dried herbs, mayo, and sour cream) mixing well.
3. Add one tablespoon of milk to the mixture - and another if it's too thick.
4. Layer the salad with vegetables, cheese, and egg slices. Scoop a spoonful of mustard in the center along with a drizzle of dressing.
5. Toss and enjoy!

Nutrition:
Calories: 336
Fat: 26.32g
Protein: 16.82g
Carbs: 7.19g
Sodium: 386mg

150. CAULIFLOWER MAC N' CHEESE

Preparation Time: 10 minutes
Cooking Time: 30 minutes
Servings: 4
Ingredients:

- 3 tablespoons unsalted butter
- 1 head cauliflower
- 1 cup cheddar cheese
- Black pepper & sea salt to taste
- ¼ cup of each:
- Unsweetened almond milk
- Heavy cream

Directions:

1. Cut the cauliflower into small florets and shred the cheese.
2. Heat the oven to 450ºF. Cover a baking sheet with aluminum foil or parchment paper.

3. Melt 2 tablespoons of butter. Toss the florets and butter. Give it a shake of pepper and salt. Place the cauliflower on the baking pan and roast for 10-15 minutes.
4. Warm up the rest of the butter, milk, heavy cream, and cheese in the microwave or double boiler. Pour in the cheese and serve.

Nutrition:
Calories: 327.61
Fat: 30.4g
Protein: 9.8g
Carbs: 5.38g
Sodium: 425mg

151. FETTUCCINE CHICKEN ALFREDO

Preparation Time: 13 minutes
Cooking Time: 30 minutes
Servings: 2
Ingredients:

- 2 tablespoon unsalted butter
- 2 minced garlic cloves
- ½ teaspoon dried basil
- ½ cup heavy cream
- 4 tablespoon grated parmesan

For the Chicken and Noodles:

- 2 chicken thighs - no bones or skin
- 1 tablespoon olive oil
- 1 bag Miracle Noodle - Fettuccini
- Salt and pepper

Directions:

1. For the Sauce: Add the cloves to a pan with the butter for 2 minutes. Empty the cream into the skillet and let it simmer for 2 additional minutes. Toss in one tablespoon of the parmesan at a time. Add the pepper, salt, and dried basil. Simmer for 3 to 5 minutes on the low heat setting.
2. For the Chicken: Pound the chicken with a meat tenderizer hammer until it is approximately ½-inch thick. Warm up the oil in a skillet using the medium heat setting and put the chicken in to cook for about seven minutes per side. Shred and set aside.
3. For the Noodles: Prepare the package of noodles. Rinse, and boil them for 2 minutes in a pot of water.
4. Fold in the noodles along with the sauce and shredded chicken. Cook slowly for 2 minutes and enjoy.

Nutrition:
Calories: 585
Fat: 51g
Carbs: 25g
Sodium: 641mg
Protein: 25g

152. LEMON GARLIC SHRIMP PASTA

Preparation Time: 16 minutes
Cooking Time: 32 minutes
Servings: 8
Ingredients:

- 2 bags of angel hair pasta
- 4 garlic cloves
- 2 tablespoons each: Olive oil & Unsalted butter
- ½ lemon
- 1 lb. large raw shrimp
- ½ teaspoon paprika
- Fresh basil
- Pepper and salt

Directions:

1. Drain the water from the package of noodles and rinse them in cold water.
2. Add them to a pot of boiling water for 2 minutes. Transfer them to a hot skillet over medium heat to remove the excess liquid (dry roast). Set them to the side.
3. Use the same pan to warm the oil, butter, and smashed garlic. Sauté a few minutes but don't brown.
4. Slice the lemon into rounds and add them to the garlic along with the shrimp. Sauté for approximately 3 minutes per side.
5. Add the noodles and spices and stir to blend the flavors.

Nutrition:
Calories: 540
Fat: 9.12g
Protein: 22g
Carbs: 93g
Sodium: 251mg

153. BBQ MEAT LOVER'S PIZZA

Preparation Time: 9 minutes
Cooking Time: 30 minutes
Servings: 4
Ingredients:

- 2 cups (8 oz.) mozzarella
- 1 tablespoon psyllium husk powder
- ¾ cup almond flour
- 3 tablespoons (1½ oz.) cream cheese
- 1 large egg

- ½ teaspoon of each: Black pepper & Salt
- 1 tablespoon Italian seasoning

For the Topping:
- 1 cup (4 oz.) mozzarella cheese
- To Taste: BBQ sauce
- Sliced Kabana/hard salami
- Bacon slices
- Sprinkled oregano - optional

Directions:
1. Set the temperature of the oven to 400ºF.
2. Melt the cheese in the microwave – about 45 seconds. Toss in the cream cheese and egg, mixing well.
3. Blend in the psyllium husk, flour, salt, pepper, and Italian seasoning. Make the dough as circular as possible. Bake for ten minutes. Flip it onto a piece of parchment paper.
4. Cover the crust with the toppings and some more cheese. Bake until the cheese is golden, slice, and serve.

Nutrition:
Calories: 205
Fat: 27g
Protein: 18g
Sodium: 897mg
Carbs: 10.24g

154. SPAGHETTI SQUASH AND CHICKPEA BOLOGNESE

Preparation Time: 5 minutes
Cooking Time: 25 minutes
Servings: 4
Ingredients:
- 1 3-4-pound spaghetti squash
- ½ teaspoon ground cumin
- 1 cup no-sugar-added spaghetti sauce
- 1 15-ounce/425-g can low-sodium chickpeas, drained and rinsed
- 6 ounces (170 g) extra-firm tofu

Directions:
1. Preheat the oven to 400ºF (205ºC).
2. Cut the squash in half lengthwise. Scoop out the seeds and discard them.
3. Season both halves of the squash with the cumin and place them on a baking sheet cut side down. Roast for 25 minutes.
4. Meanwhile, heat a medium saucepan over low heat, and pour in the spaghetti sauce and chickpeas.

5. Press the tofu between 2 layers of paper towels, and gently squeeze out any excess water.
6. Crumble the tofu into the sauce and cook for 15 minutes.
7. Remove the squash from the oven, and comb through the flesh of each half with a fork to make thin strands.
8. Divide the "spaghetti" into 4 portions and top each portion with one-quarter of the sauce.

Nutrition:
Calories: 193
Fat: 5.28g
Protein: 9.84g
Carbs: 29g
Sodium: 319mg

155. ZUCCHINI AND PINTO BEAN CASSEROLE

Preparation Time: 15 minutes
Cooking Time: 15 minutes
Servings: 4
Ingredients:
- 1 zucchini, peeled
- 1 15-ounce/425-g can pinto beans
- 1⅓ cups salsa
- 1⅓ cups shredded Mexican cheese blend
- Non-stick cooking spray

Directions:
1. Slice the zucchini into rounds. You'll need at least 16 slices.
2. Spray a 6-inch cake pan with nonstick spray.
3. Put the beans into a medium bowl and mash some of them with a fork.
4. Cover the bottom of the pan with about 4 zucchini slices. Add about ⅓ of the beans, ⅓ cup of salsa, and ⅓ cup of cheese. Press down. Repeat for 2 more layers. Add the remaining zucchini, salsa, and cheese. (There are no beans in the top layer.)
5. Cover the pan loosely with foil.
6. 1 cup of water should be added to an electric pressure cooker.
7. Place the pan on the wire rack and drop it into the pot with care. Close and secure the pressure cooker lid. Set the valve to the sealing position.
8. Cook for 15 minutes on high pressure.
9. When the cooking is finished, let the pressure drop normally.
10. Unlock and remove the cover after the pin has dropped.

11. Carefully remove the pan from the pot, lifting it by the handles of the wire rack. Let the casserole sit for 5 minutes before slicing into quarters and serving.

Nutrition:
Calories: 300
Fat: 13.31g
Protein: 18g
Carbs: 29.27g
Sodium: 953.8mg

156. EGGPLANT-ZUCCHINI PARMESAN

Preparation Time: 10 minutes
Cooking Time: 2 hours
Servings: 6
Ingredients:
- 1 medium eggplant, peeled and cut into 1-inch cubes
- 1 medium zucchini, cut into 1-inch pieces
- 1 medium onion, cut into thin wedges
- 1½ cups purchased light spaghetti sauce
- ⅔ cup reduced-fat Parmesan cheese, grated

Directions:
1. Place the vegetables, spaghetti sauce, and ⅓ cup Parmesan in the crockpot. Stir to combine. Cover and cook on high for 2 to 2 ½ hours, or on low for 4 to 5 hours.
2. Sprinkle remaining Parmesan on top before serving.

Nutrition:
Calories: 92
Fat: 3.0g
Protein: 4.2g
Carbs: 12.5g
Sodium: 463.74mg

157. GRILLED PORTOBELLO AND ZUCCHINI BURGER

Preparation Time: 5 minutes
Cooking Time: 10 minutes
Servings: 4
Ingredients:
- 2 large portabella mushroom caps
- ½ small zucchini, sliced
- 2 slices low-fat cheese
- 2 whole wheat sandwich thins
- 2 teaspoons roasted red bell peppers
- 2 teaspoons olive oil

Directions:
1. Heat grill, or charcoal, to medium-high heat.

2. Lightly brush mushroom caps with olive oil. Grill mushroom caps and zucchini slices until tender, about 3 to 4 minutes per side.
3. Place on sandwich thin. Top with sliced cheese and roasted red bell pepper. Serve.

Nutrition:
Calories: 128.63
Fat: 4.59g
Protein: 7.76g
Carbs: 13g
Sodium: 236mg

158. LEMON WAX BEANS

Preparation Time: 5 minutes
Cooking Time: 15 minutes
Servings: 4
Ingredients:
- 2 pounds wax beans
- Juice of ½ lemon
- 2 tablespoons extra-virgin olive oil
- Freshly ground black pepper and sea salt, to taste

Directions:
1. Preheat the oven to 400°F (205°C).
2. Line a baking sheet with aluminum foil.
3. Toss the beans and olive oil in a large mixing basin. Season with salt and pepper to taste.
4. Place the beans on a baking pan and spread them out evenly.
5. Roast the beans until caramelized and tender, about 10 to 12 minutes.
6. Place the beans on a serving plate and top with lemon juice.

Nutrition:
Calories: 135
Fat: 7.4g
Protein: 4.17g
Carbs: 16.7g
Sodium: 183mg

159. WILTED DANDELION GREENS WITH SWEET ONION

Preparation Time: 15 minutes
Cooking Time: 12 minutes
Servings: 4
Ingredients:
- 1 Vidalia onion, thinly sliced
- 2 garlic cloves, minced
- 2 bunches dandelion greens, roughly chopped
- ½ cup low-sodium vegetable broth

- 1 tablespoon extra-virgin olive oil
- Freshly ground black pepper, to taste

Directions:
1. Heat the olive oil in a large skillet over low heat.
2. Cook the onion and garlic for 2 to 3 minutes until tender, stirring occasionally.
3. Add the dandelion greens and broth and cook for 5 to 7 minutes, stirring frequently, or until the greens are wilted.
4. Transfer to a plate and season with black pepper. Serve warm.

Nutrition:
Calories: 63
Fat: 3.8g
Protein: 0.8g
Carbs: 6.7g
Sodium: 26.31mg

160. ASPARAGUS WITH SCALLOPS

Preparation Time: 10 minutes
Cooking Time: 15 minutes
Servings: 4
Ingredients:
- 1 pound asparagus, trimmed and cut into 2-inch segments
- 1 pound sea scallops
- ¼ cup dry white wine
- Juice of 1 lemon
- 2 garlic cloves, minced
- 3 teaspoons extra-virgin olive oil, divided
- 1 tablespoon unsalted butter
- ¼ teaspoon freshly ground black pepper

Directions:
1. In a large pan, heat 1½ teaspoons oil over medium heat.
2. Add the asparagus and sauté for 5 to 6 minutes until just tender, stirring regularly. Remove from the skillet and cover with aluminum foil to keep warm.
3. Add the remaining 1½ teaspoons of oil and the butter to the skillet. When the butter is sizzling and melted, place the scallops in a single layer in the skillet. Cook for approx. 3 minutes on one side until nicely browned. Use tongs to gently loosen and flip the scallops and cook on the other side for 3 minutes more until browned and cooked through. Remove and cover with foil to keep warm.

4. In the same skillet, combine the wine, lemon juice, garlic, and pepper. Bring to a simmer for 1 to 2 minutes, stirring to mix in any browned pieces left in the pan.
5. Return the asparagus and the cooked scallops to the skillet to coat with the sauce. Serve warm.

Nutrition:
Calories: 170
Fat: 7.1g
Protein: 15.8g
Carbs: 8.82g
Sodium: 447.18mg

161. BUTTER COD WITH ASPARAGUS

Preparation Time: 5 minutes
Cooking Time: 10 minutes
Servings: 4
Ingredients:
- 4 4-ounce cod fillets
- ¼ teaspoon garlic powder
- 24 asparagus spears, woody ends trimmed
- ½ cup brown rice, cooked
- 1 tablespoon freshly squeezed lemon juice
- ¼ teaspoon salt
- ¼ teaspoon freshly ground black pepper
- 2 tablespoons unsalted butter

Directions:
1. In a large bowl, season the cod fillets with garlic powder, salt, and pepper. Set aside.
2. Melt the butter in a skillet over medium-low heat.
3. Place the cod fillets and asparagus in the skillet in a single layer. Cook covered for 8 minutes, or until the cod is cooked through.
4. Divide the cooked brown rice, cod fillets, and asparagus among 4 plates. Serve drizzled with lemon juice.

Nutrition:
Calories: 180.5
Fat: 6.64g
Protein: 22.1g
Carbs: 8.93g
Sodium: 238.77mg

162. CREAMY COD FILLET WITH QUINOA AND ASPARAGUS

Preparation Time: 5 minutes
Cooking Time: 15 minutes
Servings: 4
Ingredients:

- ½ cup uncooked quinoa
- 4 4-ounce cod fillets
- ½ teaspoon garlic powder, divided
- 24 asparagus spears, cut the bottom 1½ inches off
- 1 cup half-and-half
- ¼ teaspoon salt
- ¼ teaspoon freshly ground black pepper
- 1 tablespoon avocado oil

Directions:
1. Put the quinoa in a pot of salted water. Bring to a boil. Reduce the heat to low and simmer for 15 minutes or until the quinoa is soft and has a white "tail." Cover and turn off the heat. Let sit for 5 minutes.
2. On a clean work surface, rub the cod fillets with ¼ teaspoon of garlic powder, salt, and pepper.
3. Heat the avocado oil in a nonstick skillet over medium-low heat.
4. Add the cod fillets and asparagus to the skillet and cook for 8 minutes or until they are tender. Flip the cod and shake the skillet halfway through the cooking time.
5. Pour the half-and-half in the skillet, and sprinkle with remaining garlic powder. Turn up the heat to high and simmer for 2 minutes until creamy.
6. Divide the quinoa, cod fillets, and asparagus into 4 bowls and serve warm.

Nutrition:
Calories: 288
Fat: 11.87g
Protein: 27g
Carbs: 19.86g
Sodium: 275mg

163. ASPARAGUS AND SCALLOP SKILLET WITH LEMON

Preparation Time: 10 minutes
Cooking Time: 15 minutes
Servings: 4
Ingredients:
- 1 pound asparagus, trimmed and cut into 2-inch segments
- 1 pound sea scallops
- ¼ cup dry white wine
- 2 garlic cloves, minced
- Juice of 1 lemon
- 3 teaspoons extra-virgin olive oil, divided
- 1 tablespoon unsalted butter

- ¼ teaspoon freshly ground black pepper

Directions:
1. Heat half of olive oil in a nonstick skillet over medium heat until shimmering.
2. Add the asparagus to the skillet and sauté for 6 minutes until soft. Transfer the cooked asparagus to a large plate and cover it with aluminum foil.
3. Heat the remaining half of olive oil and butter in the skillet until the butter is melted.
4. Add the scallops to the skillet and cook for 6 minutes or until opaque and browned. Flip the scallops with tongs halfway through the cooking time. Transfer the scallops to the plate and cover with aluminum foil.
5. Combine the wine, garlic, lemon juice, and black pepper in the skillet. Simmer over medium-low heat for 2 minutes. Keep stirring during the simmering.
6. Pour the sauce over the asparagus and scallops to coat well, then serve warm.

Nutrition:
Calories: 169.74
Fat: 7g
Protein: 15.8g
Sodium: 447mg
Carbs: 8.82g

164. CAULIFLOWER RICE WITH CHICKEN

Preparation Time: 15 Minutes
Cooking Time: 15 Minutes
Servings: 4
Ingredients:
- ½ large cauliflower
- ¾ cup cooked meat
- ½ bell pepper
- 1 carrot
- 2 ribs celery
- 1 tablespoon stir fry sauce (low-carb)
- 1 tablespoon extra-virgin olive oil
- Salt and pepper, to taste

Directions:
1. Chop cauliflower in a processor to "rice." Place in a bowl.
2. Properly chop all vegetables in a food processor into thin slices.
3. Add cauliflower and other plants to wok with heated oil. Fry until all veggies are tender.

4. Add chopped meat and sauce to the wok and fry for 10 Minutes.
5. Serve. This dish is very mouth-watering!

Nutrition:
Calories: 122.42
Protein: 12.39 g
Fat: 5.29 g
Carbohydrates: 6.11 g
Sodium: 340.55mg

165. TURKEY WITH FRIED EGGS

Preparation Time: 10 minutes
Cooking Time: 20 minutes
Servings: 4
Ingredients:
- 4 large potatoes
- 1 cooked turkey thigh
- 1 large onion (about 2 cups diced)
- Unsalted butter
- Chile flakes
- 4 eggs
- Salt and pepper to taste

Directions:
1. Rub the cold boiled potatoes on the coarsest holes of a box grater. Dice the turkey.
2. Cook the onion in as much unsalted butter as you feel comfortable with until it's just fragrant and translucent.
3. Add the rubbed potatoes and a cup of diced cooked turkey, salt, and pepper to taste, and cook for 20 Minutes.
4. Top each with a fried egg. Yummy!

Nutrition:
Calories: 514.7
Protein: 32.5g
Fat: 17g
Carbohydrates: 59.7g
Sodium: 354.21mg

166. SWEET POTATO, KALE, AND WHITE BEAN STEW

Preparation Time: 15 minutes
Cooking Time: 25 minutes
Servings: 4
Ingredients:
- 1 15-ounce can low-sodium cannellini beans, rinsed and drained, divided
- 1 tablespoon olive oil
- 1 medium onion, chopped
- 2 garlic cloves, minced
- 2 celery stalks, chopped
- 3 medium carrots, chopped

- 2 cups low-sodium vegetable broth
- 1 teaspoon apple cider vinegar
- 2 medium sweet potatoes (about 1¼ pounds)
- 2 cups chopped kale
- 1 cup shelled edamame
- ¼ cup quinoa
- 1 teaspoon dried thyme
- ½ teaspoon cayenne pepper
- ½ teaspoon salt
- ¼ teaspoon freshly ground black pepper

Directions:
1. Put half the beans into a blender and blend until smooth. Set aside.
2. In a large soup pot over medium heat, heat the oil. When the oil is hot, include the onion and garlic, and cook until the onion softens and the garlic is sweet for about 3 minutes.
3. Add the celery and carrots and continue cooking until the vegetables soften for about 5 minutes.
4. Add the broth, vinegar, sweet potatoes, unblended beans, kale, edamame, and quinoa, and bring the mixture to a boil. Turn down the heat and simmer until the vegetables soften for about 10 minutes.
5. Add the blended beans, thyme, cayenne, salt, and black pepper, increase the heat to medium-high, and bring the mixture to a boil. Turn down the heat and simmer, uncovered, until the flavors combine, about 5 minutes.
6. Into each of 4 containers, scoop 1¾ cup of stew.

Nutrition:
Calories: 373
Total Fat: 7g
Saturated Fat: 1g
Protein: 15g
Total Carbohydrates: 65g
Fiber: 15g
Sugar: 13g
Sodium: 540mg

167. SLOW COOKER 2-BEAN SLOPPY JOES

Preparation Time: 10 minutes
Cooking Time: 6 hours
Servings: 4
Ingredients:
- 1 15-ounce can low-sodium black beans

- 1 15-ounce can low-sodium pinto beans
- 1 15-ounce can no-salt-added diced tomatoes
- 1 medium green bell pepper, chopped, cored, and seeded
- 1 medium yellow onion, chopped
- ¼ cup low-sodium vegetable broth
- 2 garlic cloves, minced
- 2 servings (¼ cup) meal prep barbecue sauce or bottled barbecue sauce
- ¼ teaspoon salt
- ¼ teaspoon freshly ground black pepper
- 4 whole wheat buns

Directions:
1. In a slow cooker, combine the black beans, pinto beans, diced tomatoes, bell pepper, onion, broth, garlic, meal prep barbecue sauce, salt, and black pepper. Stir the ingredients, then cover and cook on low for 6 hours.
2. Into each of 4 containers, spoon 1¼ cups of sloppy joe mix. Serve with 1 whole-wheat bun.
3. Refrigerate sealed containers for up to a week in the refrigerator. Place freezer-safe containers in the freezer for up to 2 months to freeze. Refrigerate overnight to thaw. Microwave uncovered on high for 2 to 2 1/2 minutes to reheat individual pieces. Alternatively, reheat the entire dish in a saucepan on the stovetop. Bring the sloppy joes to a boil, then reduce the heat and simmer until heated through, 10 to 15 minutes. Serve with a whole wheat bun.

Nutrition:
Calories: 392
Total Fat: 3g
Protein: 17g
Total Carbohydrates: 79g
Fiber: 19g
Sugar: 15g
Sodium: 759mg

168. LIGHTER EGGPLANT PARMESAN

Preparation Time: 15 minutes
Cooking Time: 35 minutes
Servings: 4
Ingredients:
- Non-stick cooking spray
- 3 eggs, beaten

- 1 tablespoon dried parsley
- 2 teaspoons ground oregano
- ⅛ teaspoon freshly ground black pepper
- 1 cup panko breadcrumbs, preferably whole-wheat
- 1 large eggplant (about 2 pounds)
- 5 servings (2½ cups) chunky tomato sauce or jarred low-sodium tomato sauce
- 1 cup part-skim mozzarella cheese
- ¼ cup grated parmesan cheese

Directions:
1. Preheat the oven to 450ºF. Coat a baking sheet with cooking spray.
2. In a medium bowl, whisk together the eggs, parsley, oregano, and pepper.
3. Pour the panko into a separate medium bowl.
4. Slice the eggplant into ¼-inch-thick slices. Shake off any excess egg mixture from each eggplant slice. Then dredge both sides of the eggplant in the panko breadcrumbs. Place the coated eggplant on the baking sheet that has been prepared, leaving a ½-inch space between each slice.
5. Bake for about 15 minutes until soft and golden brown. Now remove from the oven and set aside to slightly cool.
6. Pour ½ cup of chunky tomato sauce on the bottom of an 8x15-inch baking dish. Using a spatula or the back of a spoon spread the tomato sauce evenly. Place half the slices of cooked eggplant, slightly overlapping, in the dish, and top with 1 cup of chunky tomato sauce, ½ cup of mozzarella, and 2 tablespoons of grated parmesan. Repeat the layer, ending with the cheese.
7. Bake uncovered for 20 minutes until the cheese is bubbling and slightly browned.
8. Remove from the oven and allow cooling for 15 minutes before dividing the eggplant equally into 4 separate containers.

Nutrition:
Calories: 333
Total Fat: 14g
Saturated Fat: 6g
Protein: 20g
Total Carbohydrates: 35g
Fiber: 11g

Sugar: 15g
Sodium: 994mg

169. COCONUT-LENTIL CURRY

Preparation Time: 15 minutes
Cooking Time: 35 minutes
Servings: 4
Ingredients:

- 1 tablespoon olive oil
- 1 medium yellow onion, chopped
- 1 garlic clove, minced
- 1 medium red bell pepper, diced
- 1 15-ounce can green or brown lentils, rinsed and drained
- 2 medium sweet potatoes, washed, peeled, and cut into bite-size chunks (about 1¼ pounds)
- 1 15-ounce can no-salt-added diced tomatoes
- 2 tablespoons tomato paste
- 4 teaspoons curry powder
- ⅛ teaspoon ground cloves
- 1 15-ounce can light coconut milk
- ¼ teaspoon salt
- 2 pieces whole wheat naan bread, halved, or 4 slices crusty bread

Directions:

1. In a large saucepan over medium heat, heat the olive oil. When the oil is shimmering, add both the onion and garlic and cook until the onion softens and the garlic is sweet, for about 3 minutes.
2. Add the bell pepper and continue cooking until it softens, about 5 minutes more. Add the lentils, sweet potatoes, tomatoes, tomato paste, curry powder, and cloves, and bring the mixture to a boil. Reduce the heat to medium-low, cover, and simmer until the potatoes are softened about 20 minutes.
3. Add the coconut milk and salt and return to a boil. Reduce the heat and simmer until the flavors combine for about 5 minutes.
4. Into each of 4 containers, spoon 2 cups of curry.
5. Enjoy each serving with half of a piece of naan bread or 1 slice of crusty bread.

Nutrition:
Calories: 559
Total Fat: 16g
Saturated Fat: 7g

Protein: 16g
Total Carbohydrates: 86g
Fiber: 16g
Sugar: 18g
Sodium: 819mg

170. STUFFED PORTOBELLO WITH CHEESE

Preparation Time: 15 minutes
Cooking Time: 25 minutes
Servings: 4
Ingredients:

- 4 Portobello mushroom caps
- 1 tablespoon olive oil
- ½ teaspoon salt, divided
- ¼ teaspoon freshly ground black pepper, divided
- 1 cup baby spinach, chopped
- 1½ cups part-skim ricotta cheese
- ½ cup part-skim shredded mozzarella cheese
- ¼ cup grated parmesan cheese
- 1 garlic clove, minced
- 1 tablespoon dried parsley
- 2 teaspoons dried oregano
- 4 teaspoons unseasoned breadcrumbs, divided
- 4 servings (4 cups) roasted broccoli with shallots

Directions:

1. Preheat the oven to 375°F. Line a baking sheet with aluminum foil.
2. Brush the mushroom caps with olive oil, and sprinkle with ¼ teaspoon salt and ⅛ teaspoon pepper. Put the mushroom caps on the prepared baking sheet and bake until soft, about 12 minutes.
3. Combine the spinach, ricotta, mozzarella, parmesan, garlic, parsley, oregano, and the remaining salt and pepper in a medium mixing bowl.
4. Spoon ½ cup of cheese mixture into each mushroom cap, and sprinkle each with 1 teaspoon of breadcrumbs. Return the mushrooms to the oven for 8 to 10 minutes more, or until warmed through.
5. Take the mushrooms from the oven and set aside for 10 minutes before placing each in a separate container. Add 1 cup of roasted broccoli with shallots to each container.

Nutrition:
Calories: 419
Total Fat: 30g
Saturated Fat: 10g
Protein: 23g

Total Carbohydrates: 19g
Fiber: 2g
Sugar: 3g
Sodium: 790mg

171. LIGHTER SHRIMP SCAMPI

Preparation Time: 15 minutes
Cooking Time: 15 minutes
Servings: 4
Ingredients:

- 1½ pounds large peeled and deveined shrimp
- ¼ teaspoon salt
- ⅛ teaspoon freshly ground black pepper
- 2 tablespoons olive oil
- 1 shallot, chopped
- 2 garlic cloves, minced
- ¼ cup cooking white wine
- Juice of ½ lemon (1 tablespoon)
- ½ teaspoon sriracha
- 2 tablespoons unsalted butter, at room temperature
- ¼ cup chopped fresh parsley
- 4 servings (6 cups) zucchini noodles with lemon vinaigrette

Directions:

1. Season the shrimp with salt and pepper.
2. Heat the oil in a medium saucepan over medium heat. Cook for approximately 3 minutes, or until the shallot softens and the garlic is aromatic, before adding the shallot and garlic. Cover and cook until the shrimp are opaque, 2 to 3 minutes on each side. Transfer the shrimp to a large platter using a slotted spoon.
3. Stir together the wine, lemon juice, and sriracha in a saucepan. Bring the mixture to a boil, then lower to a low heat and simmer for 3 minutes, or until the liquid is reduced by half. Stir in the butter for 3 minutes, or until it is melted. Toss the shrimp back into the pot to coat. Stir in the parsley to mix.
4. Into each of 4 containers, place 1½ cups of zucchini noodles with lemon vinaigrette, and top with ¾ cup of scampi.

Nutrition:
Calories: 364
Total Fat: 21g
Saturated Fat: 6g
Protein: 37g
Total Carbohydrates: 10g

Fiber: 2g
Sugar: 6g
Sodium: 557mg

172. MAPLE-MUSTARD SALMON

Preparation Time: 10 minutes, plus 30 minutes marinating time
Cooking Time: 20 minutes
Servings: 4
Ingredients:

- Nonstick cooking spray
- ½ cup 100% maple syrup
- 2 tablespoons Dijon mustard
- ¼ teaspoon salt
- 4 5-ounce salmon fillets
- 4 servings (4 cups) roasted broccoli with shallots
- 4 servings (2 cups) parleyed whole-wheat couscous

Directions:

1. Preheat the oven to 400°F. Line a baking sheet with aluminum foil and coat with cooking spray.
2. In a medium bowl, whisk together the maple syrup, mustard, and salt until smooth.
3. Put the salmon fillets into the bowl and toss to coat. Cover and place in the refrigerator to marinate for at least 30 minutes and up to overnight.
4. Shake off excess marinade from the salmon fillets and place them on the prepared baking sheet, leaving a 1-inch space between each fillet. Discard the extra marinade.
5. Bake for about 20 minutes until the salmon is opaque and a thermometer inserted in the thickest part of a fillet reads 145°F.
6. Into each of 4 resealable containers, place 1 salmon fillet, 1 cup of roasted broccoli with shallots, and ½ cup of whole wheat couscous.

Nutrition:
Calories: 601
Total Fat: 29g
Saturated Fat: 4g
Protein: 36g
Total Carbohydrates: 51g
Fiber: 3g
Sugar: 23g
Sodium: 610mg

173. CHICKEN SALAD WITH GRAPES AND PECANS

Preparation Time: 15 Minutes

Cooking Time: 5 Minutes
Servings: 4
Ingredients:

- ⅓ cup unsalted pecans, chopped
- 10 ounces cooked skinless, boneless chicken breast or rotisserie chicken, finely chopped
- ½ medium yellow onion, finely chopped
- 1 celery stalk, finely chopped
- ¾ cup red or green seedless grapes, halved
- ¼ cup light mayonnaise
- ¼ cup non-fat plain Greek yogurt
- 1 tablespoon Dijon mustard
- 1 tablespoon dried parsley
- ¼ teaspoon salt
- ⅛ teaspoon freshly ground black pepper
- 1 cup shredded romaine lettuce
- 4 8-inch whole wheat pitas

Directions:

1. Heat a small skillet over medium-low heat to toast the pecans. Cook the pecans until fragrant, about 3 minutes. Remove from the heat and set aside to cool.
2. In a medium bowl, mix the chicken, onion, celery, pecans, and grapes.
3. In a small bowl, whisk together the mayonnaise, yogurt, mustard, parsley, salt, and pepper. Spoon the sauce over the chicken mixture and stir until well combined.
4. Into each of 4 containers, place ¼ cup of lettuce and top with 1 cup of chicken salad. Store the pitas separately until ready to serve.
5. When ready to eat, stuff the serving of salad and lettuce into 1 pita.

Nutrition:
Calories: 314
Total Fat: 12.8g
Saturated Fat: 2g
Protein: 22.4g
Sodium: 508mg
Total Carbohydrates: 28.54g
Fiber: 4g

174. MILLET PILAF

Preparation Time: 10 minutes
Cooking Time: 15 minutes
Servings: 4
Ingredients:

- 1 cup millet
- 2 tomatoes, rinsed, seeded, and chopped
- 1¾ cups filtered water
- 2 tablespoons extra-virgin olive oil
- ¼ cup chopped dried apricot
- Zest of 1 lemon
- Juice of 1 lemon
- ½ cup fresh parsley, rinsed and chopped
- Himalayan pink salt
- Freshly ground black pepper

Directions:

1. In an electric pressure cooker, combine the millet, tomatoes, and water. Lock the lid into place, select Manual and High Pressure, and cook for 7 minutes.
2. When the beep sounds, quickly release the pressure by pressing Cancel and twisting the steam valve to the Venting position. Carefully remove the lid.
3. Stir in olive oil, apricot, lemon zest, lemon juice, and parsley. Taste, season with salt and pepper and serve.

Nutrition:
Calories: 270
Total Fat: 8g
Total Carbohydrates: 42g
Sodium: 202.86mg
Fiber: 5g
Sugar: 3g
Protein: 6g

175. SWEET AND SOUR ONIONS

Preparation Time: 10 minutes
Cooking Time: 11 minutes
Servings: 4
Ingredients:

- 4 large onions, halved
- 2 garlic cloves, crushed
- 3 cups vegetable stock
- 1½ tablespoon balsamic vinegar
- ½ teaspoon Dijon mustard
- 1 tablespoon sugar

Directions:

1. Combine onions and garlic in a pan. Fry for 3 minutes, or till softened.
2. Pour stock, vinegar, Dijon mustard, and sugar. Bring to a boil.
3. Reduce heat. Cover and let the combination simmer for 10 minutes.

4. Turn off heat. Continue stirring until the liquid is reduced and the onions are brown. Serve.

Nutrition:
Calories: 203
Total Fat: 41.2g
Saturated Fat: 0.8g
Sodium: 861mg
Total Carbohydrates: 29.5g
Fiber: 16.3g
Sugar 29.3g
Protein: 19.2g

176. SAUTÉED APPLES AND ONIONS

Preparation Time: 14 minutes
Cooking Time: 16 minutes
Servings: 3
Ingredients:
- 2 cups dry cider
- 1 large onion, halved
- 2 cups vegetable stock
- 4 apples, sliced into wedges
- Pinch of salt
- Pinch of pepper

Directions:
1. Combine cider and onion in a saucepan. Bring to a boil until the onions are cooked and the liquid is almost gone.
2. Pour the stock and the apples. Season with salt and pepper. Stir occasionally. Cook for about 10 minutes or until the apples are tender but not mushy. Serve.

Nutrition:
Calories: 343
Total Fat: 51.2g
Saturated Fat: 0.8g
Sodium: 861mg
Total Carbohydrates: 22.5g
Fiber: 6.3g
Sugar 2.3g
Protein: 9.2g

177. ZUCCHINI NOODLES WITH PORTABELLA MUSHROOMS

Preparation Time: 14 minutes
Cooking Time: 16 minutes
Servings: 3
Ingredients:
- 1 zucchini, processed into spaghetti-like noodles
- 3 garlic cloves, minced
- 2 white onions, thinly sliced
- 1 thumb-sized ginger, julienned
- 1 lb. chicken thighs
- 1 lb. portabella mushrooms, sliced into thick slivers
- 2 cups chicken stock

- 3 cups water
- Pinch of sea salt, add more if needed
- Pinch of black pepper, add more if needed
- 2 teaspoon sesame oil
- 4 tablespoons coconut oil, divided
- ¼ cup fresh chives, minced, for garnish

Directions:
1. Pour 2 tablespoons of coconut oil into a large saucepan. Fry mushroom slivers in batches for 5 minutes or until seared brown. Set aside. Transfer these to a plate.
2. Sauté the onion, garlic, and ginger for 3 minutes or until tender. Add in chicken thighs, cooked mushrooms, chicken stock, water, salt, and pepper stir mixture well. Bring to a boil.
3. Decrease gradually the heat and allow simmering for 20 minutes or until the chicken is forking tender. Tip in sesame oil.
4. Serve by placing an equal amount of zucchini noodles into bowls. Ladle soup and garnish with chives.

Nutrition:
Calories: 163
Total Fat: 4.2g
Saturated Fat: 0.8g
Sodium: 86 mg
Total Carbohydrates: 22.5g
Fiber: 6.3g
Sugar 2.3g
Protein: 9.2g

178. GRILLED TEMPEH WITH PINEAPPLE

Preparation Time: 12 minutes
Cooking Time: 16 minutes
Servings: 3
Ingredients:
- 10 oz. tempeh, sliced
- 1 red bell pepper, quartered
- ¼ pineapple, sliced into rings
- 6 oz. green beans
- 1 tablespoon coconut aminos
- 2½ tablespoon orange juice, freshly squeezed
- 1½ tablespoon lemon juice, freshly squeezed
- 1 tablespoon extra-virgin olive oil
- ¼ cup hoisin sauce

Directions:
1. Blend together the olive oil, orange and lemon juices,

coconut aminos or soy sauce, and hoisin sauce in a bowl. Add the diced tempeh and set aside.
2. Heat up the grill or place a grill pan over medium-high flame. Once hot, lift the marinated tempeh from the bowl with a pair of tongs and transfer them to the grill or pan.
3. Grill for 2 to 3 minutes, or until browned all over.
4. Grill the sliced pineapples alongside the tempeh, then transfer them directly onto the serving platter.
5. Place the grilled tempeh beside the grilled pineapple and cover with aluminum foil to keep warm.
6. Meanwhile, place the green beans and bell peppers in a bowl and add just enough of the marinade to coat.
7. Prepare the grill pan and add the vegetables. Grill until fork tender and slightly charred.
8. Transfer the grilled vegetables to the serving platter and arrange artfully with the tempeh and pineapple. Serve at once.

Nutrition:
Calories: 163
Total Fat: 4.2g
Saturated Fat: 0.8g
Sodium: 861mg
Total Carbohydrates: 22.5g
Fiber: 6.3g
Sugar 2.3g
Protein: 9.2g

179. COURGETTES IN CIDER SAUCE

Preparation Time: 13 minutes
Cooking Time: 17 minutes
Servings: 3
Ingredients:
- 2 cups baby courgettes
- 3 tablespoons vegetable stock
- 2 tablespoons apple cider vinegar
- 1 tablespoon light brown sugar
- 4 spring onions, finely sliced
- 1 piece fresh ginger root, grated
- 1 teaspoon chickpea flour
- 2 teaspoons water

Directions:
1. Bring a pan with salted water to a boil. Add courgettes. Bring to a boil for 5 minutes.
2. Meanwhile, in a pan, combine vegetable stock, apple cider

vinegar, brown sugar, onions, ginger root, lemon juice and rind, and orange juice and rind. Take to a boil. Lower the heat and allow simmering for 3 minutes.
3. Mix the chickpea flour with water. Stir well. Pour into the sauce. Continue stirring until the sauce thickens.
4. Drain courgettes. Transfer to the serving dish. Spoon over the sauce. Toss to coat courgettes. Serve.

Nutrition:
Calories: 173
Total Fat: 9.2g
Saturated Fat: 0.8g
Sodium: 861mg
Total Carbohydrates: 22.5g
Fiber: 6.3g
Sugar: 2.3g
Protein: 9.2g

180. BAKED MIXED MUSHROOMS

Preparation Time: 8 minutes
Cooking Time: 20 minutes
Servings: 3
Ingredients:
- 2 cups mixed wild mushrooms
- 1 cup chestnut mushrooms
- 2 cups dried porcini
- 2 shallots
- 4 garlic cloves
- 3 cups raw pecans
- ½ bunch fresh thyme
- 1 bunch flat-leaf parsley
- 2 tablespoons olive oil
- 2 fresh bay leaves
- 1½ cups stale bread

Directions:
1. Remove skin and finely chop garlic and shallots. Roughly chop the wild mushrooms and chestnut mushrooms. Pick the leaves of the thyme and tear the bread into small pieces. Put inside the pressure cooker.
2. Place the pecans and roughly chop the nuts. Pick the parsley leaves and roughly chop.
3. Place the porcini in a bowl then add 300ml of boiling water. Set aside until needed.
4. Heat oil in the pressure cooker. Add the garlic and shallots. Cook for 3 minutes while stirring occasionally.
5. Drain porcini and reserve the liquid. Add the porcini into the pressure cooker together with the wild mushrooms and chestnut mushrooms. Add the bay leaves and thyme.
6. Position the lid and lock it in place. Put to high heat and bring to high pressure. Adjust heat to stabilize. Cook for 10 minutes. Adjust taste if necessary.
7. Transfer the mushroom mixture into a bowl and set aside to cool completely.
8. Once the mushrooms are completely cool, add the bread, pecans, a pinch of black pepper and sea salt, and half of the reserved liquid into the bowl. Mix well. Add more reserved liquid if the mixture seems dry.
9. Add more than half of the parsley into the bowl and stir. Transfer the mixture into a 20cm x 25cm lightly greased baking dish and cover with tin foil.
10. Bake in the oven for 35 minutes. Then, get rid of the foil and cook for another 10 minutes. Once done, sprinkle the remaining parsley on top and serve with bread or crackers. Serve.

Nutrition:
Calories: 343
Total Fat: 4.2g
Saturated Fat: 0.8g
Sodium: 861mg
Total Carbohydrates: 22.5g
Fiber: 6.3g
Sugar 2.3g
Protein: 9.2g

181. SPICED OKRA

Preparation Time: 14 minutes
Cooking Time: 16 minutes
Servings: 3
Ingredients:
- 2 cups okra
- ¼ teaspoon Stevia
- 1 teaspoon chili powder
- ½ teaspoon ground turmeric
- 1 tablespoon ground coriander
- 2 tablespoons fresh coriander, chopped
- 1 tablespoon ground cumin
- ¼ teaspoon salt
- 1 tablespoon desiccated coconut
- 3 tablespoons vegetable oil
- ½ teaspoon black mustard seeds
- ½ teaspoon cumin seeds
- Fresh tomatoes, to garnish

Directions:
1. Trim okra. Wash and dry.
2. Combine Stevia, chili powder, turmeric, ground coriander, fresh coriander, cumin, salt, and desiccated coconut in a bowl.
3. Heat the oil in a pan. Cook mustard and cumin seeds for 3 minutes. Stir continuously. Add okra. Tip in the spice mixture. Cook on low heat for 8 minutes.
4. Transfer to a serving dish. Garnish with fresh tomatoes.

Nutrition:
Calories: 163
Total Fat: 4.2g
Saturated Fat: 0.8g
Sodium: 861mg
Total Carbohydrates: 22.5g
Fiber: 6.3g
Sugar 2.3g
Protein: 9.2g

182. LEMONY SALMON BURGERS

Preparation Time: 10 minutes
Cooking Time: 10 minutes
Servings: 4
Ingredients:
- 2 3-oz cans boneless, skinless pink salmon
- ¼ cup panko breadcrumbs
- 4 teaspoon lemon juice
- ¼ cup red bell pepper
- ¼ cup sugar-free yogurt
- 1 egg
- 2 1.5-oz whole wheat hamburger buns, toasted

Directions:
1. Mix drained and flaked salmon, finely chopped bell pepper, panko breadcrumbs.
2. Combine 2 tablespoons sugar-free yogurt, 3 teaspoons fresh lemon juice, and egg in a bowl. Shape mixture into 2 3-inch patties, bake on the skillet over medium heat for 4 to 5 minutes per side.
3. Stir together 2 tablespoons sugar-free yogurt and 1 teaspoon lemon juice; spread over bottom halves of buns.
4. Top each with 1 patty, and cover with bun tops. This dish is very mouth-watering, enjoy!

Nutrition:
Calories: 144.48
Protein: 12.54g
Fat: 3.9g
Carbohydrates: 14.41g
Sodium: 300.42mg

183. CAPRESE TURKEY BURGERS

Preparation Time: 10 Minutes
Cooking Time: 10 Minutes
Servings: 4
Ingredients:
- ½ lb. 93% lean ground turkey
- 2 1.5-oz whole wheat hamburger buns, toasted
- ¼ cup shredded mozzarella cheese (part-skim)
- 1 egg
- 1 big tomato
- 1 small clove garlic
- 4 large basil leaves
- ⅛ teaspoon salt
- ⅛ teaspoon pepper

Directions:
1. Combine turkey, white egg, Minced garlic, salt, and pepper (mix until combined);
2. Shape into 2 cutlets. Put cutlets into a skillet; cook 5 to 7 minutes per side.
3. Top cutlets properly with cheese and sliced tomato at the end of cooking.
4. Put 1 cutlet on the bottom of each bun.
5. Top each patty with 2 basil leaves. Cover with bun tops.

My guests enjoy this dish every time they visit my home.
Nutrition:
Calories: 152
Protein: 19g
Fat: 4g
Carbohydrates: 10.39g
Sodium: 265mg

184. PASTA SALAD

Preparation Time: 15 minutes
Cooking Time: 15 minutes
Servings: 4
Ingredients:
- 8 oz. whole wheat pasta
- 2 tomatoes
- 1 5-oz pkg spring mix
- 9 slices bacon
- ⅓ cup mayonnaise (reduced fat)
- 1 tablespoon Dijon mustard
- 3 tablespoon apple cider vinegar
- ¼ teaspoon salt
- ½ teaspoon pepper

Directions:
1. Cook and drain pasta.
2. Put chilled pasta, chopped tomatoes, and spring mix in a bowl.
3. Crumble the cooked bacon over pasta.

4. Combine mayonnaise, mustard, vinegar, salt, and pepper in a small bowl.
5. Pour dressing over pasta, stirring to coat.
6. Serve and enjoy! Remember, understanding diabetes is the first step in curing it.

Nutrition:
Calories: 536.65
Protein: 16.7g
Fat: 32.97g
Carbohydrates: 46g
Sodium: 693.94mg

185. CHICKEN, STRAWBERRY, AND AVOCADO SALAD

Preparation Time: 10 minutes
Cooking Time: 5 minutes
Servings: 4
Ingredients:
- 1½ cups chicken (skin removed)
- ¼ cup almonds
- 2 5-oz pkg salad greens
- 1 16-oz pkg strawberries
- 1 avocado
- ¼ cup green onion
- ¼ cup lime juice
- 3 tablespoon extra-virgin olive oil
- 2 tablespoon honeys
- ¼ teaspoon salt
- ¼ teaspoon pepper

Directions:

1. Toast almonds until golden and fragrant.
2. Mix lime juice, oil, honey, salt, and pepper.
3. Mix greens, sliced strawberries, chicken, diced avocado, and sliced green onion, and sliced almonds, drizzle with dressing. Toss to coat. Yummy!

Nutrition:
Calories: 384
Protein: 13.4g
Fat: 27.5 g
Carbohydrates: 25.53g
Sodium: 203mg

186. BEEF PIZZA

Preparation Time: 14 minutes
Cooking Time: 30 minutes
Servings: 4
Ingredients:
- 2 large eggs
- 1 pkg. (20 oz.) ground beef
- 28 pepperoni slices

- ½ cup of each: Shredded cheddar cheese & Pizza sauce
- 4 oz. mozzarella cheese
- Also Needed: 1 cast iron skillet

Directions:
1. Combine the eggs, beef, and seasonings. Place in the skillet to form the crust. Bake until the meat is done or about 15 minutes.
2. Take it out and add the sauce, cheese, and toppings. Place the pizza in the oven for a few minutes until the cheese has melted. Remove and enjoy!

Nutrition:
Calories: 722
Fat: 58g
Protein: 44g
Carbs: 2.84g
Sodium: 1014mg

187. BELL PEPPER BASIL PIZZA

Preparation Time: 13 minutes
Cooking Time: 30 minutes
Servings: 8
Ingredients:
For the Pizza Base:
- 6 oz. mozzarella cheese
- 2 tablespoons of each: Fresh Parmesan cheese, Cream cheese & Psyllium husk
- 1 teaspoon Italian seasoning
- 1 large egg
- ½ teaspoon of each: Black pepper & Salt

For the Toppings:
- 4 oz. shredded cheddar cheese
- ¼ cup marinara sauce
- 1 med. vine-ripened tomato
- 2-3 med. bell peppers
- 2-3 tablespoons fresh basil, chopped

Directions:
1. Set the temperature in the oven to 400°F.
2. Melt the cheese in the microwave for 40-50 seconds. Add the remainder of the pizza base fixings to the cheese, mixing well with your hands.
3. Flatten the dough to form the 2 circular pizzas. Bake ten minutes. Remove and add the toppings. Bake for about 8-10 additional minutes.
4. Let it cool and serve.

Nutrition:
Calories: 163
Fat: 11.87g
Protein: 9.87g
Carbs: 4.7g
Sodium: 446.92mg

188. EASY PIZZA FOR 2

Preparation Time: 5 minutes
Cooking Time: 10 minutes
Servings: 2
Ingredients:

- ½ cup chunky no-salt-added tomato sauce
- 1 ready-made whole wheat flatbread (about 10 inches in diameter)
- 2 slices of onion, (¼-inch wide)
- 4 sliced red bell pepper (¼-inch wide)
- ½ cup shredded low-fat mozzarella
- 2 tablespoons chopped fresh basil

Directions:

1. Heat the oven to 350°F.
2. Coat the baking pan lightly with the cooking oil.
3. Spread the tomato sauce on the flatbread. Cover with tomato, chili pepper, mozzarella, and basil.
4. Place the pizza in a baking pan and cook until the cheese melts and becomes lightly browned approximately five minutes.

Nutrition:
Calories: 277
Protein: 15.19g
Fat: 11g
Carbs: 35.49g
Sodium: 365.49mg

189. PITA PIZZA

Preparation Time: 12 minutes
Cooking Time: 30 minutes
Servings: 2
Ingredients:

- ½ cup marinara sauce
- 1 low-carb pita
- 2 oz. cheddar cheese
- 14 slices pepperoni
- 1 oz. roasted red peppers

Directions:

1. Set the oven to 450°F.
2. Slice the pita in half and put it on a foil-lined baking tray. Rub with a bit of oil and toast for one to 2 minutes.
3. Pour the sauce over the bread, sprinkle with the cheese, and other toppings. Bake for another five minutes or until the cheese melts.

Nutrition:
Calories: 408
Fat: 27g
Protein: 16.78g

Carbs: 23.29g
Sodium: 1211mg

190. CHIPOTLE FISH TACOS

Preparation Time: 10 minutes
Cooking Time: 31 minutes
Servings: 4
Ingredients:

- ½ small diced yellow onion
- 2 pressed cloves of garlic
- 1 chopped fresh jalapeño
- 2 tablespoon olive oil
- 4 oz. chipotle peppers in adobo sauce
- 2 tablespoon mayonnaise
- 2 tablespoon unsalted butter
- 4 low-carb tortillas
- 1 lb. haddock fillets

Directions:

1. In a skillet, fry the onion on med-high for five minutes.
2. Lower the temperature to the medium heat setting. Toss in the garlic, and jalapeño. Stir another 2 minutes.
3. Chop and add the chipotles, along with the adobo sauce into the pan.
4. Drop the butter, mayonnaise, and fish into the pan and cook for about eight minutes.
5. Make the Tacos: Fry the tortilla for approximately 2 minutes for each side. Chill and shape them with the prepared fixings.

Nutrition:
Calories: 344.61
Fat: 21.6g
Protein: 27.38g
Carbs: 18.5g
Sodium: 603mg

191. CUMIN SPICED BEEF WRAPS

Preparation Time: 10 minutes
Cooking Time: 35 minutes
Servings: 2
Ingredients:

- 1-2 tablespoons coconut oil
- ¼ onion, diced
- ⅔ lb. ground beef
- 2 tablespoons chopped cilantro
- 1 diced red bell pepper
- 1 teaspoon minced ginger
- 2 tsp. cumin
- 4 minced garlic cloves
- Pepper and salt, to taste
- 8 large cabbage leaves

Directions:

1. Warm up a frying pan and pour in the oil. Sauté the peppers, onions, and ground beef using

medium heat. When done, add the pepper, salt, cumin, ginger, cilantro, and garlic.
2. Fill a large pot with water (¾ full) and wait for it to boil. Cook each leaf for 20 seconds, plunge it in cold water and drain it before placing it on your serving dish.
3. Scoop the mixture onto each leaf, fold, and enjoy.

Nutrition:
Calories: 503
Fat: 37.77g
Protein: 28.6g
Carbs: 12.87g
Sodium: 511.61mg

192. BALSAMIC BEEF POT ROAST

Preparation Time: 10 minutes
Cooking Time: 33 minutes
Servings: 10
Ingredients:

- 1 boneless (approx. 3 lb.) chuck roast
- 1 teaspoon of each: Garlic powder, Black ground pepper
- 1 tablespoon kosher salt
- ¼ cup balsamic vinegar
- ½ cup chopped onion
- 2 cups water
- ¼ teaspoon xanthan gum

Directions:

1. Combine the salt, garlic powder, and pepper and rub the chuck roast with the combined fixings.
2. Use a heavy skillet to sear the roast. Add the vinegar and deglaze the pan as you continue cooking for one more minute.
3. Toss the onion into a pot with the 2 cups boiling water along with the roast. Cover with a top and simmer for 3 to 4 hours on a low setting.
4. Take the meat from the pot and add it to a cutting surface. Shred into chunks and remove any fat or bones.
5. Add the xanthan gum to the broth and whisk. Place the roast meat back in the pan to warm up.
6. Serve with a favorite side dish.

Nutrition:
Calories: 349
Fat: 25g
Protein: 26.23 g
Carbs: 2.18g
Sodium: 648.59mg

193. CHEESEBURGER CALZONE

Preparation Time: 12 minutes
Cooking Time: 33 minutes
Servings: 8
Ingredients:
- ½ yellow diced onion
- 1½ lb. ground beef – lean
- 4 thick-cut bacon strips
- 4 dill pickle spears
- 8 oz. cream cheese, divided
- 1 egg
- ½ cup mayonnaise

1 cup of each:
- Shredded cheddar cheese
- Almond flour
- Shredded mozzarella cheese

Directions:
1. Program the oven to 425°F. Prepare a cookie sheet with parchment paper.
2. Chop the pickles into spears. Set aside for now.
3. Prepare the Crust: Combine ½ of the cream cheese and the mozzarella cheese. Microwave 35 seconds. When it melts, add the egg and almond flour to make the dough. Set aside.
4. Cook the beef on the stove using medium heat.
5. Cook the bacon (microwave for five minutes or stovetop). When cool, break into bits.
6. Dice the onion and add to the beef and cook until softened. Toss in the bacon, cheddar cheese, pickle bits, the rest of the cream cheese, and mayonnaise. Stir well.
7. Roll the dough onto the prepared baking tin. Scoop the mixture into the center. Fold the ends and side to make the calzone.
8. Bake until browned or about 15 minutes. Let it rest for 10 minutes before slicing.

Nutrition:
Calories: 580
Fat: 47g
Protein: 31g
Carbs: 5.9g
Sodium: 702.23mg

194. NACHO STEAK IN THE SKILLET

Preparation Time: 11 minutes
Cooking Time: 36 minutes
Servings: 5
Ingredients:
- 1 tablespoon unsalted butter
- 8 oz. beef round tip steak
- ⅓ cup melted refined coconut oil
- ½ teaspoon turmeric
- 1 teaspoon chili powder
- 1½ pounds cauliflower

1 oz. each shredded:
- Cheddar cheese
- Monterey jack cheese

Garnish:
- 1 oz. canned jalapeño slices
- ⅓ cup sour cream
- Avocado – approx. 5 oz.

Directions:
1. Set the oven temperature to 400°F.
2. Prepare the cauliflower into chip-like shapes.
3. Combine the turmeric, chili powder, and coconut oil in a mixing dish.
4. Toss in the cauliflower and add it to a tin. Set the baking timer for 20 to 25 minutes.
5. Over med-high heat in a cast-iron skillet, add the butter. Cook until both sides are done, flipping just once. Let it rest for five to ten minutes. Thinly slice, and sprinkle with some pepper and salt to the steak.
6. When done, transfer the florets to the skillet and add the steak strips. Top it off with the cheese and bake for five to ten more minutes.
7. Serve with your favorite garnish.

Nutrition:
Calories: 350.5
Fat: 30.49g
Protein: 14.44g
Carbs: 6.49g
Sodium: 150mg

195. PORTOBELLO BUN CHEESEBURGERS

Preparation Time: 9 minutes
Cooking Time: 32 minutes
Servings: 6
Ingredients:
- 1 lb. lean ground beef
- 1 teaspoon of each:
- 1 tablespoon Worcestershire sauce
- Pink Himalayan salt
- Ground black pepper
- 1 tablespoon avocado oil
- 6 slices sharp cheddar cheese
- 6 Portobello mushroom caps

Directions:
1. Remove the stems, rinse, and dab dry the mushrooms.
2. Combine the salt, pepper, beef, and Worcestershire sauce in a mixing container. Form into patties.
3. Warm up the oil (medium heat). Let the caps simmer for about 3 to 4 minutes per side.
4. Transfer the mushrooms to a bowl. Using the same pan, cook the patties for 4 minutes, flip, and cook another five minutes until done.
5. Add the cheese to the burgers and cover for one minute to melt the cheese.
6. Add one of the mushroom caps to the burgers along with the desired garnishes and serve.

Nutrition:
Calories: 281
Fat: 19.47g
Protein: 23.47g
Carbs: 2.88g
Sodium: 387.17mg

196. STEAK-LOVER'S SLOW-COOKED CHILI IN THE SLOW COOKER

Preparation Time: 10 minutes
Cooking Time: 31 minutes
Servings: 12
Ingredients:
For the Chili:
- 1 cup beef or chicken stock
- ½ cup sliced leeks
- 2½ lbs. (1-inch cubes) of steak
- 2 cups whole tomatoes (canned with juices)
- ⅛ t. black pepper
- ½ teaspoon salt
- ½ teaspoon cumin
- ¼ teaspoon ground cayenne pepper
- 1 tablespoon chili powder

Optional Toppings:
- 1 teaspoon fresh chopped cilantro
- 2 tablespoon sour cream
- ¼ cup shredded cheddar cheese
- ½ avocado – sliced or cubed

Directions:
1. Toss all of the fixings into the cooker - except the toppings.
2. Use the cooker's high setting for about six hours.
3. Serve, add the toppings, and enjoy.

Nutrition:
Calories: 156.4
Fat: 6.27g
Carbs: 2.9g
Protein: 22.7g
Sodium: 226.56mg

197. VEGETARIAN KETO BURGER ON A BUN

Preparation Time: 10 minutes
Cooking Time: 35 minutes
Servings: 2
Ingredients:

- Mushrooms
- 1-2 tablespoon freshly chopped basil – 1 teaspoon dried
- 2 medium-large flat mushrooms – ex. Portobello
- 1 tablespoon of each:
- Coconut oil/ghee
- ½ teaspoon dried Freshly chopped oregano
- 1 crushed garlic clove
- ¼ teaspoon salt
- Black pepper

For the Garnish:

- 2 large organic eggs
- 2 slices cheddar/gouda cheese
- 2 tablespoon mayonnaise
- 2 keto buns

Directions:

1. Prepare the mushrooms for marinating by seasoning with crushed garlic, pepper, salt, ghee (melted), and fresh herbs. Save a small amount for frying the eggs. Marinate for about one hour at room temperature.
2. Arrange the mushrooms in the pan with the top side facing upwards. Cook for about five minutes on the med-high setting. Flip and continue cooking for another five minutes.
3. Remove the pan from the burner and flip the mushrooms over and add the cheese. When it is time to serve, put them under the broiler for a minute or so to melt the cheese.
4. With the remainder of the ghee, fry the eggs leaving the yolk runny. Remove from the heat.
5. Slice the buns and add them to the grill, cooking until crisp for about 2 to 3 minutes.
6. To assemble, add one tablespoon of mayonnaise to each bun and top them off with mushroom, egg, tomato, and lettuce.
7. Put the tops on the buns and serve.

Nutrition:
Calories: 497.11
Fat: 33.47g
Protein: 19.62g
Sodium: 870mg
Carbs: 32.44g

198. CALIFORNIA WRAPS

Preparation Time: 5 minutes
Cooking Time: 15 minutes
Servings: 4
Ingredients:

- 4 slices turkey breast, cooked
- 4 slices ham, cooked
- 4 lettuce leaves
- 4 slices tomato
- 4 slices avocado
- 1 teaspoon lime juice
- A handful of watercress leaves
- 4 tablespoon ranch dressing, sugar-free

Directions:

1. Top a lettuce leaf with a turkey slice, ham slice, and tomato.
2. In a bowl combine avocado and lime juice and place on top of tomatoes. Top with watercress and dressing.
3. Repeat with the remaining ingredients for 4. Topping each lettuce leaf with a turkey slice, ham slice, tomato, and dressing.

Nutrition:
Calories: 250
Carbohydrates: 13.67g
Protein: 19g
Sodium: 629mg

DINNER

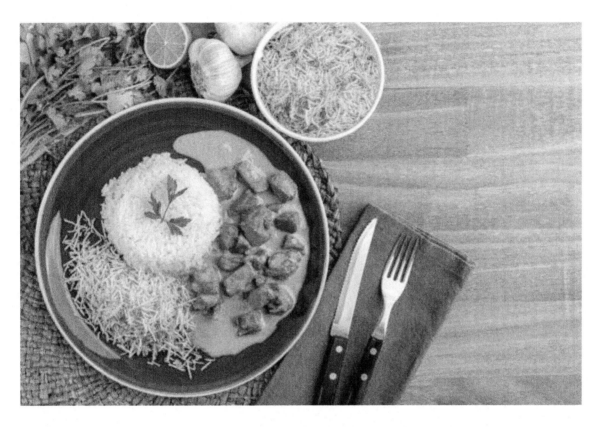

199. PORK CHOP DIANE

Preparation Time: 10 minutes
Cooking Time: 20 minutes
Servings: 4
Ingredients:

- ¼ cup low-sodium chicken broth
- 1 tablespoon freshly squeezed lemon juice
- 2 teaspoons Worcestershire sauce
- 2 teaspoons Dijon mustard
- 4 5-ounce boneless pork loin chops
- 1 teaspoon extra-virgin olive oil
- 1 teaspoon lemon zest
- 1 teaspoon unsalted butter
- 2 teaspoons chopped fresh chives

Directions:

1. Blend together the chicken broth, lemon juice, Worcestershire sauce, and Dijon mustard and set it aside.
2. Season the pork chops lightly.
3. Heat a large skillet over medium-high heat and add the olive oil.
4. Cook the pork chops, turning once, until they are no longer pink, about 8 minutes per side.
5. Put aside the chops.
6. Pour the broth mixture into the skillet and cook until warmed through and thickened, about 2 minutes.
7. Blend lemon zest, butter, and chives.
8. Garnish with a generous spoonful of sauce.

Nutrition:
Calories: 248.7
Fat: 12.37g
Carbohydrates: 1.26g
Sodium: 107mg

200. AUTUMN PORK CHOPS WITH RED CABBAGE AND APPLES

Preparation Time: 15 minutes
Cooking Time: 30 minutes
Servings: 4
Ingredients:

- ¼ cup apple cider vinegar
- 2 tablespoons granulated sweetener
- 4 4-ounce pork chops, about 1 inch thick
- 1 tablespoon extra-virgin olive oil
- ½ red cabbage, finely shredded
- 1 sweet onion, thinly sliced
- 1 apple, peeled, cored, and sliced
- 1 teaspoon chopped fresh thyme

Directions:

1. Mix together the vinegar and sweetener. Set it aside.

2. Season the pork with salt and pepper.
3. Heat a large skillet over medium-high heat and add the olive oil.
4. Cook the pork chops until no longer pink, turning once, about 8 minutes per side.
5. Put chops aside.
6. Add the cabbage and onion to the skillet and sauté until the vegetables have softened for about 5 minutes.
7. Add the vinegar mixture and the apple slices to the skillet and bring the mixture to a boil.
8. Adjust heat to low and simmer, covered, for 5 additional minutes.
9. Return the pork chops to the skillet, along with any accumulated juices and thyme, cover, and cook for 5 more minutes.

Nutrition:
Calories: 123.61
Carbohydrates: 13.25g
Fiber: 2.5g
Sodium: 36.8mg

201. CHIPOTLE CHILI PORK CHOPS

Preparation Time: 4 hours
Cooking Time: 20 minutes
Servings: 4
Ingredients:
- Juice and zest of 1 lime
- 1 tablespoon extra-virgin olive oil
- 1 tablespoon chipotle chili powder
- 2 teaspoons minced garlic
- 1 teaspoon ground cinnamon
- Pinch sea salt
- 4 5-ounce pork chops

Directions:
1. Combine the lime juice and zest, oil, chipotle chili powder, garlic, cinnamon, and salt in a resealable plastic bag. Add the pork chops. Remove as much air as possible and seal the bag.
2. Marinate the chops in the refrigerator for at least 4 hours, and up to 24 hours, turning them several times.
3. Heat the oven to 400°F and set a rack on a baking sheet. Let the chops rest at room temperature for 15 minutes, then arrange them on the rack and discard the remaining marinade.

4. Roast the chops until cooked through, turning once, about 10 minutes per side.
5. Serve with lime wedges.

Nutrition:
Calories: 204
Carbohydrates: 3.2g
Sodium: 88.76mg
Sugar: 1g

202. ORANGE-MARINATED PORK TENDERLOIN

Preparation Time: 2 hours
Cooking Time: 30 minutes
Servings: 4
Ingredients:
- ¼ cup freshly squeezed orange juice
- 2 teaspoons orange zest
- 2 teaspoons minced garlic
- 1 teaspoon low-sodium soy sauce
- 1 teaspoon grated fresh ginger
- 1 teaspoon honey
- 1½ pounds pork tenderloin roast
- 1 tablespoon extra-virgin olive oil

Directions:
1. Blend together the orange juice, zest, garlic, soy sauce, ginger, and honey.
2. Pour the marinade into a resealable plastic bag and add the pork tenderloin.
3. Remove as much air as possible and seal the bag. Marinate the pork in the refrigerator, turning the bag a few times, for 2 hours.
4. Preheat the oven to 400°F.
5. Pull out the tenderloin from the marinade and discard the marinade.
6. Position big ovenproof skillet over medium-high heat and add the oil.
7. Sear the pork tenderloin on all sides, about 5 minutes in total.
8. Position the skillet in the oven and roast for 25 minutes.
9. Put aside for 10 minutes before serving.

Nutrition:
Calories: 252.49
Carbohydrates: 4g
Sugar: 3g
Sodium: 125mg

203. HOMESTYLE HERB MEATBALLS

Preparation Time: 10 minutes

Cooking Time: 15 minutes
Servings: 4
Ingredients:
- ½ pound lean ground pork
- ½ pound lean ground beef
- 1 sweet onion, finely chopped
- ¼ cup breadcrumbs
- 2 tablespoons chopped fresh basil
- 2 teaspoons minced garlic
- 1 egg

Directions:
1. Preheat the oven to 350°F.
2. Line a baking tray with parchment paper and set it aside.
3. In a large bowl, mix together the pork, beef, onion, breadcrumbs, basil, garlic, egg, salt, and pepper until very well mixed.
4. Roll the meat mixture into 2-inch meatballs.
5. Transfer the meatballs to the baking sheet and bake until they are browned and cooked through, about 15 minutes.
6. Serve the meatballs with your favorite marinara sauce and some steamed green beans.

Nutrition:
Calories: 275.53
Carbohydrates: 7.5g
Sugar: 1.7g
Sodium: 143.23mg

204. LIME-PARSLEY LAMB CUTLETS

Preparation Time: 4 hours
Cooking Time: 10 minutes
Servings: 4
Ingredients:
- ¼ cup extra-virgin olive oil
- ¼ cup freshly squeezed lime juice
- 2 tablespoons lime zest
- 2 tablespoons chopped fresh parsley
- 12 lamb cutlets (about 1½ pounds total)

Directions:
1. Combine the oil, lime juice, zest, parsley, salt, and pepper.
2. Pour marinade into a sealable plastic bag.
3. Add cutlets to the bag, then remove as much air as possible before sealing.
4. Marinate the lamb in the refrigerator for about 4 hours.
5. Preheat oven to broil.
6. Remove from the bag and put them on an aluminum foil-lined baking sheet.

7. Broil the chops for about 4 minutes per side for.
8. Allow the chops to cool for 5 minutes before serving.

Nutrition:
Calories: 363.53
Carbohydrates: 1.99g
Protein: 30g
Sodium: 98.7mg

205. BEEF FAJITAS

Preparation Time: 6 minutes
Cooking Time: 19 minutes
Servings: 4
Ingredients:
- 1 lb beef stir-fry strips
- 1 medium red onion
- 1 red bell pepper
- 1 yellow bell pepper
- ½ teaspoon of cumin
- ½ teaspoon of chili powder
- Splash of oil
- Salt
- Pepper
- Juice of ½ a lime
- Freshly chopped cilantro (also called coriander)
- 1 avocado

Directions:
1. Over medium heat, warm a cast-iron pan.
2. Clean bell peppers and cut them to long strips of 0.5cm thick and then set aside.
3. Clean and cut the red onion into strips. Set aside.
4. Add a little bit of oil once the skillet is heated. Add 2-3 packets of stir fry strips while the oil is hot. Please ensure the strips wouldn't hit one another.
5. Inside the pan, stir fry each beef batch thoroughly with salt and pepper. Cook on each side for around 1 minute and set aside on a plate and covered to stay warm.
6. Introduce chopped onion as well as peppers to the residual meat juice. When all the beef is finished cooking, set aside. Season with chili powder and cumin, then simmer-fry until the preferred consistency is achieved.
7. Move the stir fry strips of vegetables and beef to a plate and eat alongside a chopped avocado, a sprinkling of lemon juice, and a sprig of fresh cilantro.

Nutrition:
Calories: 243

Fat: 12.97g
Carbohydrate: 7.3g
Sodium: 209mg

206. MEDITERRANEAN STEAK SANDWICHES

Preparation Time: 1 hour
Cooking Time: 10 minutes
Servings: 4
Ingredients:
- 2 tablespoons extra-virgin olive oil
- 2 tablespoons balsamic vinegar
- 2 teaspoons garlic
- 2 teaspoons lemon juice
- 2 teaspoons fresh oregano
- 1 teaspoon fresh parsley
- 1-pound flank steak
- 4 whole wheat pitas
- 2 cups shredded lettuce
- 1 red onion, thinly sliced
- 1 tomato, chopped
- 1 ounce low-sodium feta cheese

Directions:
1. Blend olive oil, balsamic vinegar, garlic, lemon juice, oregano, and parsley.
2. Add the steak to the bowl, turning to coat it completely.
3. Marinate the steak for 1 hour in the refrigerator, turning it over several times.
4. Preheat the broiler. Line a baking sheet with aluminum foil.
5. Remove steak from bowl and discard the marinade.
6. Situate steak on a baking sheet and broil for 5 minutes per side for medium.
7. Set aside for 10 minutes before slicing.
8. Stuff the pitas with the sliced steak, lettuce, onion, tomato, and feta.

Nutrition:
Calories: 360
Carbohydrates: 25g
Fiber: 3.32g
Sodium: 321.7mg

207. ROASTED BEEF WITH PEPPERCORN SAUCE

Preparation Time: 10 minutes
Cooking Time: 90 minutes
Servings: 4
Ingredients:
- 1½ pounds top rump beef roast

- 3 teaspoons extra-virgin olive oil
- 3 shallots, minced
- 2 teaspoons minced garlic
- 1 tablespoon green peppercorns
- 2 tablespoons dry sherry
- 2 tablespoons almond flour
- 1 cup sodium-free beef broth

Directions:
1. Heat the oven to 300°F.
2. Season the roast with pepper and salt.
3. Heat a huge skillet over medium-high heat and add 2 teaspoons of olive oil.
4. Brown the beef on all sides, about 10 minutes in total, and transfer the roast to a baking dish.
5. Roast until desired doneness, about 1½ hours for medium. When the roast has been in the oven for 1 hour, start the sauce.
6. In a medium saucepan over medium-high heat, sauté the shallots in the remaining 1 teaspoon of olive oil until translucent, about 4 minutes.
7. Stir in the garlic and peppercorns and cook for another minute. Whisk in the sherry to deglaze the pan.
8. Whisk in the flour to form a thick paste, cooking for 1 minute and stirring constantly.
9. Fill in the beef broth and whisk for 4 minutes. Season the sauce.
10. Serve the beef with a generous spoonful of sauce.

Nutrition:
Calories: 330
Carbohydrates: 4g
Protein: 36g
Sodium: 310.36mg

208. COFFEE-AND-HERB-MARINATED STEAK

Preparation Time: 2 hours
Cooking Time: 10 minutes
Servings: 3
Ingredients:
- ¼ cup whole coffee beans
- 2 teaspoons garlic
- 2 teaspoons rosemary
- 2 teaspoons thyme
- 1 teaspoon black pepper
- 2 tablespoons apple cider vinegar
- 2 tablespoons extra-virgin olive oil

- 1 pound flank steak, trimmed of visible fat

Directions:
1. Place the coffee beans, garlic, rosemary, thyme, and black pepper in a coffee grinder or food processor and pulse until coarsely ground.
2. Transfer the coffee mixture to a resealable plastic bag and add the vinegar and oil. Shake to combine.
3. Add the flank steak and squeeze the excess air out of the bag. Seal it. Marinate the steak in the refrigerator for at least 2 hours, occasionally turning the bag over.
4. Preheat the broiler. Line a baking sheet with aluminum foil.
5. Pull the steak out and discard the marinade.
6. Place steak on the baking sheet and broil until it is done to your liking.
7. Put aside for 10 minutes before cutting it.
8. Serve with your favorite side dish.

Nutrition:
Calories: 313
Fat: 20g
Carbs: 12g
Sodium: 143mg
Protein: 31g

209. TRADITIONAL BEEF STROGANOFF

Preparation Time: 10 minutes
Cooking Time: 30 minutes
Servings: 4
Ingredients:
- 1 teaspoon extra-virgin olive oil
- 1 pound top sirloin, cut into thin strips
- 1 cup sliced button mushrooms
- ½ sweet onion, finely chopped
- 1 teaspoon minced garlic
- 1 tablespoon whole wheat flour
- ½ cup low-sodium beef broth
- ¼ cup dry sherry
- ½ cup fat-free sour cream
- 1 tablespoon chopped fresh parsley

Directions:
1. Heat a skillet over medium-high heat and add the oil.
2. Sauté the beef until browned, about 10 minutes, then remove the beef with a slotted spoon to a plate and set it aside.
3. Add the mushrooms, onion, and garlic to the skillet and sauté until lightly browned for about 5 minutes.
4. Whisk in the flour and then whisk in the beef broth and sherry.
5. Return the sirloin to the skillet and bring the mixture to a boil.
6. Reduce the heat to low and simmer until the beef is tender, about 10 minutes.
7. Stir in the sour cream and parsley. Season with salt and pepper.

Nutrition:
Calories: 257
Carbohydrates: 6g
Fiber: 1g
Sodium: 267mg

210. CHICKEN AND ROASTED VEGETABLE WRAPS

Preparation Time: 10 minutes
Cooking Time: 20 minutes
Servings: 4
Ingredients:
- ½ small eggplant
- 1 red bell pepper
- 1 medium zucchini
- ½ small red onion, sliced
- 1 tablespoon extra-virgin olive oil
- 2 8-ounce cooked chicken breasts, sliced
- 4 whole wheat tortilla wraps

Directions:
1. Preheat the oven to 400°F.
2. Wrap a baking sheet with foil and set it aside.
3. In a large bowl, toss the eggplant, bell pepper, zucchini, and red onion with olive oil.
4. Transfer the vegetables to the baking sheet and lightly season with salt and pepper.
5. Roast the vegetables until soft and slightly charred, about 20 minutes.
6. Divide the vegetables and chicken into 4 portions.
7. Wrap 1 tortilla around each portion of chicken and grilled vegetables and serve.

Nutrition:
Calories: 199
Carbohydrates: 23.8g
Fiber: 6.1g
Sodium: 217mg

211. SPICY CHICKEN CACCIATORE

Preparation Time: 20 minutes
Cooking Time: 1 hour
Servings: 6
Ingredients:
- 1 2-pound chicken
- ¼ cup almond flour
- 2 tablespoons extra-virgin olive oil
- 3 slices bacon
- 1 sweet onion
- 2 teaspoons minced garlic
- 4 ounces button mushrooms, halved
- 1 28-ounce can of low-sodium stewed tomatoes
- ½ cup red wine
- 2 teaspoons chopped fresh oregano

Directions:
1. Cut the chicken into pieces: 2 drumsticks, 2 thighs, 2 wings, and 4 breast pieces.
2. Dredge the chicken pieces in the flour and season each piece with salt and pepper.
3. Place a large skillet over medium-high heat and add the olive oil.
4. Brown the chicken pieces on all sides, about 20 minutes in total. Transfer the chicken to a plate.
5. Cook chopped bacon to the skillet for 5 minutes. With a slotted spoon, transfer the cooked bacon to the same plate as the chicken.
6. Pour off most of the oil from the skillet, leaving just a light coating. Sauté the onion, garlic, and mushrooms in the skillet until tender, about 4 minutes.
7. Stir in the tomatoes, wine, oregano, and red pepper flakes.
8. Bring the sauce to a boil. Return the chicken and bacon, plus any accumulated juices from the plate to the skillet.
9. Reduce the heat to low and simmer until the chicken is tender, about 30 minutes.

Nutrition:
Calories: 382.77
Carbohydrates: 8.78g
Fiber: 2.34g
Sodium: 265mg

212. GINGER CITRUS CHICKEN THIGHS

Preparation Time: 15 minutes
Cooking Time: 30 minutes
Servings: 4

Ingredients:
- 4 chicken thighs, bone-in, skinless
- 1 tablespoon grated fresh ginger
- 1 tablespoon extra-virgin olive oil
- Juice and zest of ½ lemon
- Juice and zest of ½ orange
- 2 tablespoons honey
- 1 tablespoon reduced-sodium soy sauce
- 1 tablespoon chopped fresh cilantro

Directions:
1. Rub the chicken thighs with ginger and season lightly with salt.
2. Place a large skillet over medium-high heat and add the oil.
3. Brown the chicken thighs, turning once, for about 10 minutes.
4. While the chicken is browning, stir together the lemon juice and zest, orange juice and zest, honey, soy sauce, and red pepper flakes in a small bowl.
5. Add the citrus mixture to the skillet, cover, and reduce the heat to low.
6. Braise chicken for 20 minutes, adding a couple of tablespoons of water if the pan is too dry.
7. Serve garnished with cilantro.

Nutrition:
Calories: 206
Carbohydrates: 11.25g
Protein: 21.78g
Sodium: 218.4mg

213. CHICKEN WITH CREAMY THYME SAUCE

Preparation Time: 15 minutes
Cooking Time: 30 minutes
Servings: 4
Ingredients:
- 4 4-ounce chicken breasts
- 1 tablespoon extra-virgin olive oil
- ½ sweet onion, chopped
- 1 cup low-sodium chicken broth
- 2 teaspoons chopped fresh thyme
- ¼ cup heavy whipping cream
- 1 tablespoon unsalted butter
- 1 scallion

Directions:
1. Preheat the oven to 375°F.

2. Season the chicken breasts slightly.
3. Heat a large ovenproof skillet over medium-high heat and add the olive oil.
4. Brown the chicken, turning once, about 10 minutes in total. Transfer the chicken to a plate.
5. In the same skillet, sauté the onion until softened and translucent, about 3 minutes.
6. Add the chicken broth and thyme, and simmer until the liquid has reduced by half, about 6 minutes.
7. Stir in the cream and butter and return the chicken and any accumulated juices from the plate to the skillet.
8. Transfer the skillet to the oven. Bake until cooked through, about 10 minutes.
9. Serve topped with the chopped scallion.

Nutrition:
Calories: 264.42
Carbohydrates: 2.4g
Fiber: 0.26g
Sodium: 76.35mg

214. ONE-POT ROASTED CHICKEN DINNER

Preparation Time: 10 minutes
Cooking Time: 40 minutes
Servings: 6
Ingredients:
- ½ head cabbage
- 1 sweet onion
- 1 sweet potato
- 4 garlic cloves
- 2 tablespoons extra-virgin olive oil
- 2 teaspoons minced fresh thyme
- 2½ pounds bone-in chicken thighs and drumsticks

Directions:
1. Preheat the oven to 450°F.
2. Lightly grease a large roasting pan and arrange the cabbage, onion, sweet potato, and garlic in the bottom. Drizzle with 1 tablespoon of oil, sprinkle with the thyme and season the vegetables lightly with salt and pepper.
3. Season the chicken with salt and pepper.
4. Place a large skillet over medium-high heat and brown the chicken on both sides in the remaining 1 tablespoon of oil, about 10 minutes in total.

5. Situate browned chicken on top of the vegetables in the roasting pan. Roast for 30 minutes.

Nutrition:
Calories: 308
Carbohydrates: 11.5g
Fiber: 2.6g
Sodium: 163.2mg

215. MUSHROOMS WITH BELL PEPPERS

Preparation Time: 15 minutes
Cooking Time: 10 minutes
Servings: 4
Ingredients:
- 1 tablespoon grapeseed oil
- 3 cups fresh button mushrooms, sliced
- ¾ cups red bell peppers
- ¾ cups green bell peppers strips
- 1½ cup white onions strips
- 2 teaspoons fresh sweet basil
- 2 teaspoons fresh oregano
- ½ teaspoon cayenne powder
- Sea salt, as desired
- 2 teaspoons onion powder

Directions:
1. Cook the oil over medium-high heat and sauté the mushrooms, bell peppers, and onion for about 5-6 minutes.
2. Add the herbs and spices and cook for about 2-3 minutes. Stir in the lime juice and serve hot.

Nutrition:
Calories: 80
Total Fat: 3.9g
Carbs: 15.8g
Sodium: 176.5mg
Protein: 2.8g

216. BELL PEPPERS & TOMATO CASSEROLE

Preparation Time: 15 minutes
Cooking Time: 35 minutes
Servings: 6
Ingredients:
For Herb Sauce:
- 4 garlic cloves, chopped
- ½ cup fresh parsley, chopped
- ½ cup fresh cilantro, chopped
- 3 tablespoons avocado oil
- 2 tablespoons fresh key lime juice
- ½ teaspoon ground cumin
- ½ teaspoon cayenne powder
- Sea salt, as desired

For Veggies:
- 1 large green bell pepper

- 1 large yellow bell pepper
- 1 large orange bell pepper
- 1 large red bell pepper
- 1 pound plum tomato wedges
- 2 tablespoons avocado oil

Directions:
1. Lightly, grease a baking dish and preheat the oven to 350ºF. For the sauce: transfer all ingredients in the food processor and pulse till smooth. In a large bowl, add the bell peppers and herb sauce and gently toss to coat.
2. Transfer the bell pepper mixture into the prepared baking dish. Drizzle with oil. Wrap the baking dish with foil and bake for about 35 minutes. Take off the cover of the baking dish and bake for another 20-30 minutes. Serve hot.

Nutrition:
Calories: 143
Total Fat: 11.8g
Protein: 1.8g
Carbs: 9.57g
Sodium: 123mg

217. VEGGIES CASSEROLE

Preparation Time: 20 minutes
Cooking Time: 45 minutes
Servings: 5
Ingredients:
- 3 plum tomatoes
- 3 tablespoons spring water
- 3 tablespoons avocado oil, divided
- ½ onion, chopped
- 3 tablespoons garlic, minced
- Sea salt, as desired
- Cayenne powder as desired
- 1 zucchini
- 1 yellow squash
- 1 green bell pepper
- 1 red bell pepper
- 1 yellow bell pepper
- 1 tablespoon fresh thyme leaves
- 1 tablespoon fresh key lime juice

Directions:
1. Preheat oven to 375 ºF. Blend the tomatoes and water until pureed.
2. In a bowl, add the tomato puree, 1 tablespoon of oil, onion, garlic, salt, and black pepper, and blend nicely. In the bottom of a 10x10-inch baking dish, spread the tomato paste mixture evenly.

3. Arrange alternating vegetable slices, starting at the outer edge of the baking dish and working concentrically towards the center. Pour some remaining oil in the vegetables and sprinkle with salt and cayenne powder, followed by the thyme. Arrange a piece of parchment paper over the vegetables. Bake for about 45 minutes. Serve hot.

Nutrition:
Calories: 120.37
Total Fat: 8.7g
Protein: 2.3g
Carbs: 10.19g
Sodium: 146.53mg

218. SWEET & SPICY CHICKPEAS

Preparation Time: 15 minutes
Cooking Time: 1 hour 10 minutes
Servings: 4
Ingredients:
- 6 plum tomatoes
- 3 tablespoons agave nectar
- ¼ cup date sugar
- 2 teaspoons onion powder
- ½ teaspoon ground ginger
- ¼ teaspoon cayenne powder
- Sea salt, as desired
- 3 cups cooked chickpeas
- ¼ cup green bell peppers
- ¼ cup white onions, chopped

Directions:
1. In a blender, add the tomatoes, agave, date sugar, and spices and pulse until smooth. In a pan, add the tomato mixture, chickpeas, bell peppers, and onion over medium heat and bring to a boil.
2. Cook for about 5 minutes. Reduce the heat to low and simmer for about 1 hour. Serve hot.

Nutrition:
Calories: 355
Total Fat: 4.18g
Protein: 14.39g
Sodium: 186mg
Carbs: 68.37g

219. CHICKPEAS & VEGGIE STEW

Preparation Time: 20 minutes
Cooking Time: 1 hour 5 minutes
Servings: 6
Ingredients:
- 3 cups portabella mushrooms
- 4 cups spring water
- 1 cup cooked chickpeas

- 1 cup fresh kale
- 1 cup white onion
- ½ cup red onion
- 1 cup green bell peppers
- ½ cup butternut squash
- 2 plum tomatoes, chopped
- 2 tablespoons grapeseed oil
- 1 teaspoon dried oregano
- 1 teaspoon dried basil
- ½ teaspoon dried thyme
- 2 teaspoons onion powder
- 1 teaspoon cayenne powder
- ½ teaspoon ginger powder
- Sea salt, as desired

Directions:
1. Combine and cook all the ingredients over high heat and bring to a boil.
2. Reduce the heat to low and simmer, covered for about 1 hour, stirring occasionally.
3. Serve hot.

Nutrition:
Calories:138
Total Fat: 5.4g
Protein: 5.1g
Carbs: 20.18g
Sodium: 130.95mg

220. ALMOND-CRUSTED SALMON

Preparation Time: 10 minutes
Cooking Time: 15 minutes
Servings: 4
Ingredients:
- ¼ cup almond meal
- ¼ cup whole wheat breadcrumbs
- ¼ teaspoon ground coriander
- ⅛ teaspoon ground cumin
- 4 6-ounce boneless salmon fillets
- 1 tablespoon fresh lemon juice
- Salt and pepper

Directions:
1. Heat the oven to 500°F and line a small baking dish with foil.
2. Combine the almond meal, breadcrumbs, coriander, and cumin in a small bowl.
3. Rinse the fish in cool water then pat dry and brush with lemon juice.
4. Season the fish with salt and pepper then dredge in the almond mixture on both sides.
5. Situate fish in the baking dish and bake for 15 minutes.

Nutrition:
Calories: 381
Carbohydrates: 6.6g
Sugar: 0.7g
Sodium: 325mg

221. CHICKEN & VEGGIE BOWL WITH BROWN RICE

Preparation Time: 10 minutes
Cooking Time: 20 minutes
Servings: 4
Ingredients:

- 1 cup instant brown rice
- ¼ cup tahini
- ¼ cup fresh lemon juice
- 2 cloves minced garlic
- ¼ teaspoon ground cumin
- Pinch salt
- 1 tablespoon olive oil
- 4 4-ounce chicken breast halves
- ½ medium yellow onion, sliced
- 1 cup green beans, trimmed
- 1 cup chopped broccoli
- 4 cups chopped kale

Directions:

1. Bring 1-cup of water to boil in a small saucepan.
2. Stir in the brown rice and simmer for 5 minutes then cover and set aside.
3. Meanwhile, whisk together the tahini with ¼ cup water in a small bowl.
4. Stir in the lemon juice, garlic, and cumin with a pinch of salt and stir well.
5. Heat up oil in a big cast iron skillet over medium heat.
6. Season the chicken with salt and pepper then add to the skillet.
7. Cook for 3 to 5 minutes on each side until cooked through then remove to a cutting board and cover loosely with foil.
8. Reheat the skillet and cook the onion for 2 minutes then stir in the broccoli and beans.
9. Sauté for 2 minutes then stir in the kale and sauté 2 minutes more.
10. Add 2 tablespoons of water then cover and steam for 2 minutes while you slice the chicken.
11. Fill the bowls with brown rice, sliced chicken, and sautéed veggies.
12. Serve hot drizzled with the lemon tahini dressing.

Nutrition:
Calories: 405.91
Carbohydrates: 28g
Fiber: 5.46g
Sodium: 125mg

222. BEEF STEAK FAJITAS

Preparation Time: 10 minutes
Cooking Time: 15 minutes
Servings: 4
Ingredients:

- 1 lb. lean beef sirloin, sliced thin
- 1 tablespoon olive oil
- 1 medium red onion, sliced
- 1 red pepper, sliced thin
- 1 green pepper, sliced thin
- ½ teaspoon ground cumin
- ½ teaspoon chili powder
- 8 6-inch whole wheat tortillas
- Fat-free sour cream

Directions:

1. Preheat a large cast-iron skillet over medium heat then add the oil.
2. Add the sliced beef and cook in a single layer for 1 minute on each side.
3. Remove the beef to a bowl and cover to keep warm.
4. Reheat the skillet then add the onions and peppers. Season with cumin and chili powder.
5. Stir-fry the veggies to your liking then add to the bowl with the beef.
6. Serve hot in small whole wheat tortillas with sliced avocado and fat-free sour cream.

Nutrition:
Calories: 446.89
Carbohydrates: 39g
Fiber: 17g
Sodium: 308.18mg

223. ITALIAN PORK CHOPS

Preparation Time: 5 minutes
Cooking Time: 45 minutes
Servings: 4
Ingredients:

- 4 pork chops, boneless
- 3 garlic cloves, minced
- 1 teaspoon dried rosemary, crushed
- ¼ teaspoon pepper
- ¼ teaspoon sea salt

Directions:

1. Heat the oven to 425ºF / 218 C.
2. Line baking tray with cooking spray and season pork chops with pepper and salt.
3. Combine garlic and rosemary and rub all over pork chops.
4. Place pork chops in a prepared baking tray.
5. Roast pork chops in preheated oven for 10 minutes.

6. Set temperature to 350ºF and roast for 25 minutes.
7. Serve and enjoy!

Nutrition:
Calories: 259.71
Carbohydrates: 1g
Protein: 31.4g
Sodium: 201.36mg

224. CHICKEN MUSHROOM STROGANOFF

Preparation Time: 5 minutes
Cooking Time: 25 minutes
Servings: 6
Ingredients:

- 1 cup fat-free sour cream
- 2 tablespoons flour
- 1 tablespoon Worcestershire sauce
- ½ teaspoon dried thyme
- 1 chicken bouillon cube, crushed
- Salt and pepper
- ½ cup water
- 1 medium yellow onion
- 8 ounces sliced mushrooms
- 1 tablespoon olive oil
- 2 cloves minced garlic
- 12 ounces chicken breast
- 6 ounces whole wheat noodles, cooked

Directions:

1. Whisk together ⅔ cup of the sour cream with the flour, Worcestershire sauce, thyme, and crushed bouillon in a medium bowl.
2. Season with salt and pepper then slowly stir in the water until well combined.
3. Cook oil in a large skillet over medium-high heat.
4. Sauté onions and mushrooms for 3 minutes.
5. Cook garlic for 2 minutes more then add the chicken.
6. Pour in the sour cream mixture and cook until thick and bubbling.
7. Reduce heat and simmer for 2 minutes.
8. Spoon the chicken and mushroom mixture over the cooked noodles and garnish with the remaining sour cream to serve.

Nutrition:
Calories: 183
Carbohydrates: 18.43g
Fiber: 1.4g
Sodium: 557.98mg

225. GRILLED TUNA KEBABS

Preparation Time: 20 minutes
Cooking Time: 10 minutes
Servings: 4
Ingredients:

- 2½ tablespoons rice vinegar
- 2 tablespoons fresh grated ginger
- 2 tablespoons sesame oil
- 2 tablespoons soy sauce
- 2 tablespoons fresh chopped cilantro
- 1 tablespoon minced green chili
- 1 ½ pound fresh tuna
- 1 large red pepper
- 1 large red onion
- A few drops of liquid Stevia

Directions:

1. Whisk together the rice vinegar, ginger, sesame oil, soy sauce, cilantro, and chili in a medium bowl. Add a few drops of liquid Stevia extract to sweeten.
2. Toss in the tuna and chill for 20 minutes, covered.
3. Meanwhile, grease a grill pan with cooking spray and soak wooden skewers in water.
4. Slide the tuna cubes onto the skewers with red pepper and onion.
5. Grill for 4 minutes per side and serve hot.

Nutrition:
Calories: 272.25
Carbohydrates: 4.9g
Fiber: 1.7g
Sodium: 527.99mg

226. CAST IRON PORK LOIN

Preparation Time: 10 minutes
Cooking Time: 20 minutes
Servings: 6
Ingredients:

- 1 1½-pound boneless pork loin
- Salt and pepper
- 2 tablespoons olive oil
- 2 tablespoons dried herb blend

Directions:

1. Heat the oven to 425°F.
2. Cut the excess fat from the pork and season.
3. Heat the oil in a large cast-iron skillet over medium heat.
4. Add the pork and cook for 2 minutes on each side.
5. Sprinkle the herbs over the pork and transfer them to the oven.
6. Roast for 10 to 15 minutes.

7. Put aside for 10 minutes before cutting to serve.

Nutrition:
Calories: 234.5
Carbohydrates: 1g
Protein: 24g
Sodium: 183.12mg

227. CRISPY BAKED TOFU

Preparation Time: 5 minutes
Cooking Time: 25 minutes
Servings: 4
Ingredients:

- 1 14-ounce block extra-firm tofu
- 1 tablespoon olive oil
- 1 tablespoon cornstarch
- ½ teaspoon garlic powder
- Salt and pepper

Directions:

1. Spread paper towels out on a flat surface.
2. Cut the tofu into slices up to about ½-inch thick and lay them out.
3. Cover the tofu with another paper towel and place a cutting board on top.
4. Let the tofu drain for 10 to 15 minutes.
5. Preheat the oven to 400°F and line a baking sheet with foil or parchment.
6. Slice tofu into cubes and situate in a large bowl.
7. Toss with olive oil, cornstarch, and garlic powder, pepper, and salt.
8. Spread on the baking sheet and bake for 10 minutes.
9. Flip the tofu and bake for another 10 to 15 minutes. Serve hot.

Nutrition:
Calories: 140
Carbohydrates: 2.1g
Fiber: 0.1g
Sodium: 198.28mg

228. TILAPIA WITH COCONUT RICE

Preparation Time: 10 minutes
Cooking Time: 15 minutes
Servings: 4
Ingredients:

- 4 6-ounce boneless tilapia fillets
- 1 tablespoon ground turmeric
- 1 tablespoon olive oil
- 2 8.8-ounce packets of precooked whole grain rice
- 1 cup light coconut milk

- ½ cup fresh chopped cilantro
- 1½ tablespoon fresh lime juice

Directions:

1. Season the fish with turmeric, salt, and pepper.
2. Cook oil in a large skillet at medium heat and add the fish.
3. Cook for 2 to 3 minutes per side until golden brown.
4. Remove the fish to a plate and cover to keep warm.
5. Reheat the skillet and add the rice, coconut milk, and a pinch of salt.
6. Simmer on high heat until thickened, about 3 to 4 minutes.
7. Stir in the cilantro and lime juice.
8. Spoon the rice onto plates and serve with the cooked fish.

Nutrition:
Calories: 460
Carbohydrates: 27.1g
Fiber: 3.7g
Sodium: 98.76mg

229. SPICY TURKEY TACOS

Preparation Time: 5 minutes
Cooking Time: 25 minutes
Servings: 8
Ingredients:

- 1 tablespoon olive oil
- 1 medium yellow onion, diced
- 2 cloves minced garlic
- 1 pound 93% lean ground turkey
- 1 cup tomato sauce, no sugar added
- 1 jalapeño, seeded and minced
- 8 low-carb multigrain tortillas

Directions:

1. Heat up oil in a big skillet over medium heat.
2. Add the onion and sauté for 4 minutes then stir in the garlic and cook 1 minute more.
3. Stir in the ground turkey and cook for 5 minutes until browned, breaking it up with a wooden spoon.
4. Sprinkle on the taco seasoning and cayenne then stir well.
5. Cook for 30 seconds and mix in the tomato sauce and jalapeño.
6. Simmer on low heat for 10 minutes while you warm the tortillas in the microwave.
7. Serve the meat in the tortillas with your favorite taco toppings.

Nutrition:
Calories: 195

Carbohydrates: 15.4g
Fiber: 8g
Sodium: 259mg

230. QUICK AND EASY SHRIMP STIR FRY

Preparation Time: 15 minutes
Cooking Time: 15 minutes
Servings: 5
Ingredients:
- 1 tablespoon olive oil
- 1-pound uncooked shrimp
- 1 tablespoon sesame oil
- 8 ounces snow peas
- 4 ounces broccoli, chopped
- 1 medium red pepper, sliced
- 3 cloves minced garlic
- 1 tablespoon fresh grated ginger
- ½ cup soy sauce
- 1 tablespoon cornstarch
- 2 tablespoons fresh lime juice
- ¼ teaspoon liquid Stevia extract

Directions:
1. Cook olive oil in a huge skillet over medium heat.
2. Add the shrimp and season, then sauté for 5 minutes.
3. Remove the shrimp to a bowl and keep warm.
4. Reheat the skillet with the sesame oil and add the veggies.
5. Sauté until the veggies are tender, about 6 to 8 minutes.
6. Cook garlic and ginger for 1 minute more.
7. Pour the remaining ingredients into the skillet after whisking them together.
8. Toss to coat the veggies then add the shrimp and reheat. Serve hot.

Nutrition:
Calories: 157.4
Carbohydrates: 10.75g
Fiber: 1.9g
Sodium: 1685mg

231. CHICKEN BURRITO BOWL WITH QUINOA

Preparation Time: 15 minutes
Cooking Time: 10 minutes
Servings: 6
Ingredients:
- 1 tablespoon chipotle chilis in adobo
- 1 tablespoon olive oil
- ½ teaspoon garlic powder
- ½ teaspoon ground cumin
- 1 pound boneless skinless chicken breast

- 2 cups cooked quinoa
- 2 cups shredded romaine lettuce
- 1 cup black beans
- 1 cup diced avocado
- 3 tablespoons fat-free sour cream

Directions:
1. Stir together the chipotle chilis, olive oil, garlic powder, and cumin in a small bowl.
2. Preheat a grill pan to medium-high and grease with cooking spray.
3. Season the chicken with salt and pepper and add to the grill pan.
4. Grill for 5 minutes then flip it and brush with the chipotle glaze.
5. Cook for another 3 to 5 minutes until cooked through.
6. Transfer the chicken to a chopping board and chop it.
7. Assemble the bowls with 1/6 of the quinoa, chicken, lettuce, beans, and avocado.
8. Top each with a half tablespoon of fat-free sour cream to serve.

Nutrition:
Calories: 344.88
Carbohydrates: 37.4g
Fiber: 8.5g
Sodium: 65,41mg

232. BAKED SALMON CAKES

Preparation Time: 10 minutes
Cooking Time: 20 minutes
Servings: 4
Ingredients:
- 15 ounces canned salmon, drained
- 1 large egg, whisked
- 2 teaspoons Dijon mustard
- 1 small yellow onion, minced
- 1½ cups whole-wheat breadcrumbs
- ¼ cup low-fat mayonnaise
- ¼ cup nonfat Greek yogurt, plain
- 1 tablespoon fresh chopped parsley
- 1 tablespoon fresh lemon juice
- 2 green onions, sliced thin

Directions:
1. Set the oven to 450°F and prep the baking sheet with parchment.
2. Flake the salmon into a medium bowl then stir in the egg and mustard.

3. Mix in the onions and breadcrumbs by hand, blending well, then shape into 8 patties.
4. Grease a large skillet and heat it over medium heat.
5. Fry patties for 2 minutes per side.
6. Situate patties to the baking sheet and bake for 15 minutes.
7. Meanwhile, whisk together the remaining ingredients.
8. Serve the baked salmon cakes with creamy herb sauce.

Nutrition:
Calories: 312.24
Carbohydrates: 33.65g
Fiber: 2.39g
Sodium: 701.56mg

233. RICE AND MEATBALL STUFFED BELL PEPPERS

Preparation Time: 15 minutes
Cooking Time: 20 minutes
Servings: 4
Ingredients:
- 4 bell peppers
- 1 tablespoon olive oil
- 1 small onion, chopped
- 2 cloves garlic, minced
- 1 cup frozen cooked rice, thawed
- 16 to 20 small frozen precooked meatballs
- ½ cup tomato sauce
- 2 tablespoons Dijon mustard

Directions:
1. To prepare the peppers, cut off about ½ inch of the tops. Carefully take out membranes and seeds from inside the peppers. Set aside.
2. In a 6x6x2-inch pan, combine the olive oil, onion, and garlic. Bake in the air fryer for 2 to 4 minutes or until crisp and tender. Remove the vegetable mixture from the pan and set it aside in a medium bowl.
3. Add the rice, meatballs, tomato sauce, and mustard to the vegetable mixture and stir to combine.
4. Stuff the peppers with the meat-vegetable mixture.
5. Situate peppers in the air fryer basket and bake for 9 to 13 minutes or until the filling is hot and the peppers are tender.

Nutrition:
Calories: 342
Carbohydrates: 26.69g
Fiber: 4.75g

Sodium: 603mg
Sugar: 8.46

234. STIR-FRIED STEAK AND CABBAGE

Preparation Time: 15 minutes
Cooking Time: 10 minutes
Servings: 4
Ingredients:
- ½ pound sirloin steak, cut into strips
- 2 teaspoons cornstarch
- 1 tablespoon peanut oil
- 2 cups chopped red or green cabbage
- 1 yellow bell pepper, chopped
- 2 green onions, chopped
- 2 cloves garlic, sliced
- ½ cup commercial stir fry sauce

Directions:
1. Toss the steak with the cornstarch and set aside
2. In a 6-inch metal bowl, combine the peanut oil with the cabbage. Place in the basket and cook for 3 to 4 minutes.
3. Remove the bowl from the basket and add the steak, pepper, onions, and garlic. Return to the air fryer and cook for 3 to 5 minutes.
4. Add the stir fry sauce and cook for 2 to 4 minutes. Serve over brown rice.

Nutrition:
Calories:221.5
Carbohydrates: 14.4g
Fiber: 2g
Sodium: 702mg

235. NORI-BURRITOS

Preparation Time: 15 minutes
Cooking Time: 20 minutes
Servings: 2
Ingredients:
- 1 avocado, ripe
- 3 c. cucumber, chopped
- ½ mango
- 4 sheets nori seaweed
- 1 zucchini, small
- A handful of amaranth or dandelion greens
- A handful of sprouted hemp seeds
- 1 tbs. tahini
- Sesame seeds, to taste

Directions:
1. Set the nori sheet on a cutting board, gleaming side facing down. Arrange all the ingredients on the nori sheet,

leaving to the right one-inch broad margin of exposed nori.
2. Fold nori sheet from the side nearest to you, roll it up and over the fillings, use both hands. Put some sesame seeds on top and slice them into thick pieces.

Nutrition:
Calories: 545
Protein: 23.38g
Fiber: 10.7g
Sodium: 80.41mg
Carbs: 52g

236. GRILLED ZUCCHINI HUMMUS WRAP

Preparation Time: 15 minutes
Cooking Time: 25 minutes
Servings: 4
Ingredients:
- 1 zucchini, ends removed and sliced
- 1 plum tomato, sliced, or cherry tomatoes, halved
- ¼ sliced red onion
- 1 cup romaine lettuce or wild arugula
- 4 tablespoons homemade hummus (mashed garbanzo beans)
- 2 spelt tortillas
- 1 tablespoon grapeseed oil
- Sea salt and cayenne pepper to taste

Directions:
1. Heat a skillet to medium heat or grill. In grapeseed oil, mix the sliced zucchini and sprinkle with sea salt and cayenne pepper. Place tossed, sliced zucchini directly on the grill and let cook for 3 minutes, flip over and cook for another 2 minutes. Set aside zucchini.
2. Place the tortillas on the grill for around a minute, or until the grill marks are noticeable and the tortillas are foldable. Remove tortillas from the grill and prepare wraps, 2 tablespoons of hummus, slices of zucchini, ½ cup greens, slices of onion, and tomato. Wrap firmly, and instantly savor.

Nutrition:
Calories: 147.22
Protein: 4g
Fiber: 2.51g
Carbs: 18g
Sodium: 363mg

237. CLASSIC HOMEMADE HUMMUS

Preparation Time: 5 minutes
Cooking Time: 10 minutes
Servings: 3
Ingredients:
- 1 cup cooked chickpeas
- ⅓ cup homemade tahini butter
- 2 tablespoon olive oil
- 2 tablespoon key lime juice
- A dash of onion powder
- Sea salt, to taste

Directions:
1. Blend everything in a food processor or high-powered blender and serve.

Nutrition:
Calories: 368.8
Protein: 6.14g
Fiber: 5.1g
Sodium: 233mg

238. VEGGIE FAJITAS TACOS

Preparation Time: 10 minutes
Cooking Time: 15 minutes
Servings: 3
Ingredients:
- 1 onion
- Juice of ½ key lime
- 2 bell peppers
- Your choice of seasonings (onion powder, cayenne pepper)
- 6 whole wheat tortillas
- 1 tablespoon grapeseed oil
- Avocado
- 2-3 large portobello mushrooms

Directions:
1. Remove mushroom stems, spoon gills out if necessary, and clear tops clean. Slice into approximately ⅓ "thick slices. Slice the onion and bell peppers into thin slices.
2. Pour 1 tablespoon grape seed oil into a big skillet on medium heat and onions and peppers. Cook for 2 minutes. Mix in seasonings and mushrooms. Stir frequently and cook for another seven-eight minutes or until tender.
3. Heat the tortillas and spoon the fajita material into the middle of the tortilla. Serve with key lime juice and avocado.

Nutrition:
Calories: 375.75
Protein: 10.96g
Fiber: 12.32g
Sodium: 711.4mg

239. LEMON CHICKEN WITH PEPPERS

Preparation Time: 5 minutes
Cooking Time: 20 minutes
Servings: 6
Ingredients:

- 1 teaspoon cornstarch
- 1 tablespoon low-sodium soy sauce
- 12 oz. chicken breast tenders, cut in thirds
- ¼ cup fresh lemon juice
- ¼ cup low-sodium soy sauce
- ¼ cup fat-free chicken broth
- 1 teaspoon fresh ginger, minced
- 2 cloves garlic, minced
- 1 tablespoon Splenda
- 1 teaspoon cornstarch
- 1 tablespoon vegetable oil
- ¼ cup red bell pepper
- ¼ cup green bell pepper

Directions:

1. Mix 1 teaspoon cornstarch and 1 tablespoon soy sauce. Add sliced chicken tenders. Chill to marinate for 10 minutes.
2. Stir the lemon juice, ¼ cup soy sauce, chicken broth, ginger, garlic, Splenda, and 1 teaspoon cornstarch together.
3. Warm up oil in a medium frying pan. Cook chicken over medium-high heat until thoroughly cooked.
4. Add sauce and sliced peppers. Cook 1 to 2 minutes more.

Nutrition:
Calories: 150
Fiber: 1g
Sodium: 411.32mg
Carbohydrates: 6g

240. DIJON HERB CHICKEN

Preparation Time: 7 minutes
Cooking Time: 25 minutes
Servings: 4
Ingredients:

- 4 skinless, boneless chicken breast halves
- 1 tablespoon unsalted butter
- 1 tablespoon olive or vegetable oil
- 2 garlic cloves, finely minced
- ½ cup dry white wine
- ¼ cup water
- 2 tablespoons Dijon-style mustard
- ½ teaspoon dried dill weed
- ¼ teaspoon coarsely ground pepper
- ⅓ cups chopped fresh parsley

Directions:

1. Place chicken breasts between sheets of plastic wrap or waxed paper, and pound with a kitchen mallet until they are evenly about ¼-inch thick.
2. Warm up butter and oil over medium-high heat; cook chicken pieces for 3 minutes per side. Transfer chicken to a platter; keep warm and set aside.
3. Sauté garlic for 15 seconds in skillet drippings; stir in wine, water, mustard, dill weed, salt, and pepper. Boil and reduce volume by ½, stirring up the browned bits at the bottom of the skillet.
4. Drizzle sauce over chicken cutlets. Sprinkle with parsley and serve.

Nutrition:
Calories: 223
Fiber: 1g
Sodium: 112mg
Carbohydrates: 6g

241. SESAME CHICKEN STIR FRY

Preparation Time: 10 minutes
Cooking Time: 30 minutes
Servings: 6
Ingredients:

- 12 ounces skinless, boneless chicken breast
- 1 tablespoon vegetable oil
- 2 garlic cloves, finely minced
- 1 cup broccoli florets
- 1 cup cauliflowers
- ½ pound fresh mushrooms, sliced
- 4 green onions, cut into 1-inch pieces
- 2 tablespoons low-sodium soy sauce
- 3 tablespoon dry sherry
- 1 teaspoon finely minced fresh ginger
- 1 teaspoon cornstarch melted in 2 tablespoons water
- ¼ teaspoon sesame oil
- ¼ cup dry-roasted peanuts

Directions:

1. Cut off fat from chicken and thinly slice diagonally into 1-inch strips.
2. In a huge non-stick skillet, heat oil and stir fry chicken for 4 minutes. Remove; put aside and keep warm.
3. Stir fry garlic for 15 seconds; then broccoli and cauliflower, stir fry for 2 minutes. Fry

mushrooms, green onions, soy sauce, sherry, and ginger for 2 minutes.
4. Pour dissolved arrowroot, sesame oil, peanuts, and the chicken. Cook until heated through and the sauce has thickened.

Nutrition:
Calories: 256
Carbohydrates: 9g
Protein: 30g
Sodium: 364mg

242. ROSEMARY CHICKEN

Preparation Time: 9 minutes
Cooking Time: 30 minutes
Servings: 4
Ingredients:

- 1 2½-3-pound broiler-fryer chicken
- Salt and ground black pepper to taste
- 4 garlic cloves, finely minced
- 1 teaspoon dried rosemary
- ¼ cup dry white wine
- ¼ cup chicken broth

Directions:

1. Preheat broiler.
2. Season chicken with salt and pepper. Place in broiler pan. Broil 5 minutes per side.
3. Situate chicken, garlic, rosemary, wine, and broth in a Dutch oven. Cook, covered, at medium heat for about 30 minutes, turning once.

Nutrition:
Calories: 176
Carbohydrates: 1g
Fat: 1g
Sodium: 279mg

243. PEPPER CHICKEN SKILLET

Preparation Time: 10 minutes
Cooking Time: 35 minutes
Servings: 4
Ingredients:

- 1 tablespoon vegetable oil
- 12 ounces skinless, boneless chicken breasts
- 2 garlic cloves, finely minced
- 3 bell peppers (red, green, and yellow)
- 2 medium onions, sliced
- 1 teaspoon ground cumin
- 1½ teaspoon dried oregano leaves
- 2 teaspoons chopped fresh jalapeño peppers

- 3 tablespoons fresh lemon juice
- 2 tablespoons chopped fresh parsley
- ¼ teaspoon salt

Directions:

1. In a big non-stick skillet, heat oil at medium-high heat; stir-fry chicken for 4 minutes.
2. Cook garlic for 15 seconds, stirring constantly. Fry bell pepper strips, sliced onion, cumin, oregano, and jalapeño peppers for 2 to 3 minutes.
3. Toss lemon juice, parsley, salt, and pepper and serve.

Nutrition:
Calories: 174
Carbohydrates: 10.9g
Sodium: 190.88mg
Protein: 21g

244. DIJON SALMON

Preparation Time: 8 minutes
Cooking Time: 26 minutes
Servings: 6
Ingredients:

- 1 tablespoon olive oil
- 1½ pounds salmon fillets, cut into 6 pieces
- ¼ cup lemon juice
- 2 tablespoons Equal (sugar substitute)
- 2 tablespoons Dijon mustard
- 1 tablespoon unsalted butter or margarine
- 1 tablespoon capers
- 1 clove garlic, minced
- 2 tablespoons chopped fresh dill

Directions:

1. Heat up olive oil in a large non-stick skillet over medium heat. Add salmon and cook for 5 minutes, turning once. Reduce the heat to medium-low and cover the pan. Cook for 6–8 minutes, or until the salmon flakes easily with a fork.
2. Transfer the salmon to a serving platter and keep heated.
3. In a pan, combine the lemon juice, Equal, mustard, butter, capers, and garlic. Cook at medium heat for 3 minutes, stirring frequently.
4. To serve, spoon sauce over salmon. Sprinkle with dill.

Nutrition:
Calories: 252
Carbohydrates: 5.36g
Protein: 23g
Sodium: 101mg

245. PULLED PORK

Preparation Time: 10 minutes
Cooking Time: 35 minutes
Servings: 6
Ingredients:

- 1 whole pork tenderloin
- 1 teaspoon chili powder
- ½ teaspoon garlic powder
- ½ cup onion
- 1½ teaspoons garlic
- 1 14.5-ounce can tomatoes
- 1 tablespoon cider vinegar
- 1 tablespoon prepared mustard
- 1 to 2 teaspoons chili powder
- ¼ teaspoon maple extract
- ¼ teaspoon Liquid Smoke
- ⅓ cup Equal (sugar substitute)
- 6 multigrain hamburger buns

Directions:

1. Season pork with 1 teaspoon chili powder and garlic powder; place in baking pan. Bake in preheated 425°F oven for 30 to 40 minutes. Set aside for 15 minutes. Slice into 2 to 3-inch slices; shred slices into bite-size pieces with a fork.
2. Coat medium saucepan with cooking spray. Cook onion and garlic for 5 minutes. Cook tomatoes, vinegar, mustard, chili powder, maple extract, and Liquid Smoke to the saucepan. Allow to boil; decrease heat.
3. Simmer, uncovered, 10 to 15 minutes. Sprinkle Equal.
4. Season. Stir pork into sauce. Cook 2 to 3 minutes. Spoon mixture into buns.

Nutrition:
Calories: 252
Carbohydrates: 29g
Protein: 21g
Sodium: 433mg

246. HERB LEMON SALMON

Preparation Time: 10 minutes
Cooking Time: 27 minutes
Servings: 5
Ingredients:

- 2 cups water
- ⅔ cup farro
- 1 medium eggplant
- 1 red bell pepper
- 1 summer squash
- 1 small onion
- 1½ cups cherry tomatoes
- 3 tablespoons extra-virgin olive oil
- ¾ teaspoon salt, divided
- ½ teaspoon ground pepper

- 2 tablespoons capers
- 1 tablespoon red-wine vinegar
- 2 teaspoons honey
- 1¼ pounds salmon cut into 4 portions
- 1 teaspoon lemon zest
- ½ teaspoon Italian seasoning
- Lemon wedges for serving

Directions:

1. Situate racks in the upper and lower thirds of the oven; set to 450°F. Prep 2 rimmed baking sheets with foil and coat with cooking spray.
2. Boil water and farro. Adjust heat to low, cover, and simmer for 30 minutes. Drain if necessary.
3. Mix eggplant, bell pepper, squash, onion, and tomatoes with oil, ½ teaspoon salt, and ¼ teaspoon pepper. Portion between the baking sheets. Roast on the upper and lower racks for 25 minutes, stirring once half-way through. Put them back in the bowl. Mix in capers, vinegar, and honey.
4. Rub salmon with lemon zest, Italian seasoning, and the remaining ¼ teaspoon each salt and pepper and situate on one of the baking sheets.
5. Roast on the lower rack for 12 minutes, depending on thickness. Serve with farro, vegetable caponata, and lemon wedges.

Nutrition:
Calories: 422.8
Fat: 23g
Carbohydrates: 29.7g
Sodium: 494.75mg

247. GINGER CHICKEN

Preparation Time: 10 minutes
Cooking Time: 25 minutes
Servings: 5
Ingredients:

- 2 tablespoons vegetable oil - divided
- 1 pound boneless, skinless chicken breasts
- 1 cup red bell pepper strips
- 1 cup sliced fresh mushrooms
- 16 fresh pea pods, cut in half crosswise
- ½ cup sliced water chestnuts
- ¼ cup sliced green onions
- 1 tablespoon grated fresh ginger root
- 1 large clove garlic, crushed

- ⅔ cup reduced-fat, reduced-sodium chicken broth
- 2 tablespoons Equal (sugar substitute)
- 2 tablespoons light soy sauce
- 4 teaspoons cornstarch
- 2 teaspoons dark sesame oil

Directions:
1. Heat up 1 tablespoon vegetable oil in a large skillet over medium-high heat. Stir fry chicken until no longer pink. Remove chicken from skillet.
2. In a pan, heat the remaining 1 tablespoon vegetable oil. Red peppers, mushrooms, pea pods, water chestnuts, green onion, ginger, and garlic are all good additions. Stir fry the mixture for 3–4 minutes, or until the veggies are crisp-tender.
3. In the meantime, whisk together the chicken broth, Equal, soy sauce, cornstarch, and sesame oil until smooth. Add into skillet mixture. Cook over medium heat until the sauce is thick and clear. Stir in the chicken and heat thoroughly. If desired, season with salt and pepper to taste.
4. If preferred, serve over hot cooked rice.

Nutrition:
Calories: 232.8
Fat: 9g
Carbohydrates: 19g
Sodium: 601.24mg

248. TERIYAKI CHICKEN

Preparation Time: 7 minutes
Cooking Time: 26 minutes
Servings: 6
Ingredients:
- 1 tablespoon cornstarch
- 1 tablespoon cold water
- ½ cup Splenda
- ½ cup soy sauce
- ¼ cup cider vinegar
- 1 clove garlic, minced
- ½ teaspoon ground ginger
- ¼ teaspoon ground black pepper
- 12 skinless, boneless chicken breast halves

Directions:
1. Combine cornstarch, cold water, Splenda, soy sauce, vinegar, garlic, ginger, and ground black pepper in a small saucepan over low heat. Cook, stirring constantly, until the sauce thickens and bubbles.

2. Preheat oven to 425°F (220°C).
3. Position chicken pieces in a lightly greased 9x13 inch baking dish. Brush chicken with the sauce. Turn pieces over, and brush again.
4. Bake for 30 minutes in a preheated oven. Bake for another 30 minutes on the other side. During cooking, brush with sauce every 10 minutes.

Nutrition:
Calories: 553.39
Carbohydrates: 18g
Protein: 91g
Sodium: 1374mg

249. ROASTED GARLIC SALMON

Preparation Time: 8 minutes
Cooking Time: 45 minutes
Servings: 6
Ingredients:
- 14 large cloves of garlic
- ¼ cup olive oil
- 2 tablespoons fresh oregano
- 1 teaspoon salt
- ¾ teaspoon pepper
- 6 cups Brussels sprouts
- ¾ cup white wine, preferably Chardonnay
- 2 pounds wild-caught salmon fillet

Directions:
1. Heat oven to 450°F.
2. Finely chop 2 garlic cloves and combine in a small bowl with oil, 1 tablespoon oregano, ½ teaspoon salt, and ¼ teaspoon pepper. Slice remaining garlic and mix in Brussels sprouts and 3 tablespoons of the seasoned oil in a big roasting pan. Roast, stirring once, for 15 minutes.
3. Pour in wine to the remaining oil mixture. Remove from oven, stir the vegetables and place salmon on top. Dash with the wine mixture. Sprinkle with the remaining 1 tablespoon oregano and ½ teaspoon each salt and pepper.
4. Bake for 10 minutes more. Serve with lemon wedges.

Nutrition:
Calories: 388
Carbohydrates: 12g
Protein: 37g
Sodium: 479.22mg

250. LEMON SESAME HALIBUT

Preparation Time: 9 minutes

Cooking Time: 29 minutes
Servings: 4
Ingredients:
- 2 tablespoons lemon juice
- 2 tablespoons extra-virgin olive oil
- 1 clove garlic, minced
- Freshly ground pepper, to taste
- 2 tablespoons sesame seeds
- 1¼ pounds halibut or mahi-mahi, cut into 4 portions
- 1½-2 teaspoons dried thyme leaves
- ¼ teaspoon coarse sea salt or kosher salt
- Lemon wedges

Directions:
1. Preheat oven to 450°F. Line a baking sheet with foil.
2. Combine lemon juice, oil, garlic, and pepper in a shallow glass dish. Add fish and turn to coat. Wrap and marinate for 15 minutes.
3. Fry sesame seeds in a small dry skillet over medium-low heat, stirring constantly, for 3 minutes. Set aside to cool. Mix in thyme.
4. Season the fish with salt, and coat evenly with the sesame seed mixture, covering the sides as well as the top. Place the fish to the prepared baking sheet and roast until just opaque in the center, 10 to 14 minutes. Serve with lemon wedges.

Nutrition:
Calories: 142
Fat: 11g
Carbohydrates: 2g
Sodium: 160.93mg

251. TURKEY SAUSAGE CASSEROLE

Preparation Time: 12 minutes
Cooking Time: 32 minutes
Servings: 4
Ingredients:
- 5 ounces turkey breakfast sausage, casings removed
- 1 teaspoon canola oil
- 1 onion, chopped
- 1 red bell pepper, chopped
- 4 large eggs
- 4 large egg whites
- 2½ cups low-fat milk
- 1 teaspoon dry mustard
- ½ teaspoon salt
- ¼ teaspoon freshly ground pepper
- ⅔ cup low-fat cheddar cheese, divided

- 10 slices whole wheat bread, crusts removed

Directions:
1. Grease 9x13-inch baking dish with cooking spray.
2. Fry sausage in a skillet over medium heat, crumbling with a fork until browned. Transfer to a bowl.
3. Cook oil, onion, and bell pepper to skillet, stirring occasionally, for 5 minutes. Fry sausage for 5 minutes more. Remove from heat and set aside.
4. Mix eggs and egg whites in a large bowl until blended. Whisk in milk, mustard, salt, and pepper. Stir in ⅓ cup cheddar.
5. Arrange bread in a single layer in a prepared baking dish. Pour egg mixture over bread and top with reserved vegetables and sausage. Sprinkle with remaining ⅓ cup cheddar. Seal with plastic wrap and chill for at least 5 hours or overnight.
6. Preheat oven to 350°F. Bake casserole, uncovered, until set and puffed 40 to 50 minutes. Serve hot.

Nutrition:
Calories: 471.57
Carbohydrates: 42.44g
Protein: 36.64g
Sodium: 1232mg

252. SPINACH CURRY

Preparation Time: 10 minutes
Cooking Time: 22 minutes
Servings: 4
Ingredients:
- ¾ cup cooked whole wheat angel hair pasta
- ½ cup baby spinach
- ⅓ cup chopped red bell pepper
- ¼ cup grated carrot
- ¼ cup chopped fresh cilantro
- 2 cups low-sodium chicken broth
- 1 tablespoon green curry paste

Directions:
1. Combine pasta, spinach, bell pepper, carrot, and cilantro in a heatproof bowl.
2. Bring chicken broth to a boil. Stir in curry paste. Pour the broth over the pasta mixture. Serve hot.

Nutrition:
Calories: 71.62
Fiber: 1.68g

Carbohydrates: 11.81g
Sodium: 226.21mg

253. ZUCCHINI HERBED SOUP

Preparation Time: 12 minutes
Cooking Time: 34 minutes
Servings: 5
Ingredients:
- 3 cups reduced-sodium chicken broth
- 1½ pounds zucchini,
- 1 tablespoon chopped fresh tarragon
- ¾ cup shredded reduced-fat cheddar cheese
- ¼ teaspoon salt
- ¼ teaspoon freshly ground pepper

Directions:
1. Boil broth, zucchini, and tarragon in a medium saucepan over high heat. Decrease the heat to simmer and cook, uncovered, for 10 minutes. Puree in a blender until smooth.
2. Place soup back in the pan and heat over medium-high, slowly stirring in cheese until it is well-mixed.
3. Remove from heat and season. Serve hot or chilled.

Nutrition:
Calories: 94
Fiber: 1.33g
Carbohydrates: 5.49g
Sodium: 583.75mg

254. KAMUT BURGERS

Preparation Time: 20 minutes
Cooking Time: 20 minutes
Servings: 6
Ingredients:
- 3 cups cooked Kamut cereal
- 1 cup spelt flour
- ½ cup unsweetened hemp milk
- 1 cup green bell peppers, seeded and chopped
- 1 cup red onions, chopped
- 1 tablespoon fresh oregano, chopped
- 1 tablespoon fresh basil, chopped
- 1 teaspoon onion powder
- 1 teaspoon sea salt
- ½ teaspoon cayenne powder
- 4 tablespoons grapeseed oil
- 8 cups fresh baby kale

Directions:
1. In a bowl, add all the ingredients except for oil and kale and mix until well

combined. Make 12 equal-sized patties from the mixture. Cook 2 tablespoons of oil over medium-high heat in a skillet and cook 6 patties for 10 minutes on both sides. Repeat with the rest of the oil and patties. Portion the kale and top each with 2 burgers.
2. Serve immediately.

Nutrition:
Calories: 316.53
Total Fat: 14.66g
Protein: 11g
Sodium: 414.67mg

255. CHICKPEAS & MUSHROOM BURGERS

Preparation Time: 20 minutes
Cooking Time: 20 minutes
Servings: 4
Ingredients:
- 2 portobello mushrooms, chopped roughly
- ½ cup green bell peppers
- ½ cup white onion, chopped roughly
- 2 cups cooked chickpeas
- ½ cup fresh cilantro
- 2 teaspoons fresh oregano, chopped
- 2 teaspoons onion powder
- ½ teaspoon cayenne powder
- Sea salt, as desired
- ¼ cup chickpea flour
- 3 tablespoons grapeseed oil
- 6 cups fresh baby arugula

Directions:
1. Transfer all of the ingredients to a food processor and pulse for about 3 seconds. Make 8 equal-sized patties from the mixture.
2. In a large skillet, heat half of the oil over medium-high heat and cook 4 patties for 4 minutes per side. Repeat. Split the arugula and garnish each with 2 burgers.

Nutrition:
Calories: 318.99
Total Fat: 14.13g
Protein: 13.12g
Carbs: 38g
Sodium: 202.82mg

256. VEGGIE BURGERS

Preparation Time: 5 minutes
Cooking Time: 6 minutes
Servings: 2
Ingredients:
- ½ cup fresh kale, tough ribs removed and chopped

- ½ cup green bell peppers, seeded and chopped
- ½ cup onions, chopped
- 1 plum tomato, chopped
- 2 teaspoons fresh oregano, chopped
- 2 teaspoons fresh basil, chopped
- 1 teaspoon dried dill
- 1 teaspoon onion powder
- ½ teaspoon ginger powder
- ½ teaspoon cayenne powder
- Sea salt, as desired
- 1 cup chickpeas flour
- ¼-½ cup spring water
- 2 tablespoons grapeseed oil
- 3 cups fresh arugula

Directions:
1. Mix in the vegetables, herbs, spices, and salt in a bowl. Add the flour and mix well. Gradually, add in the water until a thick mixture is formed. Make patties from the mixture.
2. Cook the oil over medium-high heat and cook the patties for about 2-3 minutes per side. Divide the arugula onto serving plates and top each with 2 burgers.

Nutrition:
Calories: 364.56
Total Fat: 18g
Protein: 13.87g
Carbs: 39g
Sodium: 389.92mg

257. FALAFEL WITH TZATZIKI SAUCE

Preparation Time: 20 minutes
Cooking Time: 12 minutes
Servings: 8
Ingredients:
For Falafel:
- 1 pound dry chickpeas
- 1 small onion
- ¼ cup fresh parsley, chopped
- 4 garlic cloves, peeled
- 1½ tablespoons chickpea flour
- Sea salt, as desired
- ½ teaspoon cayenne powder
- ½ cup grapeseed oil

For Tzatziki Sauce:
- ½ cup Brazil nuts
- ½ cup spring water
- ¼ cup cucumber, chopped
- 1 tablespoon fresh key lime juice
- 1 garlic clove, minced
- 1 teaspoon fresh dill
- Pinch of sea salt
- 12 cups fresh arugula

Directions:

1. For the falafel: In a food processor, add all the ingredients and pulse until well combined and a coarse meal-like mixture forms. Transfer the falafel mixture into a bowl. With plastic wrap, cover the bowl and refrigerate for about 1-2 hours. With 2 tablespoons of the mixture, make balls.
2. Cook the oil at 375°F in a skillet. Add the falafel in 2 batches and cook for about 5-6 minutes or until golden brown on all sides. Meanwhile, for tzatziki: In a blender, add all the ingredients and pulse until smooth. With a slotted spoon, transfer the falafel onto a paper towel-lined plate to drain. Divide the arugula and falafel onto serving plates evenly.
3. Serve alongside the tzatziki.

Nutrition:
Calories: 412.64
Total Fat: 23.3g
Protein: 14.1g
Carbs: 40.24g
Sodium: 124mg

258. VEGGIE BALLS IN TOMATO SAUCE

Preparation Time: 20 minutes
Cooking Time: 15 minutes
Servings: 8
Ingredients:
- 1½ cups cooked chickpeas
- 2 cups fresh button mushrooms
- ½ cup onions, chopped
- ¼ cup green bell peppers, seeded and chopped
- 2 teaspoons oregano
- 2 teaspoons fresh basil
- 1 teaspoon dried sage
- 1 teaspoon dried dill
- 1 tablespoon onion powder
- ½ teaspoon cayenne powder
- ½ teaspoon ginger powder
- Sea salt, as desired
- ½-1 cup chickpea flour
- 6 cups homemade tomato sauce
- 2 tablespoons grapeseed oil

Directions:
1. In a food processor, add the chickpeas, veggies, herbs, and spices and pulse until well combined. Transfer the mixture into a large bowl with flour and mix until well combined. Make balls from the mixture.
2. Cook the oil over medium-high heat and let the balls cook in 2

batches for about 4-5 minutes or until golden brown from all sides. In a large pan, add the tomato sauce and veggie balls over medium heat and simmer for about 5 minutes. Serve hot.

Nutrition:
Calories: 181.48
Total Fat: 5.7g
Protein: 8.2g
Carbs: 27.9g
Sodium: 113.56mg

259. AIR FRYER BREADED PORK CHOPS

Preparation Time: 10 minutes
Cooking Time: 12 minutes
Servings: 4
Ingredients:
- 1 cup whole wheat breadcrumbs
- ¼ teaspoon salt
- 1-4 pieces pork chops (center cut and boneless)
- ½ teaspoon chili powder
- 1 tablespoon Parmesan cheese
- 1 ½ teaspoon paprika
- One egg, beaten
- ½ teaspoon onion powder
- ½ teaspoon granulated garlic
- Pepper, to taste

Directions:
1. Preheat the air fryer to 400°F.
2. Now rub kosher salt on both sides of the pork chops and let them to rest.
3. Add beaten egg in a large bowl.
4. In a mixing bowl, combine the Parmesan cheese, breadcrumbs, garlic, pepper, paprika, chilli powder, and onion powder.
5. Dip the pork chop in the egg, then in the breadcrumb mixture.
6. Spray it with oil and place it in the air fryer.
7. Allow it to cook for 12 minutes at 400°F. Halfway through, turn it over. Cook for six minutes.
8. Serve with a side of salad.

Nutrition:
Calories: 198
Fat: 6.35 g
Protein: 13.5 g
Carbs: 20.9g
Sodium: 404.3mg

260. PORK TAQUITOS IN THE AIR FRYER

Preparation Time: 10 minutes
Cooking Time: 20 minutes
Servings: 10
Ingredients:

- 3 cups pork tenderloin, cooked & shredded
- Cooking spray
- 2½ cups fat-free shredded mozzarella
- 10 small tortillas
- Salsa for dipping
- Juice of one lime

Directions:
1. Preheat the air fryer to 380°F.
2. Mix in the lime juice with the meat.
3. Microwave for 10 seconds with a moist cloth over the tortilla to soften.
4. In a tortilla, place the pork filling and cheese on top and tightly roll up the tortilla.
5. Place tortillas on a greased foil pan.
6. Spray oil over tortillas. Cook for 7-10 minutes or until tortillas are golden brown, flip halfway through.
7. Serve with fresh salad.

Nutrition:
Calories: 235.29
Fat: 3.8g
Protein: 21.08g
Carbs: 30.1g
Sodium: 275.97mg

261. AIR FRYER TASTY EGG ROLLS

Preparation Time: 10 minutes
Cooking Time: 21 minutes
Servings: 3
Ingredients:
- ½ bag coleslaw mix
- ½ onion
- ½ teaspoon Salt
- ½ cup of mushrooms
- 2 cups lean ground pork
- One stalk of celery
- Wrappers (egg roll)

Directions:
1. Cook lean ground pork and onion for 5-7 minutes in a pan over medium heat.
2. Cook for about five minutes with the coleslaw mixture, salt, mushrooms, and celery in the pan.
3. Lay out the egg roll wrapper and add the filling (1/3 cup), roll it up, and seal with water.
4. Spray the rolls with cooking spray.
5. Put in the air fryer for 6-8 minutes at 400°F, flipping once halfway through.
6. Serve hot.

Nutrition:
Calories: 245

Fat: 10g
Protein: 11g
Carbs: 8.85g
Sodium: 481.14mg

262. PORK DUMPLINGS IN AIR FRYER

Preparation Time: 30 minutes
Cooking Time: 20 minutes
Servings: 6
Ingredients:
- 18 dumpling wrappers
- 1 teaspoon olive oil
- 4 cups bok choy, chopped
- 2 tablespoon rice vinegar
- 1 tablespoon diced ginger
- ¼ teaspoon crushed red pepper
- 1 tablespoon diced garlic
- ½ cup lean ground pork
- Cooking spray
- 2 teaspoon light soy sauce
- ½ teaspoon honey
- 1 teaspoon toasted sesame oil
- Finely chopped scallions

Directions:
1. Heat the olive oil in a large skillet, then add the bok choy and sauté for 6 minutes before adding the garlic and ginger and cooking for another minute. Place this mixture on a paper towel and blot the excess oil.
2. In a mixing bowl, combine the bok choy combination, crushed red pepper, and lean ground pork.
3. Place a dumpling wrapper on a dish and fill it with one spoonful of filling. Seal and crimp the edges with water.
4. With cooking spray, spray the air fryer basket, place the dumplings in the air fryer basket, and cook at 375°F for 12 minutes, or until browned.
5. Meanwhile, to create the sauce, combine sesame oil, rice vinegar, scallions, soy sauce, and honey in a mixing dish.
6. Serve the dumplings with sauce.

Nutrition:
Calories: 128.13
Fat: 5g
Protein: 5.1g
Carbs: 17.1g
Sodium: 159.96mg

263. AIR FRYER PORK CHOP & BROCCOLI

Preparation Time: 20 minutes
Cooking Time: 22 minutes
Servings: 2
Ingredients:

- 2 cups broccoli florets
- 2 pieces bone-in pork chop
- ½ teaspoon paprika
- 2 tablespoon avocado oil
- ½ teaspoon garlic powder
- ½ teaspoon onion powder
- 2 cloves of crushed garlic
- 1 teaspoon salt, divided

Directions:
1. Let the air fryer preheat to 350°F. Spray the basket with cooking oil
2. In a mixing bowl, combine one tablespoon oil, onion powder, half teaspoon salt, garlic powder, and paprika. Rub this spice mixture over the sides of the pork chops.
3. Place the pork chops in the air fryer basket and cook for 5 minutes.
4. In the meantime, add 1 teaspoon oil, garlic, half teaspoon of salt, and broccoli to a bowl and coat well
5. Cook for another five minutes after flipping the pork chop and adding the broccoli.
6. Serve immediately after removing from the air fryer.

Nutrition:
Calories: 410
Fat: 27.5g
Protein: 33.5g
Carbs: 7.06g
Sodium: 1270.49mg

264. CHEESY PORK CHOPS IN AIR FRYER

Preparation Time: 5 minutes
Cooking Time: 8 minutes
Servings: 2
Ingredients:
- 4 lean pork chops
- ½ teaspoon salt
- ½ teaspoon garlic powder
- 4 tablespoons shredded cheese
- Chopped cilantro

Directions:
1. Let the air fryer preheat to 350°F.
2. Rub the pork chops with garlic, cilantro, and salt. Place in the air fryer. Allow it to cook for 4 minutes. Cook for another 2 minutes on the other side.
3. Cook for another 2 minutes, or until the cheese has melted, on top of them.
4. Serve with salad greens.

Nutrition:
Calories: 422.89
Protein: 69g
Fat: 13.9g

Carbs: 0.63g
Sodium: 826.17mg

265. PORK RIND NACHOS

Preparation Time: 6 minutes
Cooking Time: 5 minutes
Servings: 3
Ingredients:
- 1 cup shredded Cheddar cheese
- 1 tablespoon fresh cilantro, minced
- 1 cup 4 ounces pork rinds
- 1/3 pound ground beef
- 1/4 cup cherry tomatoes quarters cut
- 5 tablespoons taco seasoning
- 1 jalapeno pepper sliced
- 1 avocado diced

Directions:
1. First, over medium heat, brown the ground beef in a pan on the stove. When it's done, add 1/2 tablespoon taco seasoning and combine thoroughly.
2. Turn on your oven's broiler.
3. Place the pork rinds onto an oven-safe pan. Top the pork rinds with taco meat, cherry tomatoes, avocados, and shredded cheese.
4. Place the pan under the broiler until all the cheese is melted. Top the nachos garnished with cilantro.
5. Serve with sour cream or homemade guacamole.

Nutrition:
Calories: 569
Carbs: 15g
Protein: 39.76g
Fat: 40g
Sugar: 6.1g
Sodium: 1978.85mg

266. JAMAICAN JERK PORK IN AIR FRYER

Preparation Time: 10 minutes
Cooking Time: 20 minutes
Servings: 4
Ingredients:
- Pork, cut into 3-inch pieces
- 1/4 cup jerk paste

Directions:
1. Rub jerk paste all over the pork pieces.
2. Let it marinate for a minimum of 4 hours, at least, in the refrigerator..
3. Let the air fryer preheat to 390°F. Spray with olive oil
4. Before putting in the air fryer, let the meat sit for 20 minutes at room temperature.

5. Cook for 20 minutes at 390°F in the air fryer, flip halfway through.
6. Take it out from the air fryer let it rest for ten minutes before slicing.
7. Serve with microgreens.

Nutrition:
Calories: 165.86
Protein: 8.9g
Fat: 12.9g
Carbs: 3.17g
Sodium: 199mg

267. GLAZED PORK TENDERLOIN WITH MUSTARD

Preparation Time: 10 minutes
Cooking Time: 18 minutes
Servings: 4
Ingredients:
- 1/4 cup yellow mustard
- One pork tenderloin
- 1/4 teaspoon salt
- 3 tablespoon honey
- 1/8 teaspoon freshly ground black pepper
- 1 tablespoon minced garlic
- 1 teaspoon dried rosemary
- 1 teaspoon Italian seasoning

Directions:
1. With a knife, cut the top of the pork tenderloin. Add garlic (minced) to the cuts. Then sprinkle with kosher salt and pepper.
2. In a bowl, add honey, mustard, rosemary, and Italian seasoning mix until combined. Rub this mustard mix all over pork.
3. Let it marinate in the refrigerator for at least 2 hours.
4. Put pork tenderloin in the air fryer basket. Cook for 18-20 minutes at 400°F until internal temperature of pork reaches 145°F
5. Take out from the air fryer and serve with a side of salad.

Nutrition:
Calories: 211.6
Protein: 26.6g
Fat: 4.99g
Carbs: 14.8g
Sodium: 383.39mg

268. AIR-FRIED BEEF SCHNITZEL

Preparation Time: 10 minutes
Cooking Time: 15 minutes
Servings: 1
Ingredients:

- One lean beef schnitzel
- 2 tablespoon olive oil
- 1/4 cup breadcrumbs
- One egg
- One lemon

Directions:
1. Preheat the air fryer to 350°F.
2. Mix breadcrumbs and oil in a large mixing bowl until a crumbly mixture forms.
3. Coat the beef steak with the breadcrumb mixture after dipping it in the whisked egg.
4. Cook the breaded beef in the air fryer for 15 minutes or longer, or until thoroughly cooked through.
5. Remove from the air fryer and serve with salad leaves and lemon on the side.

Nutrition:
Calories: 576.7
Protein: 37.18g
Fat: 37.7g
Carbs: 22.9g
Sodium: 326.18mg

269. AIR FRYER MEATLOAF

Preparation Time: 10 minutes
Cooking Time: 40 minutes
Servings: 8
Ingredients:
- 4 cups ground lean beef
- 1 cup breadcrumbs, soft and fresh
- 1/2 cup chopped mushrooms
- Cloves of minced garlic
- 1/2 cup shredded carrots
- 1/4 cup beef broth
- 1/2 cup chopped onions
- 2 eggs beaten
- 3 tablespoon ketchup
- 1 tablespoon Worcestershire sauce
- 1 teaspoon Dijon mustard
For Glaze:
- 1/4 cup honey
- 1/2 cup ketchup
- 2 teaspoon Dijon mustard

Directions:
1. In a big bowl, add beef broth and breadcrumbs, stir well. Set it aside. In a food processor, add garlic, onions, mushrooms, and carrots, and pulse on high until finely chopped
2. In a separate bowl, add soaked breadcrumbs, Dijon mustard, Worcestershire sauce, eggs, lean ground beef, ketchup, and salt. With your hands, combine well and make it into a loaf.

3. Let the air fryer preheat to 390°F.
4. Put meatloaf in the air fryer and let it cook for 45 minutes.
5. In the meantime, add Dijon mustard, ketchup, and brown sugar to a bowl and mix. Glaze this mix over meatloaf when five minutes are left.
6. Rest the meatloaf for ten minutes before serving.

Nutrition:
Calories: 272.8
Protein: 19g
Fat: 9.9 g
Carbs: 27g
Sodium: 439.52mg

270. AIR-FRIED STEAK WITH ASPARAGUS BUNDLES

Preparation Time: 20 minutes
Cooking Time: 91 minutes
Servings: 4
Ingredients:
- Olive oil spray
- Flank steak (2 pounds) – cut into 6 pieces
- Kosher salt and black pepper
- 2 cloves of minced garlic
- 4 cups asparagus
- ½ cup tamari sauce
- 3 bell peppers, sliced thinly
- ⅓ cup beef broth
- 1 tablespoon of unsalted butter
- ¼ cup Balsamic vinegar

Directions:
1. Rub the meat with salt and pepper.
2. Toss the steak in a Ziploc bag with the garlic and tamari sauce, then close the bag.
3. Let it marinate for one hour.
4. Place bell peppers and asparagus in the center of the steak in the same way.
5. Roll the steak tightly around the veggies and fasten with toothpicks.
6. Preheat the air fryer.
7. Spray the steak with olive oil spray and place in the air fryer.
8. Cook for 15 minutes at 400°F until steaks are cooked.
9. Remove the steak from the air fryer and set it aside.
10. Allow the steak bundles to rest for 5 minutes before serving/slicing.
11. Meanwhile, heat the butter, balsamic vinegar, and broth over medium heat. Mix thoroughly and cut in half.

Season with salt and pepper to taste.
12. Pour over steaks right before serving.

Nutrition:
Calories: 477.76
Protein: 56.8g
Fat: 17.56g
Carbs: 15g
Sodium: 2413mg

271. AIR FRYER HAMBURGERS

Preparation Time: 5 minutes
Cooking Time: 16 minutes
Servings: 4
Ingredients:
- 4 whole wheat buns
- 4 cups lean ground beef chuck
- Salt to taste
- 4 slices of any cheese
- Black pepper, to taste

Directions:
1. Preheat the air fryer to 350°F.
2. Combine the lean ground beef, pepper, and salt in a mixing bowl. Form patties from the mixture.
3. Cook for 6 minutes, flipping halfway through, in a single layer in the air fryer. One minute before you take out the patties, add cheese on top.
4. Remove from the air fryer after cheese has melted.
5. Add ketchup, any dressing to your buns, add tomatoes and lettuce, and patties.
6. Serve hot.

Nutrition:
Calories: 542
Protein: 33g
Fat: 31.8g
Carbs: 25g
Sodium: 704.62mg

272. AIR FRYER BEEF STEAK KABOBS WITH VEGETABLES

Preparation Time: 30 minutes
Cooking Time: 10 minutes
Servings: 4
Ingredients:
- 2 tablespoon light soy sauce
- ⅓ cup low-fat sour cream
- 4 cups lean beef chuck ribs, cut into one-inch pieces
- Half onion
- 8 skewers – 6 inches
- One bell pepper

Directions:
1. Soy sauce and sour cream should be combined in a

mixing dish. Add the lean beef pieces, coat thoroughly, and set aside for 30 minutes or longer to marinate.
2. Cut onion and bell pepper into one-inch pieces. In water, soak skewers for ten minutes.
3. Skewer the onions, bell peppers, and meat. Sprinkle with black pepper.
4. Allow it to cook for 10 minutes in a 400°F preheated air fryer, flipping halfway through.
5. Serve with yogurt dipping sauce.

Nutrition:
Calories: 517
Protein: 19.56g
Fat: 45.88g
Carbs: 5.7g
Sodium: 618mg

273. AIR-FRIED EMPANADAS

Preparation Time: 10 minutes
Cooking Time: 21 minutes
Servings: 2
Ingredients:
- 8 pieces square gyoza wrappers
- 1 tablespoon olive oil
- ¼ cup white onion, finely diced
- ¼ cup mushrooms, finely diced
- ½ cup lean ground beef
- 2 teaspoon chopped garlic
- ¼ teaspoon paprika
- ¼ teaspoon ground cumin
- Six green olives, diced
- ⅛ teaspoon ground cinnamon
- ½ cup diced tomatoes
- One egg, lightly beaten

Directions:
1. In a skillet, over a medium flame, add oil, onions, and beef and cook for 3 minutes, until beef turns brown.
2. Add mushrooms and cook for six minutes until it starts to brown. Then add paprika, cinnamon, olives, cumin, and garlic and cook for 3 minutes or more.
3. Add in the chopped tomatoes and cook for a minute. Turn off the heat; let it cool for five minutes.
4. Lay gyoza wrappers on a flat surface. Add one and a half tablespoons of beef filling in each wrapper. Brush edges with water or egg, fold wrappers, pinch edges.
5. Put 4 empanadas in an even layer in an air fryer basket and

cook for 7 minutes at 400°F until nicely browned.

6. Serve with sauce and salad greens.

Nutrition:
Calories: 285
Fat: 14.6g
Protein: 14.37g
Carbs: 25g
Sodium: 212.37mg

274. AIR FRY RIBEYE STEAK

Preparation Time: 5 minutes
Cooking Time: 14 minutes
Servings: 2
Ingredients:
- 2 medium-sized lean ribeye steaks
- Salt & freshly ground black pepper, to taste

Directions:
1. Let the air fry preheat at 400°F. Pat dry steaks with paper towels.
2. On steaks, use any spice combination or simply salt and pepper.
3. Generously season both sides of the steak.
4. Place the steaks in an air fryer basket. Cook to the desired level of rareness. Alternatively, cook for 14 minutes and flip half-way through.
5. Remove from the air fryer and set aside for 5 minutes.
6. Serve with a microgreen salad.

Nutrition:
Calories: 725.46
Protein: 56g
Fat: 55g
Carbs: 0.92g
Sodium: 540.68mg

275. BREADED CHICKEN TENDERLOINS

Preparation Time: 10 minutes
Cooking Time: 13 minutes
Servings: 4
Ingredients:
- 8 chicken tenderloins
- 2 tablespoon olive oil
- One egg, whisked
- ¼ cup breadcrumbs

Directions:
1. Preheat the air fryer to 350°F.
2. Mix breadcrumbs and oil in a large mixing basin until a crumbly mixture forms.
3. Dip chicken tenderloin in whisked egg and coat in breadcrumbs mixture.

4. Cook the breaded chicken in the air fryer for 12 minutes.
5. Remove from the air fryer and serve with a green salad of your choice.

Nutrition:
Calories: 225.34
Protein: 24.78g
Fat: 11.15g
Carbs: 4.94g
Sodium: 110mg

276. PARMESAN CHICKEN MEATBALLS

Preparation Time: 10 minutes
Cooking Time: 13 minutes
Servings: 20
Ingredients:
- ½ cup pork rinds, ground
- 4 cups ground chicken
- ½ cup Parmesan cheese, grated
- 1 teaspoon kosher salt
- ½ teaspoon garlic powder
- One egg beaten
- ½ teaspoon paprika
- ½ teaspoon pepper

Breading
- ½ cup whole wheat breadcrumbs, ground

Directions:
1. Let the air fryer pre-heat to 400°F.
2. Add cheese, chicken, egg, pepper, ½ cup of pork rinds, garlic, salt, and paprika in a big mixing ball. Mix well into a dough, make into 1-and-a-half-inch balls.
3. Coat the meatballs in whole wheat breadcrumbs.
4. Spray the air fry basket and add meatballs in one even layer.
5. Let it cook for 12 minutes at 400°F, flipping once halfway through.
6. Serve with salad greens.

Nutrition:
Calories: 77.59
Fat: 4g
Protein: 8.1g
Carbs: 2.22g
Sodium: 173.9mg

277. LEMON ROSEMARY CHICKEN

Preparation Time: 30 minutes
Cooking Time: 21 minutes
Servings: 2
Ingredients:
For the Marinade:
- 2 ½ cups chicken
- 1 teaspoon ginger, minced
- ½ tablespoon olive oil
- 1 tablespoon soy sauce

For the Sauce:
- ½ lemon
- 3 tablespoon honey
- 1 tablespoon oyster sauce
- ½ cup fresh rosemary, chopped

Directions:
1. In a big mixing bowl, add the marinade ingredients with chicken, and mix well.
2. Keep in the refrigerator for at least half an hour.
3. Let the oven preheat to 390°F for 3 minutes.
4. Place the marinated chicken in the air fryer in a single layer. And cook for 6 minutes at 200°F.
5. Meanwhile, add all the sauce ingredients to a bowl and mix well except for lemon wedges.
6. Brush the sauce generously over half-baked chicken, add lemon juice on top.
7. Cook for another 13 minutes at 390°F. Flip the chicken halfway through. Let the chicken evenly brown.
8. Serve right away and enjoy.

Nutrition:
Calories: 486
Protein: 30.16g
Fat: 27.59g
Carbs: 30.21g
Sodium: 807mg

278. AIR FRYER CHICKEN & BROCCOLI

Preparation Time: 10 minutes
Cooking Time: 15 minutes
Servings: 4
Ingredients:
- 2 tablespoon olive oil
- 4 cups chicken breast, boneless and skinless (cut into cubes)
- ½ medium onion, roughly sliced
- 1 tablespoon low-sodium soy sauce
- ½ teaspoon garlic powder
- 2 teaspoon rice vinegar
- 1–2 cups broccoli, cut into florets
- 2 teaspoon hot sauce
- 1 tablespoon fresh minced ginger
- 1 teaspoon sesame seed oil
- Salt & black pepper, to taste

Directions:
1. In a bowl, add chicken breast, onion, and broccoli. Combine them well.
2. In another bowl, add ginger, oil, sesame oil, rice vinegar, hot sauce, garlic powder, and soy

sauce mix it well. Then add the broccoli, chicken, and onions to the marinade.
3. Coat the chicken well with the sauces. Let it rest in the refrigerator for 15 minutes.
4. Place chicken mix in one even layer in air fryer basket and cook for 16-20 minutes, at 380°F. Halfway through, toss the basket gently and cook the chicken evenly
5. Add five minutes more, if required.
6. Add salt and pepper, if needed.
7. Serve hot with lemon wedges.

Nutrition:
Calories: 259.89
Fat: 12g
Protein: 32.69g
Carbs: 3.9g
Sodium: 435.84mg

279. AIR-FRIED SECTION AND TOMATO

Preparation Time: 10 minutes
Cooking Time: 5 minutes
Servings: 2
Ingredients:
- 1 aubergine, sliced thickly into 4 disks
- 1 tomato, sliced into 2 thick disks
- 2 teaspoon feta cheese, reduced fat
- 2 fresh basil leaves, minced
- 2 balls, small buffalo mozzarella, reduced-fat, roughly torn
- Pinch of salt
- Pinch of black pepper

Directions:
1. Preheat Air Fryer to 330°F.
2. Spray a small amount of oil into the air fryer basket. Fry aubergine slices for 5 minutes or until golden brown on both sides. Transfer to a plate.
3. Fry tomato slices in batches for 5 minutes or until seared on both sides.
4. To serve, stack salad starting with an aborigine base, buffalo mozzarella, basil leaves, tomato slice, and ½ teaspoon feta cheese.
5. Top with another slice of aubergine and ½ teaspoon feta cheese. Serve.

Nutrition:
Calorie: 447.66
Carbohydrates: 15.46g
Fat: 33.4g
Protein: 23.37g

Fiber: 7.49g
Sodium: 871.94mg

280. CHEESY SALMON FILLETS

Preparation Time: 15 minutes
Cooking Time: 20 minutes
Servings: 2-3
Ingredients:
For the Salmon Fillets:
- 2 pieces, 4 oz. each salmon fillets, choose even cuts
- ½ cup sour cream, reduced-fat
- ¼ cup cottage cheese, reduced-fat
- ¼ cup Parmigiano-Reggiano cheese, freshly grated

For the Garnish:
- Spanish paprika
- ½ piece lemon, cut into wedges

Directions:
1. Preheat Air Fryer to 330°F.
2. To make the salmon fillets, mix sour cream, cottage cheese, and Parmigiano-Reggiano cheese in a bowl.
3. Layer salmon fillets in the air fryer basket. Fry for 20 minutes or until cheese turns golden brown.
4. To assemble, place a salmon fillet and sprinkle paprika. Garnish with lemon wedges and squeeze lemon juice on top. Serve.

Nutrition:
Calorie: 274
Carbohydrates: 1g
Fat: 19g
Protein: 24g
Sodium: 255mg
Fiber: 0.5g

281. SALMON WITH ASPARAGUS

Preparation Time: 5 Minutes
Cooking Time: 10 Minutes
Servings: 3
Ingredients:
- 1 lb. salmon, sliced into fillets
- 1 tablespoon olive oil
- Salt & pepper, as needed
- 1 bunch of asparagus, trimmed
- 2 cloves of garlic, minced
- Zest & juice of ½ lemon
- 1 tablespoon unsalted butter

Directions:
1. Spoon in the butter and olive oil into a large pan and heat it over medium-high heat.
2. Once it becomes hot, place the salmon and season it with salt and pepper.

3. Cook for 4 minutes per side and then cook the other side.
4. Stir in the garlic and lemon zest to it.
5. Cook for further 2 minutes or until slightly browned.
6. Off the heat and squeeze the lemon juice over it.
7. Serve it hot.

Nutrition:
Calories: 409
Carbohydrates: 2.7g
Protein: 32.8g
Fat: 28.8g
Sodium: 497mg

282. SHRIMP IN GARLIC BUTTER

Preparation Time: 5 Minutes
Cooking Time: 20 Minutes
Servings: 4
Ingredients:
- 1 lb. shrimp, peeled & deveined
- ¼ teaspoon red pepper flakes
- 6 tablespoon unsalted butter, divided
- ½ cup chicken stock
- Salt & pepper, as needed
- 2 tablespoon parsley, minced
- 5 cloves of garlic, minced
- 2 tablespoon lemonjJuice

Directions:
1. Heat a large bottomed skillet over medium-high heat.
2. Spoon in 2 tablespoons of the butter and melt it. Add the shrimp.
3. Season it with salt and pepper. Sear for 4 minutes or until shrimp gets cooked.
4. Transfer the shrimp to a plate and stir in the garlic.
5. Sauté for 30 seconds or until aromatic.
6. Pour the chicken stock and whisk it well. Allow it to simmer for 5 to 10 minutes or until it has been reduced to half.
7. Spoon the remaining butter, red pepper, and lemon juice into the sauce. Mix.
8. Continue cooking for another 2 minutes.
9. Take off the pan from the heat and add the cooked shrimp to it.
10. Garnish with parsley and transfer to the serving bowl.
11. Enjoy.

Nutrition:
Calories: 307
Carbohydrates: 3g
Protein: 27g
Fat: 20g

Sodium: 522mg

283. SEARED TUNA STEAK

Preparation Time: 10 Minutes
Cooking Time: 10 Minutes
Servings: 2
Ingredients:
- 1 teaspoon sesame seeds
- 1 tablespoon sesame oil
- 2 tablespoon soy sauce
- Salt & pepper, to taste
- 2 × 6 oz. Ahi tuna steaks

Directions:
1. Season the tuna steaks with salt and pepper. Keep them aside in a shallow bowl.
2. In another bowl, mix soy sauce and sesame oil.
3. Pour the sauce over the salmon and coat them generously with the sauce.
4. Keep it aside for 10 to 15 minutes and then heat a large skillet over medium heat.
5. Once hot, keep the tuna steaks and cook them for 3 minutes or until seared underneath.
6. Flip the fillets and cook them for 3 more minutes.
7. Transfer the seared tuna steaks to the serving plate and slice them into ½ inch slices. Top with sesame seeds.

Nutrition:
Calories: 255
Fat: 9g
Carbohydrates: 1g
Protein: 40.5g
Sodium: 293mg

284. BEEF CHILI

Preparation Time: 10 Minutes
Cooking Time: 20 Minutes
Servings: 4
Ingredients:
- ½ teaspoon garlic powder
- 1 teaspoon coriander, grounded
- 1 lb. ground beef
- ½ teaspoon sea salt
- ½ teaspoon cayenne pepper
- 1 teaspoon ground cumin
- ½ teaspoon ground pepper
- ½ cup salsa, no-sugar added

Directions:
1. Heat a large-sized pan over medium-high heat and cook the beef in it until browned.
2. Stir in all the spices and cook them for 7 minutes or until everything is combined.

3. When the beef gets cooked, spoon in the salsa.
4. Bring the mixture to a simmer and cook for another 8 minutes or until everything comes together.
5. Take it from heat and transfer it to a serving bowl.

Nutrition:
Calories: 229
Fat: 10g
Carbohydrates: 2g
Protein: 33g
Sodium: 675mg

285. GREEK BROCCOLI SALAD

Preparation Time: 10 Minutes
Cooking Time: 15 Minutes
Servings: 4
Ingredients:
- 1¼ lb. broccoli, sliced into small bites
- ¼ cup almonds, sliced
- ⅓ cup sun-dried tomatoes
- ¼ cup feta cheese, crumbled
- ¼ cup red onion, sliced

For the Dressing:
- ¼ cup olive oil
- Dash of red pepper flakes
- 1 garlic clove, minced
- ¼ teaspoon salt
- 2 tablespoon lemon juice
- ½ teaspoon Dijon mustard
- 1 teaspoon low-carb sweetener syrup
- ½ teaspoon oregano, dried

Directions:
1. Mix broccoli, onion, almonds, and sun-dried tomatoes in a large mixing bowl.
2. In another small-sized bowl, combine all the dressing ingredients until emulsified.
3. Spoon the dressing over the broccoli salad.
4. Allow the salad to rest for half an hour before serving.

Nutrition:
Calories: 272
Carbohydrates: 11.9g
Protein: 8g
Fat: 21.6g
Sodium: 321mg

286. CHEESY CAULIFLOWER GRATIN

Preparation Time: 5 Minutes
Cooking Time: 25 Minutes
Servings: 6
Ingredients:
- 6 deli slices pepper jack cheese
- 4 cups cauliflower florets

- Salt and pepper, as needed
- 4 tablespoons unsalted butter
- ⅓ cup heavy whipping cream

Directions:
1. Mix the cauliflower, cream, butter, salt, and pepper in a safe microwave bowl and combine well.
2. Microwave the cauliflower mixture for 25 minutes on high until it becomes soft and tender.
3. Remove the ingredients from the bowl and mash with the help of a fork.
4. Taste for seasonings and spoon in salt and pepper as required.
5. Arrange the slices of pepper jack cheese on top of the cauliflower mixture and microwave for 3 minutes until the cheese starts melting.
6. Serve warm.

Nutrition:
Calories: 421
Carbohydrates: 3g
Protein: 19g
Fat: 37g
Sodium: 111mg

287. STRAWBERRY SPINACH SALAD

Preparation Time: 5 Minutes
Cooking Time: 10 Minutes
Servings: 4
Ingredients:
- 4 oz. feta cheese, crumbled
- 8 strawberries, sliced
- 2 oz. almonds
- 6 slices bacon, thick-cut, crispy, and crumbled
- 10 oz. spinach leaves, fresh
- 2 Roma tomatoes, diced
- 2 oz. red onion, sliced thinly

Directions:
1. For making this healthy salad, mix all the ingredients needed to make the salad in a large-sized bowl and toss well.

Nutrition:
Calories: 255
Fat: 16g
Carbohydrates: 8g
Protein: 14g
Sodium: 27mg

288. EASY EGG SALAD

Preparation Time: 5 Minutes
Cooking Time: 15 to 20 Minutes
Effort: Easy
Servings: 4
Ingredients:
- 6 eggs
- ¼ teaspoon salt

- 2 tablespoon mayonnaise
- 1 teaspoon lemon juice
- 1 teaspoon Dijon mustard
- Pepper, to taste
- Lettuce leaves, to serve

Directions:
1. Keep the eggs in a saucepan of water and pour cold water until it covers the egg by another 1 inch.
2. Bring to a boil and then remove the eggs from heat.
3. Peel the eggs under cold running water.
4. Transfer the cooked eggs into a food processor and pulse them until chopped.
5. Stir in the mayonnaise, lemon juice, salt, Dijon mustard, and pepper and mix them well.
6. Taste for seasoning and add more if required.
7. Serve in the lettuce leaves.

Nutrition:
Calories: 166
Fat: 14g
Carbohydrates: 0.85g
Protein: 10g
Sodium: 132mg

289. BAKED CHICKEN LEGS

Preparation Time: 10 Minutes
Cooking Time: 40 Minutes
Effort: Easy
Servings: 6
Ingredients:
- 6 chicken legs
- ¼ teaspoon black pepper
- ¼ cup unsalted butter
- ½ teaspoon sea salt
- ½ teaspoon smoked paprika
- ½ teaspoon garlic powder

Directions:
1. Preheat the oven to 425°F.
2. Pat the chicken legs with a paper towel to absorb any excess moisture.
3. Marinate the chicken pieces by first applying the butter over them and then with the seasoning. Set it aside for a few minutes.
4. Bake them for 25 minutes. Turnover and bake for further 10 minutes or until the internal temperature reaches 165°F.
5. Serve them hot.

Nutrition:
Calories: 518
Fat: 41g
Protein: 34.7g
Carbs: 0.65g
Sodium: 3336mg

290. ROASTED PORK & APPLES

Preparation Time: 15 minutes
Cooking Time: 30 minutes
Servings: 4
Ingredients:
- Salt and pepper to taste
- ½ teaspoon dried, crushed
- 1 lb. pork tenderloin
- 1 tablespoon canola oil
- 1 onion, sliced into wedges
- 3 cooking apples, sliced into wedges
- ⅔ cup apple cider
- Sprigs fresh sage

Directions:
1. In a bowl, mix salt, pepper, and sage.
2. Season both sides of pork with this mixture.
3. Place a pan over medium heat.
4. Brown both sides.
5. Transfer to a roasting pan.
6. Add the onion on top and around the pork.
7. Drizzle oil on top of the pork and apples.
8. Roast in the oven at 425°F for 10 minutes.
9. Add the apples, roast for another 15 minutes.
10. In a pan, boil the apple cider and then simmer for 10 minutes.
11. Pour the apple cider sauce over the pork before serving.

Nutrition:
Calories: 239
Total Fat: 6 g
Saturated Fat: 1 g
Cholesterol: 74 mg
Sodium: 209 mg
Total Carbohydrates: 22 g
Dietary Fiber: 3 g
Total Sugar: 16 g
Protein: 24 g
Potassium: 655 mg

291. PORK WITH CRANBERRY RELISH

Preparation Time: 30 minutes
Cooking Time: 30 minutes
Servings: 4

Ingredients:
- 12 oz. pork tenderloin, fat trimmed and sliced crosswise
- Salt and pepper to taste
- ¼ cup almond flour
- 2 tablespoons olive oil
- 1 onion, sliced thinly
- ¼ cup dried cranberries

- ¼ cup low-sodium chicken broth
- 1 tablespoon balsamic vinegar

Directions:
1. Flatten each slice of pork using a mallet.
2. In a dish, mix the salt, pepper, and flour.
3. Dip each pork slice into the flour mixture.
4. Add oil to a pan over medium-high heat.
5. Cook pork for 3 minutes per side or until golden crispy.
6. Transfer to a serving plate and cover with foil.
7. Cook the onion in the pan for 4 minutes.
8. Stir in the rest of the ingredients.
9. Simmer until the sauce has thickened.

Nutrition:
Calories: 211
Total Fat: 9 g
Saturated Fat: 2 g
Cholesterol: 53 mg
Sodium: 116 mg
Total Carbohydrates: 15 g
Dietary Fiber: 1 g
Total Sugar: 6 g
Protein: 18 g
Potassium: 378 mg

292. SESAME PORK WITH MUSTARD SAUCE

Preparation Time: 25 minutes
Cooking Time: 25 minutes
Servings: 4
Ingredients:
- 2 tablespoons low-sodium teriyaki sauce
- ¼ cup chili sauce
- 2 cloves garlic, minced
- 2 teaspoons ginger, grated
- 2 pork tenderloins
- 2 teaspoons sesame seeds
- ¼ cup low-fat sour cream
- 1 teaspoon Dijon mustard
- Salt to taste
- 1 scallion, chopped

Directions:
1. Preheat your oven to 425°F.
2. Mix the teriyaki sauce, chili sauce, garlic, and ginger.
3. Put the pork on a roasting pan.
4. Brush the sauce on both sides of the pork.
5. Bake in the oven for 15 minutes.
6. Brush with more sauce.
7. Top with sesame seeds.
8. Roast for 10 more minutes.

9. Mix the rest of the ingredients.
10. Serve the pork with mustard sauce.

Nutrition:
Calories: 135
Total Fat: 3 g
Saturated Fat: 1 g
Cholesterol: 56 mg
Sodium: 302 mg
Total Carbohydrates: 7 g
Dietary Fiber: 1 g
Total Sugar: 15 g
Protein: 20 g
Potassium: 755 mg

293. STEAK WITH MUSHROOM SAUCE

Preparation Time: 20 minutes
Cooking Time: 5 minutes
Servings: 4
Ingredients:

- 12 oz. sirloin steak, sliced and trimmed
- 2 teaspoons grilling seasoning
- 2 teaspoons oil
- 6 oz. broccoli, trimmed
- 2 cups frozen peas
- 3 cups fresh mushrooms, sliced
- 1 cup beef broth (unsalted)
- 1 tablespoon mustard
- 2 teaspoons cornstarch
- Salt to taste

Directions:
1. Preheat your oven to 350°F.
2. Season meat with grilling seasoning.
3. In a pan over medium-high heat, cook the meat and broccoli for 4 minutes.
4. Sprinkle the peas around the steak.
5. Put the pan inside the oven and bake for 8 minutes.
6. Remove both meat and vegetables from the pan.
7. Add the mushrooms to the pan.
8. Cook for 3 minutes.
9. Mix the broth, mustard, salt, and cornstarch.
10. Add to the mushrooms.
11. Cook for 1 minute.
12. Pour sauce over meat and vegetables before serving.

Nutrition:
Calories: 226
Total Fat: 6 g
Saturated Fat: 2 g
Cholesterol: 51 mg
Sodium: 356 mg
Total Carbohydrates: 16 g
Dietary Fiber: 5 g
Total Sugar: 6 g
Protein: 26 g

Potassium: 780 mg

294. STEAK WITH TOMATO & HERBS

Preparation Time: 30 minutes
Cooking Time: 30 minutes
Servings: 2
Ingredients:

- 8 oz. beef loin steak, sliced in half
- Salt and pepper to taste
- Cooking spray
- 1 teaspoon fresh basil, snipped
- ¼ cup green onion, sliced
- ½ cup tomato, chopped

Directions:
1. Season the steak with salt and pepper.
2. Spray oil on your pan.
3. Put the pan over medium-high heat.
4. Once hot, add the steaks.
5. Reduce heat to medium.
6. Cook for 10 to 13 minutes for medium, turning once.
7. Add the basil and green onion.
8. Cook for 2 minutes.
9. Add the tomato.
10. Cook for 1 minute.
11. Let cool a little before slicing.

Nutrition:
Calories: 170
Total Fat: 6 g
Saturated Fat: 2 g
Cholesterol: 66 mg
Sodium: 207 mg
Total Carbohydrates: 3 g
Dietary Fiber: 1 g
Total Sugar: 5 g
Protein: 25 g
Potassium: 477 mg

295. BARBECUE BEEF BRISKET

Preparation Time: 25 minutes
Cooking Time: 10 hours
Servings: 10
Ingredients:

- 4 lb. beef brisket (boneless), trimmed and sliced
- 1 bay leaf
- 2 onions, sliced into rings
- ½ teaspoon dried thyme, crushed
- ¼ cup chili sauce
- 1 clove garlic, minced
- Salt and pepper to taste
- 2 tablespoons light brown sugar
- 2 tablespoons cornstarch
- 2 tablespoons cold water

Directions:
1. Put the meat in a slow cooker.

2. Add the bay leaf and onion.
3. In a bowl, mix the thyme, chili sauce, salt, pepper, and sugar.
4. Pour the sauce over the meat.
5. Mix well.
6. Seal the pot and cook on low heat for 10 hours.
7. Discard the bay leaf.
8. Pour cooking liquid into a pan.
9. Add the mixed water and cornstarch.
10. Simmer until the sauce has thickened.
11. Pour the sauce over the meat.

Nutrition:
Calories: 182
Total Fat: 6 g
Saturated Fat: 2 g
Cholesterol: 57 mg
Sodium: 217 mg
Total Sugar: 4 g
Protein: 20 g
Potassium: 383 mg

296. BEEF & ASPARAGUS

Preparation Time: 15 minutes
Cooking Time: 10 minutes
Servings: 4
Ingredients:

- 2 teaspoons olive oil
- 1 lb. lean beef sirloin, trimmed and sliced
- 1 carrot, shredded
- Salt and pepper to taste
- 12 oz. asparagus, trimmed and sliced
- 1 teaspoon dried herbes de Provence, crushed
- ½ cup Marsala
- ¼ teaspoon lemon zest

Directions:
1. Pour oil in a pan over medium heat.
2. Add the beef and carrot.
3. Season with salt and pepper.
4. Cook for 3 minutes.
5. Add the asparagus and herbs.
6. Cook for 2 minutes.
7. Add the Marsala and lemon zest.
8. Cook for 5 minutes, stirring frequently.

Nutrition:
Calories: 327
Total Fat: 7 g
Saturated Fat: 2 g
Cholesterol: 69 mg
Sodium: 209 mg
Total Carbohydrates: 29 g
Dietary Fiber: 2 g
Total Sugar: 3 g
Protein: 28 g
Potassium: 576 mg

297. ITALIAN BEEF

Preparation Time: 20 minutes
Cooking Time: 1 hour and 20 minutes
Servings: 4
Ingredients:

- Cooking spray
- 1 lb. beef round steak, trimmed and sliced
- 1 cup onion, chopped
- 2 cloves garlic, minced
- 1 cup green bell pepper, chopped
- ½ cup celery, chopped
- 2 cups mushrooms, sliced
- 14½ oz. canned diced tomatoes
- ½ teaspoon dried basil
- ¼ teaspoon dried oregano
- ⅛ teaspoon crushed red pepper
- 2 tablespoons Parmesan cheese, grated

Directions:

1. Spray oil on the pan over medium heat.
2. Cook the meat until brown on both sides.
3. Transfer meat to a plate.
4. Add the onion, garlic, bell pepper, celery, and mushroom to the pan.
5. Cook until tender.
6. Add the tomatoes, herbs, and pepper.
7. Put the meat back in the pan.
8. Simmer while covered for 1 hour and 15 minutes.
9. Stir occasionally.
10. Sprinkle Parmesan cheese on top of the dish before serving.

Nutrition:
Calories: 212
Total Fat: 4 g
Saturated Fat: 1 g
Cholesterol: 51 mg
Sodium: 296 mg
Total Sugar: 6 g
Protein: 30 g
Potassium: 876 mg

298. LAMB WITH BROCCOLI & CARROTS

Preparation Time: 20 minutes
Cooking Time: 10 minutes
Servings: 4
Ingredients:

- 2 cloves garlic, minced
- 1 tablespoon fresh ginger, grated
- ¼ teaspoon red pepper, crushed
- 2 tablespoons low-sodium soy sauce
- 1 tablespoon white vinegar
- 1 tablespoon cornstarch

- 12 oz. lamb meat, trimmed and sliced
- 2 teaspoons cooking oil
- 1 lb. broccoli, sliced into florets
- 2 carrots, sliced into strips
- ¾ cup low-sodium beef broth
- 4 green onions, chopped
- 2 cups cooked spaghetti squash pasta

Directions:

1. Combine the garlic, ginger, red pepper, soy sauce, vinegar, and cornstarch in a bowl.
2. Add lamb to the marinade.
3. Marinate for 10 minutes.
4. Discard marinade.
5. In a pan over medium heat, add the oil.
6. Add the lamb and cook for 3 minutes.
7. Transfer lamb to a plate.
8. Add the broccoli and carrots. Cook for 1 minute.
9. Pour in the beef broth. Cook for 5 minutes.
10. Put the meat back in the pan. Sprinkle with green onion and serve on top of spaghetti squash.

Nutrition:
Calories: 205
Total Fat: 6 g
Saturated Fat: 1 g
Cholesterol: 40 mg
Sodium: 659 mg
Total Carbohydrates: 17 g

299. ROSEMARY LAMB

Preparation Time: 15 minutes
Cooking Time: 2 hours
Servings: 14
Ingredients:

- Salt and pepper to taste
- 2 teaspoons fresh rosemary, snipped
- 5 lb. whole leg of lamb, trimmed and cut with slits on all sides
- 3 cloves garlic, slivered
- 1 cup water

Directions:

1. Preheat your oven to 375°F.
2. Mix salt, pepper, and rosemary in a bowl.
3. Sprinkle mixture all over the lamb.
4. Insert slivers of garlic into the slits.
5. Put the lamb on a roasting pan.
6. Add water to the pan.
7. Roast for 2 hours.

Nutrition:

Calories: 136
Total Fat: 4 g
Saturated Fat: 1 g
Cholesterol: 71 mg
Sodium: 218 mg
Protein: 23 g
Potassium: 248 mg

300. MEDITERRANEAN LAMB MEATBALLS

Preparation Time: 10 minutes
Cooking Time: 20 minutes
Servings: 8
Ingredients:

- 12 oz. roasted red peppers
- 1½ cups whole wheat breadcrumbs
- 2 eggs, beaten
- ⅓ cup tomato sauce
- ½ cup fresh basil
- ¼ cup parsley snipped
- Salt and pepper to taste
- 2 lb. lean ground lamb

Directions:

1. Preheat your oven to 350°F.
2. In a bowl, mix all the ingredients and then form them into meatballs.
3. Put the meatballs on a baking pan.
4. Bake in the oven for 20 minutes.

Nutrition:
Calories: 94
Total Fat: 3 g
Saturated Fat: 1 g
Cholesterol: 35 mg
Sodium: 170 mg
Total Carbohydrates: 2 g
Dietary Fiber: 1 g

301. FISH WITH FRESH TOMATO-BASIL SAUCE

Preparation Time: 10 minutes
Cooking Time: 15 minutes
Servings: 2
Ingredients:

- 2 4-oz. tilapia fillets
- 1 tablespoon fresh basil, chopped
- ⅛ teaspoon salt
- 1 pinch of crushed red pepper
- 1 cup cherry tomatoes, chopped
- 2 teaspoons extra virgin olive oil

Directions:

1. Preheat oven to 400°F.
2. Arrange rinsed and patted dry fish fillets on foil (coat a foil baking sheet with cooking spray).

3. Sprinkle tilapia fillets with salt and red pepper.
4. Bake 12 - 15 minutes.
5. Meanwhile, mix leftover ingredients in a saucepan.
6. Cook over medium-high heat until tomatoes are tender.
7. Top fish fillets properly with tomato mixture.

Nutrition:
Calories: 167.55
Protein: 23.57g
Carbohydrates: 3.47g
Sodium: 208.45mg

302. BAKED CHICKEN

Preparation Time: 15 minutes
Cooking Time: 25 minutes
Servings: 4
Ingredients:
- 2 6-oz. bone-in chicken breasts
- ⅛ teaspoon salt
- ⅛ teaspoon pepper
- 3 teaspoons extra virgin olive oil
- ½ teaspoon dried oregano
- 7 pitted kalamata olives
- 1 cup cherry tomatoes
- ½ cup onion
- 1 9-oz. pkg frozen artichoke hearts
- 1 lemon

Directions:
1. Preheat oven to 400°F.
2. Sprinkle chicken with pepper, salt, and oregano.
3. Heat oil, add chicken, and cook until it browned.
4. Place chicken in a baking dish. Arrange tomatoes, coarsely chopped olives, and onion, artichokes and lemon cut into wedges around the chicken.
5. Bake for 20 minutes, or until the chicken is cooked through and the veggies are soft.

Nutrition:
Calories: 189.4
Fat: 10.89g
Carbohydrates:8.08g
Sodium: 376.43mg

303. SEARED CHICKEN WITH ROASTED VEGETABLES

Preparation Time: 20 minutes
Cooking Time: 30 minutes
Servings: 1
Ingredients:
- 1 8-oz. boneless, skinless chicken breasts
- ¾ lb. small Brussels sprouts

- 2 large carrots
- 1 large red bell pepper
- 1 small red onion
- 2 cloves garlic halved
- 2 tablespoons extra virgin olive oil
- ½ teaspoon dried dill
- ¼ teaspoon pepper
- ¼ teaspoon salt

Directions:
1. Preheat oven to 425°F.
2. Combine Brussels sprouts cut in half, red onion cut into wedges, sliced carrots, bell pepper cut into pieces, and halved garlic. Spread on a baking sheet.
3. Sprinkle with 1 tablespoon oil and ⅛ teaspoon salt and ⅛ teaspoon pepper. Bake until well-roasted, cool slightly.
4. In the Meantime, sprinkle chicken with dill, remaining ⅛ teaspoon salt, and ⅛ teaspoon pepper. Cook until the chicken is done. Put roasted vegetables with drippings over chicken.

Nutrition:
Calories: 779
Fat: 36g
Protein:66.7g
Sodium: 863mg
Carbs: 54g

304. FISH SIMMERED IN TOMATO-PEPPER SAUCE

Preparation Time: 5 minutes
Cooking Time: 10 minutes
Servings: 2
Ingredients:
- 2 4-oz. cod fillets
- 1 big tomato
- ⅓ cup red peppers, roasted
- 3 tablespoons almonds
- 2 cloves garlic
- 2 tablespoons fresh basil leaves
- 2 tablespoons extra virgin olive oil
- ¼ teaspoon salt
- ⅛ teaspoon pepper

Directions:
1. Toast sliced almonds in a pan until fragrant.
2. Grind almonds, basil, minced garlic, 1-2 teaspoons oil in a food processor until finely ground.
3. Add coarsely chopped tomato and red peppers, grind until smooth.
4. Season fish with salt and pepper.

5. Cook in hot oil in a large pan over medium-high heat until fish is browned. Pour sauce around fish. Cook 6 minutes more.

Nutrition:
Calories: 329.27
Fat: 23g
Carbohydrates:8.4g
Sodium: 434.91mg

305. PARMESAN BROILED FLOUNDER

Preparation Time: 10 minutes
Cooking Time: 7 minutes
Servings: 2
Ingredients:
- 2 4-oz. flounder
- 1.5 tablespoons Parmesan cheese
- 1.5 tablespoons mayonnaise
- ⅛ teaspoon soy sauce
- ¼ teaspoon chili sauce
- ⅛ teaspoon salt-free lemon-pepper seasoning

Directions:
1. Preheat the over to 425 F.
2. Mix cheese, reduced-fat mayonnaise, soy sauce, chili sauce, seasoning.
3. Put fish on a baking sheet coated with cooking spray, sprinkle with salt and pepper.
4. Spread Parmesan mixture over flounder.
5. Broil for 6 to 8 minutes or until a crust appears on the fish.

Nutrition:
Calories: 114
Fat: 9.67g
Carbohydrates: 0.37g
Sodium: 254.57mg

306. CHEESE POTATO AND PEA CASSEROLE

Preparation Time: 10 minutes
Cooking Time: 35 minutes
Servings: 3
Ingredients:
- 1 tablespoon olive oil
- ¾ lb. red potatoes
- ¾ cup green peas
- ½ cup red onion
- ¼ teaspoon dried rosemary
- ¼ teaspoon salt
- ⅛ teaspoon pepper

Directions:
1. Prepare oven to 350°F.
2. Cook 1 teaspoon oil in a skillet. Stir in thinly sliced onions and cook. Remove from pan.

3. Situate half of the thinly sliced potatoes and onions in the bottom of the skillet; top with peas, crushed dried rosemary, and ⅛ teaspoon each salt and pepper.
4. Place remaining potatoes and onions on top. Season with remaining ⅛ teaspoon salt.
5. Bake 35 minutes, pour the remaining 2 teaspoons of oil and sprinkle with cheese.

Nutrition:
Calories:144
Protein: 4.08g
Carbohydrates: 21.27g
Sodium: 213mg

307. OVEN-FRIED TILAPIA

Preparation Time: 7 minutes
Cooking Time: 15 minutes
Servings: 2
Ingredients:
- 2 4-oz. tilapia fillets
- ¼ cup yellow cornmeal
- 2 tablespoons light ranch dressing
- 1 tablespoon canola oil
- 1 teaspoon dill (dried)
- ⅛ teaspoon salt

Directions:
1. Preheat oven to 425°F. Brush both sides of rinsed and patted dry tilapia fish fillets with dressing.
2. Combine cornmeal, oil, dill, and salt.
3. Sprinkle fish fillets with cornmeal mixture.
4. Put fish on a prepared baking sheet.
5. Bake 15 minutes.

Nutrition:
Calories: 271
Protein: 24.43g
Fat:11.5g
Sodium: 360.53mg

308. JUICY GROUND BEEF CASSEROLE

Preparation Time: 10 minutes
Cooking Time: 35 minutes
Servings: 6
Ingredients:
- 2 teaspoons onion flakes
- 1 tablespoon gluten-free Worcestershire sauce
- 2 pounds ground beef
- 2 garlic cloves, peeled and minced
- Salt and pepper to taste
- 1 cup mozzarella cheese, shredded

- 2 cups cheddar cheese, shredded
- 1 cup Russian dressing
- 2 tablespoons sesame seeds, toasted
- 20 dill pickle slices
- 1 romaine lettuce head, torn

Directions:
1. Take a pan and place it on medium heat
2. Add beef, onion flakes, Worcestershire sauce, salt, pepper, and garlic.
3. Stir for 5 minutes
4. Transfer to a baking dish and add 1 cup each of cheddar and mozzarella cheese, and half of the dressing
5. Stir and spread evenly
6. Arrange pickle slices on top
7. Sprinkle remaining cheddar and sesame seeds
8. Transfer to oven and bake for 20 minutes at 350°F
9. Turn oven to broil and broil for 5 minutes
10. Divide lettuce between serving platters and top with remaining dressing
11. Enjoy!

Nutrition:
Calories: 780
Fat: 59g
Carbohydrates: 20.67g
Protein: 41g
Sodium: 1291mg

309. SKILLET TURKEY PATTIES

Preparation Time: 7 minutes
Cooking Time: 8 minutes
Servings: 2
Ingredients:
- ½ lb. lean ground turkey
- ½ cup low-sodium chicken broth
- ¼ cup red onion
- ½ teaspoon Worcestershire sauce
- 1 teaspoon extra virgin olive oil
- ¼ teaspoon oregano (dried)
- ⅛ teaspoon pepper

Directions:
1. Combine turkey, chopped onion, Worcestershire sauce, dried oregano, and pepper; make 2 patties.
2. Warm up the oil and cook patties 4 minutes per side; set aside.
3. Add broth to skillet, bring to a boil. Boil 2 minutes, spoon sauce over patties.

Nutrition:
Calories: 243.22
Fat: 16.99g
Carbohydrates:2.19g
Sodium: 93.9mg

310. TURKEY LOAF

Preparation Time: 10 minutes
Cooking Time: 50 minutes
Servings: 2
Ingredients:
- ½ lb. 93% lean ground turkey
- ⅓ cup panko breadcrumbs
- ½ cup green onion
- 1 egg
- ½ cup green bell pepper
- 1 tablespoon ketchup
- ¼ cup picante sauce
- ½ teaspoon ground cumin

Directions:
1. Preheat oven to 350°F.
2. Mix lean ground turkey, 3 tablespoons Picante sauce, panko breadcrumbs, egg, chopped green onion, chopped green bell pepper, and cumin in a bowl (mix well);
3. Put the mixture into a baking sheet; shape into an oval (about 1,5 inches thick). Bake 45 minutes.
4. Mix remaining picante sauce and the ketchup; apply over the loaf. Bake 5 minutes longer. Let stand 5 minutes.

Nutrition:
Calories: 233
Protein: 31g
Fat:3.8g
Carbs: 19g
Sodium: 782mg

311. MUSHROOM PASTA

Preparation Time: 7 minutes
Cooking Time: 10 minutes
Servings: 4
Ingredients:
- 4 oz whole grain linguine
- 1 teaspoon extra virgin olive oil
- ½ cup light sauce
- 2 tablespoons green onion
- 1 8-oz. pkg mushrooms
- 1 clove garlic
- ⅛ teaspoon salt
- ⅛ teaspoon pepper

Directions:
1. Cook pasta according to package directions, drain.
2. Fry sliced mushrooms for 4 minutes.

3. Stir in fettuccine minced garlic, salt, and pepper. Cook 2 minutes.
4. Heat light sauce until heated; top pasta mixture with sauce and with finely chopped green onion.

Nutrition:
Calories: 381.54
Fat: 14.87g
Carbohydrates:54.6g
Sodium: 572mg

312. CHICKEN TIKKA MASALA

Preparation Time: 5 minutes
Cooking Time: 15 minutes
Servings: 2
Ingredients:
- ½ lb. chicken breasts
- ¼ cup onion
- 1½ teaspoons extra-virgin olive oil
- 1 14.5-oz. can tomatoes
- 1 teaspoon ginger
- 1 teaspoon fresh lemon juice
- ⅓ cup plain Greek yogurt (fat-free)
- 1 tablespoon garam masala
- ¼ teaspoon salt
- ¼ teaspoon pepper

Directions:
1. Flavor chicken cut into 1-inch cubes with 1.5 teaspoons garam masala, ⅛ teaspoon salt, and pepper.
2. Cook chicken and diced onion for 4 to 5 minutes.
3. Add diced tomatoes, grated ginger, 1½ teaspoon garam masala, ⅛ teaspoon salt. Cook 8 to 10 minutes.
4. Add lemon juice and yogurt until blended.

Nutrition:
Calories: 305
Protein: 25g
Fat:14.57g
Carbs: 21.69g
Sodium: 744mg

313. TOMATO AND ROASTED COD

Preparation Time: 10 minutes
Cooking Time: 35 minutes
Servings: 2
Ingredients:
- 2 4-oz. cod fillets
- 1 cup cherry tomatoes
- ⅔ cup onion
- 2 teaspoons orange rind
- 1 tablespoon extra-virgin olive oil

- 1 teaspoon thyme (dried)
- ¼ teaspoon salt, divided
- ¼ teaspoon pepper, divided

Directions:
1. Preheat oven to 400°F. Mix in half tomatoes, sliced onion, grated orange rind, extra virgin olive oil, dried thyme, and ⅛ salt and pepper. Fry 25 minutes. Remove from oven.
2. Arrange fish on pan, and flavor with remaining ⅛ teaspoon of each salt and pepper. Put reserved tomato mixture over fish. Bake 10 minutes.

Nutrition:
Calories: 189.45
Protein: 21.7g
Fat:8.2g
Carbs: 8.7g
Sodium: 387.85mg

314. BACON AND CHICKEN GARLIC WRAP

Preparation Time: 15 minutes
Cooking Time: 10 minutes
Servings: 4
Ingredients:
- 1 chicken fillet, cut into small cubes
- 8-9 thin slices bacon, cut to fit cubes
- 6 garlic cloves, minced

Directions:
1. Preheat your oven to 400°F
2. Line a baking tray with aluminum foil
3. Add minced garlic to a bowl and rub each chicken piece with it
4. Wrap bacon piece around each garlic chicken bite
5. Secure with toothpick
6. Transfer bites to the baking sheet, keeping a little bit of space between them
7. Bake for about 15-20 minutes until crispy
8. Serve and enjoy!

Nutrition:
Calories: 244.36
Fat: 20.62g
Carbohydrates: 2.13g
Protein: 11.84g
Sodium: 350.64mg

315. GRILLED CHICKEN PLATTER

Preparation Time: 5 minutes
Cooking Time: 10 minutes
Servings: 6
Ingredients:
- 3 large chicken breasts, sliced in half lengthwise

- 10 ounces of frozen spinach, thawed and drained
- 3 ounces of mozzarella cheese, part-skim
- ½ a cup of roasted red peppers, cut in long strips
- 1 teaspoon of olive oil
- 2 garlic cloves, minced
- Salt and pepper as needed

Directions:
1. Preheat your oven to 400°F
2. Slice 3 chicken breast lengthwise
3. Take a non-stick pan and grease with cooking spray
4. Bake for 2-3 minutes on each side
5. Take another skillet and cook spinach and garlic in oil for 3 minutes
6. Place chicken on an oven pan and top with spinach, roasted peppers, and mozzarella
7. Bake until the cheese is melted.

Nutrition:
Calories: 264.38
Fat: 14.7g
Net Carbohydrates: 3.56g
Protein: 30g
Sodium: 349.53mg

316. PARSLEY CHICKEN BREAST

Preparation Time: 10 minutes
Cooking Time: 40 minutes
Servings: 4
Ingredients:
- 1 tablespoon dry parsley
- 1 tablespoon dry basil
- 4 chicken breast halves, boneless and skinless
- ½ teaspoon salt
- ½ teaspoon red pepper flakes, crushed
- 2 tomatoes, sliced

Directions:
1. Preheat your oven to 350°F
2. Take a 9x13 baking dish and grease it up with cooking spray
3. Sprinkle 1 tablespoon of parsley, 1 teaspoon of basil, and spread the mixture over your baking dish
4. Arrange the chicken breast halves over the dish and sprinkle garlic slices on top
5. Take a small bowl and add 1 teaspoon parsley, 1 teaspoon of basil, salt, basil, red pepper and mix well. Pour the mixture over the chicken breast
6. Top with tomato slices and cover, bake for 25 minutes

7. Remove the cover and bake for 15 minutes more
8. Serve and enjoy!

Nutrition:
Calories: 252.21
Fat: 5.4g
Carbohydrates: 2.9g
Protein: 45.58g
Sodium: 385.43mg

317. MUSTARD CHICKEN

Preparation Time: 10 minutes
Cooking Time: 40 minutes
Servings: 4
Ingredients:
- 4 chicken breasts
- ½ cup chicken broth
- 3-4 tablespoons mustard
- 3 tablespoons olive oil
- 1 teaspoon paprika
- 1 teaspoon chili powder
- 1 teaspoon garlic powder

Directions:
1. Take a small bowl and mix mustard, olive oil, paprika, chicken broth, garlic powder, chicken broth, and chili
2. Add chicken breast and marinate for 30 minutes
3. Take a lined baking sheet and arrange the chicken
4. Bake for 35 minutes at 375 Fahrenheit
5. Serve and enjoy!

Nutrition:
Calories: 499.68
Fat: 32.31g
Carbohydrates: 2g
Protein: 48g
Sodium: 403.6mg

318. BALSAMIC CHICKEN

Preparation Time: 10 minutes
Cooking Time: 25 minutes
Servings: 6
Ingredients:
- 6 chicken breast halves, skinless and boneless
- 1 teaspoon garlic salt
- Ground black pepper
- 2 tablespoons olive oil
- 1 onion, thinly sliced
- 14½ ounces tomatoes, diced
- ½ cup balsamic vinegar
- 1 teaspoon dried basil
- 1 teaspoon dried oregano
- 1 teaspoon dried rosemary
- ½ teaspoon dried thyme

Directions:

1. Season both sides of your chicken breasts thoroughly with pepper and garlic salt
2. Take a skillet and place it over medium heat
3. Add some oil and cook your seasoned chicken for 3-4 minutes per side until the breasts are nicely browned
4. Add some onion and cook for another 3-4 minutes until the onions are browned
5. Pour the diced-up tomatoes and balsamic vinegar over your chicken and season with some rosemary, basil, thyme, and rosemary
6. Simmer the chicken for about 15 minutes until they are no longer pink
7. Take an instant-read thermometer and check if the internal temperature gives a reading of 165°F.
8. If yes, then you are good to go!

Nutrition:
Calories: 319.52
Fat: 10.17g
Carbohydrates: 8.2g
Protein: 45.7g
Sodium: 421mg

319. MEATLOAF

Preparation Time: 15 Minutes
Cooking Time: 30 Minutes
Servings: 4
Ingredients:
- ½ lb. ground beef
- 1 egg
- 1 onion
- ¼ lb. carrots
- 1 teaspoon black pepper
- 1 teaspoon chili pepper
- 2 teaspoon olive oil

Directions:
1. Take the ground beef and put it in the big bowl.
2. Add egg, black pepper, and chili pepper. Stir the mixture very carefully.
3. Peel the carrot and onion and chop both.
4. Add the chopped carrot and onion to the bowl with meat and stir it carefully.
5. Preheat the oven air fryer to 390°F (200°C).
6. Meanwhile, take the tray and spray it inside with olive oil. Make the loaf from the meat and put it on the tray.
7. Lay the tray in the oven and cook it for 30 minutes.

Nutrition:
Calories: 198
Protein: 24.7 g
Fat: 8.1 g
Sodium: 71.65mg
Carbohydrates: 5.6 g

320. BEEF WITH MUSHROOMS

Preparation Time: 15 Minutes
Cooking Time: 40 Minutes
Servings: 4
Ingredients:
- ½ lb. beef
- 1/3 lb. mushrooms
- 1 onion
- 1 teaspoon olive oil
- ½ c. vegetable broth
- 1 teaspoon basil
- 1 teaspoon chili
- 2 tablespoons tomato juice

Directions:
1. For this recipe, you should take a solid piece of beef. Take the beef and pierce the meat with a knife.
2. Rub it with olive oil, basil, and chili, and lemon juice.
3. Chop the onion and mushrooms and pour them with vegetable broth.
4. Cook the vegetables for 5 minutes.
5. Take a big tray and put the meat on it. Add vegetable broth to the tray too.
6. Preheat the air fryer oven to 350°F and cook it for 35 minutes.

Nutrition:
Calories: 102.67
Protein: 13.79 g
Fat: 3.8 g
Carbohydrates: 4.16 g
Sodium: 140.35mg

321. QUICK & JUICY PORK CHOPS

Preparation Time: 10 minutes
Cooking Time: 12 minutes
Servings: 4
Ingredients:
- 4 pork chops
- 1 teaspoon olive oil
- 1 teaspoon onion powder
- 1 teaspoon paprika
- Pepper
- Salt

Directions:
1. Cover pork chops with olive oil and season with paprika, onion powder, pepper, and salt.

2. Set a dehydrating tray in a multi-level air fryer basket and place the basket in the instant pot.
3. Place pork chops on dehydrating tray.
4. Seal the pot with the air fryer cover, then set the temperature to 400°F and set the timer for 12 minutes. Turn pork chops halfway through.
5. Serve and enjoy.

Nutrition:
Calories: 270
Fat: 21.1 g
Carbohydrates: 0.8 g
Sugar 0.3 g
Sodium: 277.19mg
Protein: 18.1 g
Cholesterol: 69 mg

322. DELICIOUS & TENDER PORK CHOPS

Preparation Time: 10 minutes
Cooking Time: 12 minutes
Servings: 2
Ingredients:
- 2 pork chops
- 1 tablespoon olive oil
- ¼ teaspoon garlic powder
- ½ teaspoon onion powder
- 1 teaspoon ground mustard
- 1½ teaspoon pepper
- 1 tablespoon paprika
- 2 tablespoons brown sugar
- 1½ teaspoon salt

Directions:
1. In a small container, mix garlic powder, onion powder, mustard, paprika, pepper, brown sugar, and salt.
2. Cover pork chops with olive oil and rub with spice mixture.
3. Set a dehydrating tray in a multi-level air fryer basket and place the basket in the instant pot.
4. Place pork chops on dehydrating tray.
5. Seal the pot with the air fryer cover, then set the temperature to 400°F and the timer for 12 minutes. Turn pork chops halfway through.
6. Serve and enjoy.

Nutrition:
Calories: 375
Fat: 27.9 g
Carbohydrates: 13.1 g
Sugar 9.5 g
Protein: 19.2 g
Sodium: 1833mg
Cholesterol: 69 mg

323. PERFECT PORK CHOPS

Preparation Time: 10 minutes
Cooking Time: 15 minutes
Servings: 4
Ingredients:
- 4 pork chops
- Pepper
- Salt

Directions:
1. Season pork chops with pepper and salt.
2. Set a dehydrating tray in a multi-level air fryer basket and place the basket in the instant pot.
3. Place pork chops on dehydrating tray.
4. Seal the pot with the air fryer cover, then set the temperature to 400°F and the timer for 15 minutes. Turn pork chops halfway through.
5. Serve and enjoy.

Nutrition:
Calories: 256
Fat: 19.9 g
Protein: 18 g
Sodium: 276.34mg
Cholesterol: 69 mg

324. HERB BUTTER LAMB CHOPS

Preparation Time: 10 minutes
Cooking Time: 5 minutes
Servings: 4
Ingredients:
- 4 lamb chops
- 1 teaspoon rosemary, diced
- 1 tablespoon unsalted butter
- Pepper
- Salt

Directions:
1. Season lamb chops with pepper and salt.
2. Set the dehydrating tray in a multi-level air fryer basket and place the basket in the instant pot.
3. Place lamb chops on dehydrating tray.
4. Seal the pot with the air fryer cover, then set the temperature to 400°F and the timer for 5 minutes.
5. Spread butter and rosemary mixture over cooked lamb chops.
6. Serve and enjoy.

Nutrition:
Calories: 256.35
Fat: 20.69 g
Carbohydrates: 0.34 g
Protein: 17.49 g
Cholesterol: 129 mg

Sodium: 267.26mg

325. ZA'ATAR LAMB CHOPS

Preparation Time: 10 minutes
Cooking Time: 10 minutes
Servings: 4
Ingredients:
- 4 lamb loin chops
- ½ tablespoon Za'atar
- 1 tablespoon fresh lemon juice
- 1 teaspoon olive oil
- 2 garlic cloves, minced
- Pepper
- Salt

Directions:
1. Rub the lamb chops with Za'atar, garlic, pepper, and salt after coating them with oil and lemon juice.
2. Set a dehydrating tray in a multi-level air fryer basket, then in the instant pot.
3. Place lamb chops on dehydrating tray.
4. Seal the pot with the air fryer cover, then set the temperature to 400°F and the timer for 10 minutes. Halfway through, turn the lamb chops.
5. Serve and enjoy.

Nutrition:
Calories: 316.8
Fat: 27.71 g
Carbohydrates: 1.3 g
Sugar: 0.1 g
Protein: 15.68 g
Cholesterol: 69 mg
Sodium: 259.56mg

326. PORK CHOPS WITH GRAPE SAUCE

Preparation Time: 15 minutes
Cooking Time: 25 minutes
Servings: 4
Ingredients:
- Cooking spray
- 4 pork chops
- ¼ cup onion, sliced
- 1 clove garlic, minced
- ½ cup low-sodium chicken broth
- ¾ cup apple juice
- 1 tablespoon cornstarch
- 1 cup seedless red grapes, sliced in half
- 1 tablespoon balsamic vinegar
- 1 teaspoon honey

Directions:
1. Spray oil on your pan.
2. Put it over medium heat.
3. Add the pork chops to the pan.
4. Cook for 5 minutes per side.

5. Remove and set aside.
6. Add onion and garlic.
7. Cook for 2 minutes.
8. Pour in the broth and apple juice.
9. Bring to a boil.
10. Reduce heat to simmer.
11. Put the pork chops back to the skillet.
12. Simmer for 4 minutes.
13. In a bowl, mix the cornstarch, vinegar, and honey.
14. Add to the pan.
15. Cook until the sauce has thickened.
16. Add the grapes.
17. Pour sauce over the pork chops before serving.

Nutrition:
Calories: 188
Total Fat: 4 g
Saturated Fat: 1 g
Cholesterol: 47 mg
Sodium: 117 mg
Total Carbohydrates: 18 g
Dietary Fiber: 1 g
Total Sugar: 13 g
Protein: 19 g
Potassium: 759 mg

327. PORK CHOPS WITH APPLE STUFFING

Preparation Time: 20 minutes
Cooking Time: 45–60 minutes
Servings: 6
Ingredients:
- ¼ cup chopped celery
- ¼ cup chopped onion
- ¼ cup sugar
- ¼ teaspoon pepper
- ¼ teaspoon salt
- ½ cup breadcrumbs or cracker crumbs
- 1 tablespoon canola oil
- 2 teaspoon chopped parsley
- 3 apples, peeled, cored, and diced
- 6 bone-in pork chops, at least 1 inch thick, and Approximately 2 lbs. total

Directions:
1. Chop a pocket approximately 1½-inch deep into the side of each chop for stuffing.
2. Heat oil in a frying pan.
3. Stir celery and onion into oil in a frying pan. Cook over moderate until soft, stirring regularly.
4. Mix in diced apples. Drizzle with sugar.
5. Cover frying pan. Cook apples over low heat until soft and glazed.

6. Mix in breadcrumbs.
7. Mix in salt, pepper, and parsley.
8. Spreading open the pocket in each chop with your fingers, stuff with mixture.
9. Place half of the stuffed chops in a frying pan. Brown on both sides over moderate to high heat.
10. Take out browned chops to the platter. Cover to keep warm.
11. Repeat Step 9 with residual chops.
12. Return other chops to the frying pan.
13. Reduce heat. Put in a few tablespoons of water.
14. Cover. Cook slowly over low heat until done, approximately 20–25 minutes.

Nutrition:
Calories: 270
Total Fat: 9 g
Cholesterol: 65 mg
Total Carb 24 g
Dietary Fiber: 1 g
Sodium: 232mg
Sugars 16 g
Protein: 24 g

328. SIMPLE BARBECUE PORK CHOPS

Preparation Time: 5 minutes
Cooking Time: 5 hours
Servings: 4
Ingredients:
- 3 lbs. bone-in thick-cut pork chops
- 2–3 tablespoons barbecue seasoning
- ¼ cup water

Directions:
1. Cover each side of each pork chop with barbecue seasoning. Put them in the slow cooker.
2. Pour the water around the outside of the pork chops.
3. Close the lid and cook on low for approximately 5 hours.

Nutrition:
Calories: 446
Total Fat: 23 g
Cholesterol: 176 mg
Total Carb: 1.8 g
Protein: 53.27 g
Sodium: 541.53mg

329. SWEET-SOUR PORK

Preparation Time: 30 minutes
Cooking Time: 5–7 hours
Servings: 6
Ingredients:

- ¼ cup cider vinegar
- ¼ cup water
- ½ medium onion, thinly sliced
- ¾ cup shredded carrots
- 1 cup pineapple juice (reserved from pineapple chunks)
- 1 green bell pepper, cut into strips
- 1 tablespoon soy sauce
- 2 lbs. boneless pork shoulder, cut in strips, trimmed of fat
- 2 tablespoon brown sugar substitute to equal 1 tablespoon sugar
- 2 tablespoons coarsely chopped sweet pickles
- 2 tablespoons cornstarch
- 20-oz. can pineapple chunks in juice

Directions:
1. Place pork strips in the crockpot.
2. Put in green pepper, onion, carrots, and pickles.
3. In a vessel, combine brown sugar and cornstarch. Put in water, pineapple juice, vinegar, and soy sauce. Stir until smooth.
4. Pour over ingredients in crockpot.
5. Cover. Cook on low for approximately 5–7 hours. One hour before serving, add pineapple chunks. Stir.

Nutrition:
Calories: 270
Total Fat: 8 g
Cholesterol: 75 mg
Sodium: 285 mg
Total Carb 27 g
Dietary Fiber: 2 g
Sugars 21 g
Protein: 22 g

330. YUMMY PULLED PORK

Preparation Time: 20 minutes
Cooking Time: 4½–10¾ hours
Servings: 10
Ingredients:
- ½ cup water
- 1 cup barbecue sauce of your choice
- 1 teaspoon cumin
- 2 tablespoons Worcestershire sauce
- 2½ lb. boneless pork shoulder roast, or pork sirloin roast
- 3 tablespoons cider vinegar
- Salt and pepper, to taste

Directions:
1. Trim fat from roast. Fit roast into crockpot.

2. Sprinkle meat with salt and pepper.
3. In a small vessel, mix water, vinegar, Worcestershire sauce, and cumin. Spoon over roast, being cautious not to wash off the seasonings.
4. Cover. Cook on low for approximately 8–10 hours, or on High for 4–5 hours, just until pork is very soft but not dry.
5. Take out meat onto a platter. Discard liquid.
6. Shred meat using 2 forks. Put back into the crockpot.
7. Mix in barbecue sauce.
8. Cover. Cook on high heat for approximately 30–45 minutes

Nutrition:
Calories: 190
Total Fat: 3 g
Cholesterol: 70 mg
Sodium: 280 mg
Total Carbohydrates 12 g
Sugar: 10 g
Protein: 26 g

331. SPICY BRISKET

Preparation Time: 5 minutes
Cooking Time: 110 minutes
Servings: 10
Ingredients:
- 3 teaspoon salt
- 2 teaspoons pepper
- 1 teaspoon garlic powder
- 1 teaspoon dried thyme
- ½ teaspoon dried rosemary
- 1 5-pound beef brisket
- 1 tablespoon avocado oil
- 1 cup beef broth
- ½ cup pickled jalapeño juice
- ½ cup pickled jalapeños
- ½ onion, chopped

Directions:
1. In a bowl, combine rosemary, thyme, garlic powder, pepper, and salt.
2. Rub the brisket with the mixture and set it aside.
3. Warm the avocado oil over Sauté in the Instant Pot.
4. Sear each side of the brisket for 5 minutes.
5. Add onions, jalapeños, jalapeño juice, and broth to the Instant Pot.
6. Close the lid and press Manual.
7. Cook for 100 minutes.
8. Do a natural release for 30 to 40 minutes. Avoid quick release.
9. Remove brisket and slice.

10. Pour with the strained broth and serve.

Nutrition:
Calories: 506
Fat: 38g
Carbohydrates: 2.89g
Protein: 35.7g
Sodium: 1109mg
Sugar: 0.22g

332. LIME PULLED PORK

Preparation Time: 5 minutes
Cooking Time: 30 minutes
Servings: 4
Ingredients:
- 1 tablespoon chili adobo sauce
- 1 tablespoon chili powder
- 2 teaspoon salt
- 1 teaspoon garlic powder
- 1 teaspoon cumin
- ½ teaspoon pepper
- 2½ to 3 pounds cubed pork butt
- 1 tablespoon coconut oil
- 2 cups beef broth
- 1 lime, cut into wedges
- ¼ cup chopped cilantro

Directions:
1. In a bowl, mix pepper, cumin, garlic powder, salt, chili powder, and sauce.
2. Melt the oil on Sauté in the Instant Pot.
3. Rub the pork with a spice mixture.
4. Place pork and sear for 3 to 5 minutes per side.
5. Add broth and close the lid.
6. Press the Manual and cook for 30 minutes.
7. Do a natural release and open.
8. Shred pork.
9. If you want crispy pork, then heat in a skillet until the pork is crisp.
10. Serve warm with cilantro garnish and fresh lime wedges.

Nutrition:
Calories: 537
Fat: 35g
Carbohydrates: .47g
Protein: 46.9g
Sodium: 1976mg

333. CHIPOTLE PORK CHOPS

Preparation Time: 7 minutes
Cooking Time: 15 minutes
Servings: 4
Ingredients:
- 2 tablespoon coconut oil
- 3 chipotle chilies
- 2 tablespoon adobo sauce

- 2 teaspoon cumin
- 1 teaspoon dried thyme
- 1 teaspoon salt
- 4 5-ounce boneless pork chops
- ½ onion, chopped
- 2 bay leaves
- 1 cup chicken broth
- ½ 7-ounce can fire-roasted diced tomatoes
- ⅓ cup chopped cilantro

Directions:
1. Melt the oil on Sauté in the Instant Pot.
2. In a food processor, add salt, thyme, cumin, sauce, and chilies. Pulse to make a paste.
3. Rub paste into the pork chops.
4. Sear the chops for 5 minutes on each side.
5. Add cilantro, tomatoes, broth, bay leaves, and onion to the Instant Pot.
6. Close the lid and press Manual.
7. Cook 15 minutes on High.
8. Do a natural release when done.
9. Serve warm with cilantro garnish.

Nutrition:
Calories: 364
Fat: 20.2g
Sodium: 985.4mg
Carbohydrates: 12.15g
Protein: 31.3g

334. BUTTERY POT ROAST

Preparation Time: 5 minutes
Cooking Time: 90 minutes
Servings: 4
Ingredients:
- 4 teaspoon onion powder
- 2 teaspoon dried parsley
- 1 teaspoon salt
- 1 teaspoon garlic powder
- ½ teaspoon dried oregano
- ½ teaspoon pepper
- 1 2-pound chuck roast
- 1 tablespoon coconut oil
- 1 cup beef broth
- ½ packet dry ranch seasoning
- 1 stick butter
- 10 pepperoncini

Directions:
1. Press Sauté and heat Instant Pot.
2. In a bowl, mix pepper, oregano, garlic powder, salt, parsley, and onion powder.
3. Rub the seasoning onto the roast.
4. Add oil to the pot and place roast.

5. Sear for 5 minutes on each side.
6. Remove roast and set aside.
7. Add broth and deglaze.
8. Place roast back into the Instant Pot.
9. Sprinkle with ranch powder.
10. Place butter on top and add pepperoncini.
11. Close the lid and press Manual.
12. Cook 90 minutes.
13. Do a natural release.
14. Remove lid and remove the roast.
15. Slice and serve.

Nutrition:
Calories: 765
Fat: 63g
Carbohydrates: 8.6g
Protein: 40.5g
Sodium: 1206mg

335. CREAMY MUSHROOM POT ROAST

Preparation Time: 10 minutes
Cooking Time: 90 minutes
Servings: 6
Ingredients:
- 1 cup button mushrooms, sliced
- ½ cup onion, sliced
- 1 tablespoon coconut oil
- 2 tablespoons dried minced onion
- 2 teaspoons dried parsley
- 1 teaspoon pepper
- 1 teaspoon garlic powder
- ½ teaspoon dried oregano
- 1 teaspoon salt
- 1 2-3 pound Chuck roast
- 1 cup beef broth
- 4 tablespoons unsalted butter
- 2 oz. cream cheese
- ¼ cup heavy cream

Directions:
1. Press the Sauté button in your Instant Pot and add oil, onion, and mushrooms.
2. Cook for 5 minutes.
3. In a bowl, mix salt, oregano, garlic, pepper, parsley, and minced onion and rub into the chuck roast.
4. Press Cancel and add the roast and broth into the pot.
5. Place butter and cream cheese on top.
6. Close the lid and press Meal.
7. Cook for 90 minutes.
8. Do a natural release when done.
9. Stir in heavy cream.
10. Remove roast and press Sauté.

11. Reduce the sauce for 10 minutes.
12. Serve roast with the sauce.

Nutrition:
Calories: 504
Fat: 41g
Carbohydrates: 4.9g
Protein: 27.6g
Sodium: 656.06mg

336. SALISBURY STEAK IN MUSHROOM SAUCE

Preparation Time: 10 minutes
Cooking Time: 15 minutes
Servings: 4
Ingredients:
- 1 pound 85% lean ground beef
- 1 teaspoon steak seasoning
- 1 egg
- 2 tablespoons unsalted butter
- ½ onion, sliced
- ½ cup button mushrooms, sliced
- 1 cup beef broth
- 2 oz. cream cheese
- ¼ cup heavy cream
- ¼ teaspoon Xanthan gum

Directions:
1. Mix egg, steak seasoning, and ground beef in a bowl. Make 4 patties and set them aside.
2. Press Sauté and melt the butter.
3. Add mushrooms and onion and cook for 3 to 5 minutes.
4. Press Cancel and add beef patties, broth, and cream cheese to the Instant Pot.
5. Close the lid and press Manual.
6. Cook 15 minutes on High.
7. Do a natural release when done.
8. Remove the patties and set them aside.
9. Add xanthan gum and heavy cream. Whisk to mix.
10. Reduce the sauce on Sauté for 5 to 10 minutes.
11. Press Cancel and add patties back to the Instant Pot.
12. Serve.

Nutrition:
Calories: 382.19
Fat: 28.51g
Carbohydrates: 2.4g
Protein: 24.6g
Sodium: 416.33mg

337. BRISKET WITH CAULIFLOWER

Preparation Time: 5 minutes
Cooking Time: 15 minutes
Servings: 4

Ingredients:
- 1 cup water
- 2 cups fresh cauliflower, chopped
- 3 tablespoons unsalted butter
- ¼ onion, diced
- ¼ cup pickled jalapeño slices
- 2 cups cooked brisket
- 2 oz. softened cream cheese
- 1 cup shredded sharp cheddar cheese
- ¼ cup heavy cream
- ¼ cup cooked crumbled bacon
- 2 tablespoons sliced green onions

Directions:
1. Add water to the Instant Pot.
2. Steam the cauliflower on a steamer basket for 1 minute.
3. Do a quick release and set aside.
4. Pour out water and press Sauté.
5. Add butter, jalapeño slices, and onion.
6. Sauté for 4 minutes, add cream cheese and cooked brisket.
7. Cook 2 minutes more.
8. Add cauliflower, heavy cream, and sharp cheddar.
9. Press Cancel and gently mix until mixed well.
10. Sprinkle with green onions, and crumbled bacon.
11. Serve.

Nutrition:
Calories: 535.58
Fat: 46.4g
Carbohydrates: 7.9g
Protein: 24.07g
Sodium: 383.82mg

338. PORK CHOPS IN MUSHROOM GRAVY

Preparation Time: 5 minutes
Cooking Time: 15 minutes
Servings: 4
Ingredients:
- 4 5-ounce pork chops
- 1 teaspoon salt
- ½ teaspoon pepper
- 2 tablespoons Avocado oil
- 1 cup button mushrooms, chopped
- ½ onion, sliced
- 1 clove minced garlic
- 1 cup chicken broth
- ¼ cup heavy cream
- 4 tablespoon unsalted butter
- ¼ teaspoon Xanthan gum
- 1 tablespoon chopped fresh parsley

Directions:

1. Rub the pork chops with salt and pepper.
2. Heat the avocado oil in the Instant Pot and Sauté.
3. Add mushroom and sauté for 3 to 5 minutes.
4. Add pork chops and onion and sauté for 3 minutes.
5. Add broth and garlic and close the lid.
6. Press Manual and cook 15 minutes on High.
7. Do a natural release.
8. Remove lid and place pork chops on a plate.
9. Press Sauté and add xanthan gum, butter, and heavy cream.
10. Reduce the sauce for 5 to 10 minutes.
11. Add pork chops back into the pot.
12. Serve chops topped with parsley and sauce.

Nutrition:
Calories: 411.8
Fat: 33.23g
Carbohydrates: 4.55g
Protein: 24g

Sodium: 874.47mg

339. BEEF AND SPAGHETTI SQUASH CASSEROLE

Preparation Time: 10 minutes
Cooking Time: 20 minutes
Servings: 4
Ingredients:

- 6 pounds spaghetti squash, cooked and scraped out into long strands with a fork
- 1 cup no sugar added tomato sauce
- ½ cup whole milk ricotta
- ¼ cup grated Parmesan cheese
- 3 tablespoons unsalted butter
- ½ teaspoon dried parsley
- ½ teaspoon garlic powder
- ¼ teaspoon dried basil
- ½ teaspoon salt
- ¼ teaspoon pepper
- 1 pound 85% lean ground beef, cooked
- 1 cup shredded mozzarella cheese, divided

- 1 cup water

Directions:
1. Place the squash into a oven-safe bowl.
2. Add remaining ingredients except for water (reserve ½ mozzarella) and mix.
3. Sprinkle the remaining cheese on top and cover with a foil.
4. Pour water into the Instant Pot and place steam rack.
5. Place bowl on the steam rack and close the lid.
6. Press the Manual and cook for 10 minutes.
7. Do a natural release.
8. You can broil the dish in the oven for a few minutes to brown the top.
9. Serve.

Nutrition:
Calories: 580
Fat: 33.28g
Carbohydrates: 37.6g
Protein: 36.5g
Sodium: 957mg

SIDES

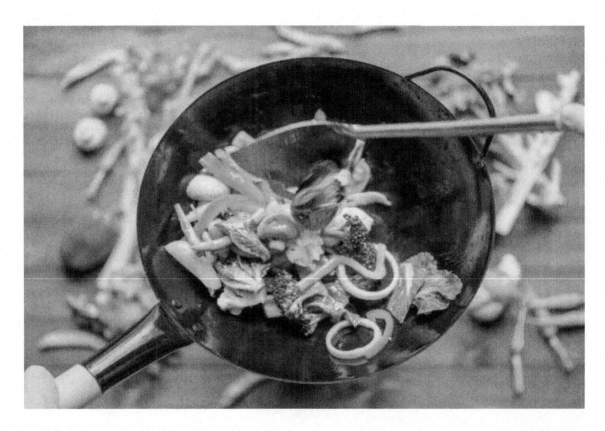

340. ROASTED TOMATO BRUSSELS SPROUTS

Preparation Time: 15 minutes
Cooking Time: 20 minutes
Servings: 4
Ingredients:
- 1 pound (454 g) Brussels sprouts
- 1 tablespoon extra-virgin olive oil
- ½ cup sun-dried tomatoes
- 2 tablespoons lemon juice
- 1 teaspoon lemon zest

Directions:
1. Set oven to 400°F (205ºC). Prep large baking sheet with aluminum foil.
2. Toss the Brussels sprouts in the olive oil in a large bowl until well coated. Sprinkle with salt and pepper.
3. Spread out the seasoned Brussels sprouts on the prepared baking sheet in a single layer.
4. Roast for 20 minutes, shaking halfway through.
5. Remove from the oven then pour in a bowl. Whisk tomatoes, lemon juice, and lemon zest and add. Serve immediately.

Nutrition:
Calories:96.8
Carbohydrates: 13.9g
Fiber: 4.1g
Sodium: 34.11mg

341. SIMPLE SAUTÉED GREENS

Preparation Time: 10 minutes
Cooking Time: 10 minutes
Servings: 4
Ingredients:
- 2 tablespoons extra-virgin olive oil
- 1 pound (454 g) Swiss chard
- 1 pound (454 g) kale
- ½ teaspoon ground cardamom
- 1 tablespoon lemon juice

Directions:
1. Heat up olive oil in a big skillet over medium-high heat.
2. Stir in Swiss chard, kale, cardamom, lemon juice to the skillet, and stir to combine. Cook for about 10 minutes, stirring continuously, or until the greens are wilted.
3. Sprinkle with salt and pepper and stir well.
4. Serve the greens on a plate while warm.

Nutrition:
Calories: 125.61
Carbohydrates: 11.69g
Fiber: 4.78g
Sodium: 254.56mg

342. GARLICKY MUSHROOMS

Preparation Time: 10 minutes
Cooking Time: 12 minutes
Servings: 4
Ingredients:
- 1 tablespoon unsalted butter
- 2 teaspoons extra-virgin olive oil
- 2 pounds button mushrooms
- 2 teaspoons minced fresh garlic
- 1 teaspoon chopped fresh thyme

Directions:
1. Warm up butter and olive oil in a large skillet over medium-high heat.
2. Add the mushrooms and sauté for 10 minutes, stirring occasionally.
3. Stir in the garlic and thyme and cook for an additional 2 minutes.
4. Season and serve on a plate.

Nutrition:
Calories: 111.98
Carbohydrates: 12.31g
Fiber: 5g
Sodium: 5.22mg

343. GREEN BEANS IN OVEN

Preparation Time: 5 minutes
Cooking Time: 17 minutes
Servings: 3
Ingredients:
- 12 oz. green beans
- 1 tablespoon olive oil
- ½ teaspoon onion powder
- ⅛ teaspoon pepper
- ⅛ teaspoon salt

Directions:
1. Preheat oven to 350°F. Mix green beans with onion powder, pepper, and oil.
2. Spread the seeds on the baking sheet.
3. Bake for 17 minutes or until you have a delicious aroma in the kitchen.
4. Serve straight away.

Nutrition:
Calories: 78.75
Fat: 5g
Protein: 2.13g
Sodium: 104.11mg
Carbs: 8.28g

344. CAULIFLOWER RICE

Preparation Time: 10 minutes
Cooking Time: 27 minutes
Servings: 3

Ingredients:
For the Tofu:
- 1 cup diced carrot
- 6 ounces tofu, extra-firm, drained
- ½ cup diced white onion
- 2 tablespoons soy sauce
- 1 teaspoon turmeric

For the Cauliflower:
- ½ cup chopped broccoli
- 3 cups cauliflower rice
- 1 tablespoon minced garlic
- ½ cup frozen peas
- 1 tablespoon minced ginger
- 2 tablespoons soy sauce
- 1 tablespoon apple cider vinegar
- 1½ teaspoon toasted sesame oil

Directions:
1. Switch on the air fryer, insert fryer pan, grease it with olive oil, then shut the lid. Set the fryer at 370°F and preheat for 5 minutes.
2. Meanwhile, place tofu in a bowl, crumble it, then add remaining ingredients and stir until mixed.
3. Open the fryer, add tofu mixture in it, spray with oil, close with its lid and cook for 10 minutes until nicely golden and crispy, stirring halfway through the frying.
4. Meanwhile, place all the ingredients for cauliflower in a bowl and toss until mixed.
5. When the air fryer beeps, open its lid, add cauliflower mixture, shake the pan gently to mix, and continue cooking for 12 minutes, shaking halfway through the frying.
6. Serve straight away.

Nutrition:
Calories: 153
Fat: 5.59g
Protein: 9.78g
Carbs: 18.99g
Sodium: 691mg

345. AIR-FRIED BRUSSELS SPROUTS

Preparation Time: 5 minutes
Cooking Time: 10 minutes
Servings: 2
Ingredients:
- 2 cups Brussels sprouts
- ¼ teaspoon sea salt
- 1 tablespoon olive oil
- 1 tablespoon apple cider vinegar

Directions:
1. Switch on the air fryer, insert fryer basket, grease it with olive oil, then shut its lid. Set the fryer to 400°F and preheat for 5 minutes.
2. Meanwhile, cut the sprouts lengthwise into ¼-inch pieces, add them to a bowl, add remaining ingredients and toss until well-coated.
3. Open the fryer, add sprouts to it, close its lid and cook for 10 minutes until crispy and cooked, shaking halfway through the frying.
4. When the air fryer beeps, open the lid, transfer sprouts onto a serving plate, and serve.

Nutrition:
Calories: 102.38
Fat: 7.39g
Protein: 2.97g
Sodium: 259mg
Carbs: 7.9g

346. GREEN BEANS

Preparation Time: 5 minutes
Cooking Time: 13 minutes
Servings: 4
Ingredients:
- 1 pound green beans
- ¾ teaspoon garlic powder
- ¾ teaspoon ground black pepper
- 1¼ teaspoon salt
- ½ teaspoon paprika

Directions:
1. Switch on the air fryer, insert fryer basket, grease it with olive oil, then close the lid, set the fryer at 400°F, and preheat for 5 minutes.
2. Meanwhile, place beans in a bowl, spray generously with olive oil, sprinkle with garlic powder, black pepper, salt, and paprika and toss until well-coated.
3. Open the fryer, add green beans to it, close with its lid and cook for 8 minutes until nicely golden and crispy, shaking halfway through the frying.
4. When the air fryer beeps, open the lid, transfer green beans onto a serving plate and serve.

Nutrition:
Calories: 38.97
Fat: 0.3g
Protein: 2.26g
Carbs: 8.76g
Sodium: 734mg

347. ASPARAGUS AVOCADO SOUP

Preparation Time: 10 minutes
Cooking Time: 20 minutes
Servings: 4
Ingredients:

- 1 avocado, peeled, pitted, cubed
- 12 ounces asparagus
- ½ teaspoon ground black pepper
- 1 teaspoon garlic powder
- 1 teaspoon sea salt
- 2 tablespoons olive oil, divided
- ½ of a lemon, juiced
- 2 cups vegetable stock

Directions:

1. Switch on the air fryer, insert fryer basket, grease it with olive oil, then shut its lid. Set the fryer at 425°F and preheat for 5 minutes.
2. Meanwhile, place asparagus in a shallow dish, drizzle with 1 tablespoon oil, sprinkle with garlic powder, salt, and black pepper, and toss until well-mixed.
3. Open the fryer, add asparagus to it and cook for 10 minutes until nicely golden and roasted, shaking halfway through the frying.
4. When the air fryer beeps, open its lid and transfer asparagus to a food processor.
5. Add remaining ingredients into a food processor and pulse until well combined and smooth.
6. Tip the soup into a saucepan, pour in water if the soup is too thick, and heat it over medium-low heat for 5 minutes until thoroughly heated.
7. Ladle soup into bowls and serve.

Nutrition:
Calories: 131.48
Fat: 11.39g
Protein: 2.5g
Sodium: 829.94mg
Carbs: 7.25g

348. COFFEE-STEAMED CARROTS

Preparation Time: 10 minutes
Cooking Time: 3 minutes
Servings: 4
Ingredients:

- 1 cup brewed coffee
- 1 teaspoon light brown sugar
- ½ teaspoon kosher salt
- Freshly ground black pepper

- 1 pound baby carrots
- Chopped fresh parsley
- 1 teaspoon grated lemon zest

Directions:

1. Pour the coffee into an electric pressure cooker. Stir in the brown sugar, salt, and pepper. Add the carrots.
2. Close the pressure cooker. Set to sealing.
3. Cook on high pressure for 3 minutes.
4. Once complete, click Cancel and quickly release the pressure.
5. Once the pin drops, open and remove the lid.
6. Using a slotted spoon, portion carrots to a serving bowl. Topped with the parsley and lemon zest and serve.

Nutrition:
Calories: 45.81
Carbohydrates: 10.7g
Fiber: 3.45g
Sodium: 322.64mg

349. ROSEMARY POTATOES

Preparation Time: 5 minutes
Cooking Time: 25 minutes
Servings: 2
Ingredients:

- 1 lb red potatoes
- 1 cup vegetable stock
- 2 tablespoons olive oil
- 2 tablespoons rosemary sprigs

Directions:

1. Place potatoes in the steamer basket and add the stock into the Instant Pot.
2. Steam the potatoes in your Instant Pot for 15 minutes.
3. Depressurize and pour away the remaining stock.
4. Set to sauté and add the oil, rosemary, and potatoes.
5. Cook until brown.

Nutrition:
Calories: 263
Carbohydrates: 31g
Fat: 14.7g
Sodium: 386.61mg

350. CORN ON THE COB

Preparation Time: 10 minutes
Cooking Time: 5 minutes
Servings: 12
Ingredients:

- 6 ears corn
- 1 Cup water

Directions:

1. Take off husks and silk from the corn. Cut or break each ear in half.
2. Pour 1 cup of water into the bottom of the electric pressure cooker. Insert a wire rack or trivet.
3. Place the corn upright on the rack, cut side down. Seal lid of the pressure cooker.
4. Cook on high pressure for 5 minutes.
5. When it's complete, select Cancel and quick release the pressure.
6. When the pin drops, unlock and take off the lid.
7. Pull out the corn from the pot. Season as desired and serve immediately.

Nutrition:
Calories: 15.79
Carbohydrates: 3.4g
Fiber: 0.37g
Sodium: 3.15mg

351. CHILI LIME SALMON

Preparation Time: 6 minutes
Cooking Time: 10 minutes
Servings: 2
Ingredients:
For Sauce:

- 1 jalapeño pepper
- 1 tablespoon chopped parsley
- 1 teaspoon minced garlic
- ½ teaspoon cumin
- ½ teaspoon paprika
- ½ teaspoon lime zest
- 1 tablespoon honey
- 1 tablespoon lime juice
- 1 tablespoon olive oil
- 1 tablespoon water

For Fish:

- 2 salmon fillets, each about 5 ounces
- 1 cup water
- ½ teaspoon salt
- ⅛ teaspoon ground black pepper

Directions:

1. Prepare salmon and for this, season salmon with salt and black pepper until evenly coated.
2. Plug in Instant Pot, insert the inner pot, pour in water, then place steamer basket and place seasoned salmon on it.
3. Close lid, press the steam button, then press the timer to set the cooking time to 5 minutes and cook on high pressure, for 5 minutes.

4. Transfer all the ingredients for the sauce to a bowl, whisk until combined, and set aside.
5. When the timer beeps, press the cancel button and do a quick pressure release until the pressure nob drops down.
6. Open the Instant Pot, then transfer salmon to a serving plate and drizzle generously with prepared sauce.
7. Serve immediately.

Nutrition:
Calories: 370
Carbohydrates: 11g
Fiber: 0.6g
Sodium: 655.48mg

352. COLLARD GREENS

Preparation Time: 5 minutes
Cooking Time: 6 hours
Servings: 12
Ingredients:
- 2 pounds chopped collard greens
- ¾ cup chopped white onion
- 1 teaspoon onion powder
- 1 teaspoon garlic powder
- 1 teaspoon salt
- 2 teaspoons brown sugar
- ½ teaspoon ground black pepper
- ½ teaspoon red chili powder
- ¼ teaspoon crushed red pepper flakes
- 3 tablespoons apple cider vinegar
- 2 tablespoons olive oil
- 14.5 ounces vegetable broth
- ½ cup water

Directions:
1. Plug in Instant Pot, insert the inner pot, add onion and collard, and then pour in vegetable broth and water.
2. Close lid, seal, press the slow cook button, then set the cooking time to 6 hours at high heat setting.
3. When the timer beeps, press the cancel button and do a natural pressure release until the pressure nob drops down.
4. Open the pot, add remaining ingredients and stir until mixed.
5. Then press the sauté/simmer button and cook for 3 minutes or more until collards reach to desired texture.
6. Serve straight away.

Nutrition:
Calories: 41.28
Carbohydrates: 4.88g

Fiber: 0.98g
Sodium: 309.35mg

353. MASHED PUMPKIN

Preparation Time: 9 minutes
Cooking Time: 15 minutes
Servings: 2
Ingredients:
- 2 cups chopped pumpkin
- ½ cup water
- 2 tablespoons powdered sugar-free sweetener of choice
- 1 tablespoon cinnamon

Directions:
1. Place the pumpkin and water in your Instant Pot.
2. Seal and cook on stew setting for 15 minutes.
3. Remove and combine with the sweetener and cinnamon.

Nutrition:
Calories: 70.1
Carbohydrates: 18.44g
Sugar: 10.9g
Sodium: 2.9mg

354. AROMATIC TOASTED PUMPKIN SEEDS

Preparation Time: 5 minutes
Cooking Time: 45 minutes
Servings: 4
Ingredients:
- 1 cup pumpkin seeds
- 1 teaspoon cinnamon
- 2 packets Stevia
- 1 tablespoon canola oil
- ¼ teaspoon sea salt

Directions:
1. Prep the oven to 300°F (150°C).
2. Combine the pumpkin seeds with cinnamon, Stevia, canola oil, and salt in a bowl. Stir to mix well.
3. Pour the seeds in a single layer on a baking sheet, then arrange the sheet in the preheated oven.
4. Bake for 45 minutes or until well toasted and fragrant. Shake the sheet twice to bake the seeds evenly.
5. Serve immediately.

Nutrition:
Calories: 121
Carbohydrates: 3.23g
Sodium: 119.48mg
Fiber: 1.3g

355. BACON-WRAPPED SHRIMP

Preparation Time: 10 minutes

Cooking Time: 6 minutes
Servings: 10
Ingredients:
- 20 shrimps, peeled and deveined
- 7 slices bacon
- 4 leaves romaine lettuce

Directions:
1. Set the oven to 400° F (205°C).
2. Wrap each shrimp with each bacon strip, then arrange the wrapped shrimps in a single layer on a baking sheet, seam side down.
3. Broil for 6 minutes. Flip the shrimp halfway through the cooking time.
4. Take out from the oven and serve on lettuce leaves.

Nutrition:
Calories: 80.91
Fat: 7g
Protein: 3.61g
Sodium: 167mg
Carbs: 0.6g

356. CHEESY BROCCOLI BITES

Preparation Time: 10 minutes
Cooking Time: 25 minutes
Servings: 6
Ingredients:
- 2 tablespoons olive oil
- 2 heads broccoli, trimmed
- 1 egg
- ⅓ cup reduced-fat shredded Cheddar cheese
- 1 egg white
- ½ cup onion, chopped
- ⅓ cup breadcrumbs
- ¼ teaspoon salt
- ¼ teaspoon black pepper

Directions:
1. Preheat the oven to 400°F (205°C). Coat a large baking sheet with olive oil.
2. Arrange a colander in a saucepan, then place the broccoli in the colander. Pour the water into the saucepan to cover the bottom. Boil, then reduce the heat to low. Close and simmer for 6 minutes. Allow cooling for 10 minutes.
3. Blend broccoli and the remaining ingredients in a food processor. Let sit for 10 minutes.
4. Make the bites: Drop 1 tablespoon of the mixture on the baking sheet. Repeat with the remaining mixture.
5. Bake in the preheated oven for 25 minutes. Flip the bites

halfway through the cooking time.

6. Serve immediately.

Nutrition:
Calories: 116.8
Carbohydrates: 7.9g
Fiber: 1.3g
Sodium: 216mg

357. EASY CAPRESE SKEWERS

Preparation Time: 5 minutes
Cooking Time: 0 minute
Servings: 10
Ingredients:

- 12 cherry tomatoes
- 8 1-inch pieces Mozzarella cheese
- 12 basil leaves
- ¼ cup Italian vinaigrette, for serving

Directions:

1. Thread the tomatoes, cheese, and bay leave alternatively through the skewers.
2. Place the skewers on a plate and baste with the Italian Vinaigrette. Serve immediately.

Nutrition:
Calories: 304
Carbohydrates: 3.02g
Fiber:0.27g
Sodium: 628mg

358. GRILLED TOFU WITH SESAME SEEDS

Preparation Time: 45 minutes
Cooking Time: 20 minutes
Servings: 6
Ingredients:

- 1½ tablespoons brown rice vinegar
- 1 scallion
- 1 tablespoon ginger root
- 1 tablespoon no-sugar-added applesauce
- 2 tablespoons naturally brewed soy sauce
- ¼ teaspoon dried red pepper flakes
- 2 teaspoons sesame oil, toasted
- 1 (14-ounce/397g) package extra-firm tofu
- 2 tablespoons fresh cilantro
- 1 teaspoon sesame seeds

Directions:

1. Combine the vinegar, scallion, ginger, applesauce, soy sauce, red pepper flakes, and sesame oil in a large bowl. Stir to mix well.

2. Dunk the tofu pieces in the bowl, then refrigerate to marinate for 30 minutes.
3. Preheat a grill pan over medium-high heat.
4. Place the tofu on the grill pan with tongs, reserve the marinade, then grill for 8 minutes or until the tofu is golden brown and have deep grilled marks on both sides. Flip the tofu halfway through the cooking time. You may need to work in batches to avoid overcrowding.
5. Transfer the tofu to a large plate and sprinkle with cilantro leaves and sesame seeds. Serve with the marinade alongside.

Nutrition:
Calories: 90
Carbohydrates: 3g
Sodium: 302.34mg
Fiber: 1g

359. KALE CHIPS

Preparation Time: 5 minutes
Cooking Time: 15 minutes
Servings: 1
Ingredients:

- ¼ teaspoon garlic powder
- Pinch of cayenne to taste
- 1 tablespoon extra-virgin olive oil
- ½ teaspoon sea salt, or to taste
- 1 8-ounce bunch of kale

Directions:

1. Preheat oven to 350ºF. Line 2 baking sheets with parchment paper.
2. Toss the garlic powder, cayenne pepper, olive oil, and salt in a large bowl, then dunk the kale in the bowl.
3. Situate kale in a single layer on one of the baking sheets.
4. Put the sheet in the preheated oven and bake for 7 minutes. Remove the sheet from the oven and put the kale into the single layer of the other baking sheet.
5. Move the sheet of kale back to the oven and bake for another 7 minutes.
6. Serve immediately.

Nutrition:
Calories: 211
Carbohydrates: 15.31g
Fiber: 6g
Sodium: 1010.96mg

360. SIMPLE DEVILED EGGS

Preparation Time: 5 minutes
Cooking Time: 8 minutes
Servings: 12
Ingredients:

- 6 large eggs
- ⅛ teaspoon mustard powder
- 2 tablespoons light mayonnaise

Directions:

1. Set the eggs in a saucepan, then pour in enough water to cover them. Bring to a boil, then boil the eggs for another 8 minutes. Turn off the heat and cover, then let sit for 15 minutes.
2. Transfer the boiled eggs to a pot of cold water and peel them under the water.
3. Transfer the eggs to a large plate, then cut them in half. Remove the egg yolks and place them in a bowl, then mash with a fork.
4. Add the mustard powder, mayo, salt, and pepper to the bowl of yolks, then stir to mix well.
5. Spoon the yolk mixture in the egg white on the plate. Serve immediately.

Nutrition:
Calories: 41.28
Carbohydrates: 2.9g
Fiber: 0g
Sodium: 55.6mg

361. SAUTÉED COLLARD GREENS AND CABBAGE

Preparation Time: 10 minutes
Cooking Time: 10 minutes
Servings: 8
Ingredients:

- 2 tablespoons extra-virgin olive oil
- 1 bunch collard greens
- ½ small green cabbage
- 6 garlic cloves
- 1 tablespoon low-sodium soy sauce

Directions:

1. Cook olive oil in a large skillet over medium-high heat.
2. Sauté the collard greens in the oil for about 2 minutes, or until the greens start to wilt.
3. Toss in the cabbage and mix well. Set to medium-low, cover, and cook for 5 to 7 minutes, stirring occasionally, or until the greens are softened.
4. Fold in the garlic and soy sauce and stir to combine. Cook for

about 30 seconds more until fragrant.

5. Remove from the heat to a plate and serve.

Nutrition:
Calories: 49
Carbohydrates: 4g
Fiber: 1.19g
Sodium: 65.77mg

362. ROASTED DELICATA SQUASH WITH THYME

Preparation Time: 10 minutes
Cooking Time: 20 minutes
Servings: 4
Ingredients:

- 1-1½ pounds Delicata squash
- 1 tablespoon extra-virgin olive oil
- ½ teaspoon dried thyme
- ¼ teaspoon salt
- ¼ teaspoon freshly ground black pepper

Directions:

1. Prep the oven to 400ºF (205ºC). Ready baking sheet with parchment paper and set aside.
2. Add the squash strips, olive oil, thyme, salt, and pepper in a large bowl, and toss until the squash strips are fully coated.
3. Place the squash strips on the prepared baking sheet in a single layer. Roast for about 20 minutes, flipping the strips halfway through.
4. Remove from the oven and serve on plates.

Nutrition:
Calories: 60.31
Carbohydrates: 6.8g
Fiber: 2.1g
Sodium: 146.33mg

363. ROASTED ASPARAGUS AND RED PEPPERS

Preparation Time: 5 minutes
Cooking Time: 15 minutes
Servings: 4
Ingredients:

- 1 pound (454 g) asparagus
- 2 red bell peppers, seeded
- 1 small onion
- 2 tablespoons Italian dressing

Directions:

1. Ready oven to 400°F (205ºC). Wrap baking sheet with parchment paper and set aside.
2. Combine the asparagus with the peppers, onion, dressing in a large bowl, and toss well.

3. Arrange the vegetables on the baking sheet and roast for about 15 minutes. Flip the vegetables with a spatula once during cooking.
4. Transfer to a large platter and serve.

Nutrition:
Calories: 54.7
Carbohydrates: 8.81g
Fiber: 3.2g
Sodium: 77.3mg

364. TARRAGON SPRING PEAS

Preparation Time: 10 minutes
Cooking Time: 12 minutes
Servings: 6
Ingredients:

- 1 tablespoon unsalted butter
- ½ Vidalia® onion
- 1 cup low-sodium vegetable broth
- 3 cups fresh shelled peas
- 1 tablespoon minced fresh tarragon

Directions:

1. Cook butter in a pan at medium heat.
2. Sauté the onion in the melted butter for about 3 minutes, stirring occasionally.
3. Pour in the vegetable broth and whisk well. Add the peas and tarragon to the skillet and stir to combine.
4. Reduce the heat to low, cover, cook for about 8 minutes more, or until the peas are tender.
5. Let the peas cool for 5 minutes and serve warm.

Nutrition:
Calories: 98.56
Carbohydrates: 15.38g
Fiber: 3.8g
Sodium: 30.22mg

365. BUTTER-ORANGE YAMS

Preparation Time: 7 minutes
Cooking Time: 45 minutes
Servings: 8
Ingredients:

- 2 medium jewel yams
- 2 tablespoons unsalted butter
- Juice of 1 large orange
- 1½ teaspoons ground cinnamon
- ¼ teaspoon ground ginger
- ¾ teaspoon ground nutmeg
- ⅛ teaspoon ground cloves

Directions:

1. Set oven to 350°F (180ºC).

2. Arrange the yam dices on a rimmed baking sheet in a single layer. Set aside.
3. Add the butter, orange juice, cinnamon, ginger, nutmeg, and garlic cloves to a medium saucepan over medium-low heat. Cook for 3 to 5 minutes, stirring continuously.
4. Spoon the sauce over the yams and toss to coat well.
5. Bake in the prepared oven for 40 minutes.
6. Let the yams cool for 8 minutes on the baking sheet before removing and serving.

Nutrition:
Calories: 130.76
Carbohydrates: 25g
Fiber: 3.79g
Sodium: 8.23mg

366. CHICKEN WITH COCONUT SAUCE

Preparation Time: 15 minutes
Cooking Time: 20 minutes
Servings: 2
Ingredients:

- ½ lb. chicken breasts
- ⅓ cup red onion
- 1 tablespoon paprika (smoked)
- 2 teaspoons cornstarch
- ½ cup light coconut milk
- 1 teaspoon extra-virgin olive oil
- 2 tablespoons fresh cilantro
- 1 10-oz. can tomatoes and green chilis
- ¼ cup water

Directions:

1. Cut chicken into little cubes; sprinkle with 1.5 teaspoons paprika.
2. Heat oil, add chicken and cook for 3 to 5 minutes.
3. Remove from skillet and fry the finely chopped onion for 5 minutes.
4. Return chicken to pan. Add tomatoes, 1.5 teaspoons paprika, and water. Bring to a boil, and then simmer for 4 minutes.
5. Mix cornstarch and coconut milk; stir into chicken mixture and cook until it has done.
6. Sprinkle with chopped cilantro.

Nutrition:
Calories: 249.95
Protein: 19.4g
Fat: 14g
Carbs: 10.11g
Sodium: 627.71mg

367. FISH WITH FRESH HERB SAUCE

Preparation Time: 10 minutes
Cooking Time: 10 minutes
Servings: 2
Ingredients:

- 2 4-oz. cod fillets
- ⅓ cup fresh cilantro
- ¼ teaspoon cumin
- 1 tablespoon red onion
- 2 teaspoons extra virgin olive oil
- 1 teaspoon red wine vinegar
- 1 small clove garlic
- ⅛ teaspoon salt
- ⅛ black pepper

Directions:

1. Combine chopped cilantro, finely chopped onion, oil, red wine vinegar, minced garlic, and salt.
2. Sprinkle both sides of fish fillets with cumin and pepper.
3. Cook fillets 4 minutes per side. Top each fillet with cilantro mixture.

Nutrition:
Calories: 136
Fat: 5.6g
Carbohydrates: 0.97g
Sodium: 238.45mg

368. RAVIOLI

Preparation Time: 5 minutes
Cooking Time: 16 minutes
Servings: 4
Ingredients:

- 8 ounces frozen vegan ravioli, thawed
- 1 teaspoon dried basil
- 1 teaspoon garlic powder
- ⅛ teaspoon ground black pepper
- ¼ teaspoon salt
- 1 teaspoon dried oregano
- 2 teaspoons nutritional yeast flakes
- ½ cup marinara sauce, unsweetened
- ½ cup panko breadcrumbs
- ¼ cup liquid from chickpeas can

Directions:

1. Place breadcrumbs in a bowl, sprinkle with salt, basil, oregano, and black pepper, add garlic powder and yeast and stir until mixed.
2. Take a bowl and then pour in chickpeas liquid in it.
3. Working on one ravioli at a time, first dip a ravioli in chickpeas liquid and then coat with breadcrumbs mixture.
4. Prepare remaining ravioli in the same manner, then take a fryer basket, grease it well with oil, and place ravioli in it in a single layer.
5. Switch on the air fryer, insert fryer basket, sprinkle oil on ravioli, shut with its lid, set the fryer at 390°F, then cook for 6 minutes, turn the ravioli and continue cooking 2 minutes until nicely golden and heated thoroughly.
6. Cook the remaining ravioli in the same manner and serve with marinara sauce.

Nutrition:
Calories: 204
Fat: 5.3g
Protein: 10.7g
Carbs: 27.77g
Sodium: 468.36mg

369. ONION RINGS

Preparation Time: 10 minutes
Cooking Time: 32 minutes
Servings: 4
Ingredients:

- 1 large white onion, peeled
- ⅔ cup pork rinds
- 3 tablespoons almond flour
- ½ teaspoon garlic powder
- ½ teaspoon paprika
- ¼ teaspoon sea salt
- 3 tablespoons coconut flour
- 2 eggs

Directions:

1. Switch on the air fryer, insert fryer basket, grease it with olive oil, then shut with its lid, set the fryer at 400°F, and preheat for 10 minutes.
2. Meanwhile, slice the peeled onion into ½ inch thick rings.
3. Take a shallow dish, add almond flour and stir in garlic powder, paprika, and pork rinds; take another shallow dish, add coconut flour and salt and stir until mixed.
4. Crack eggs in a bowl and then whisk until combined.
5. Working on one onion ring at a time, first coat onion ring in coconut flour mixture, then it in egg, and coat with pork rind mixture by scooping over the onion until evenly coated.
6. Open the fryer, place coated onion rings in it in a single layer, spray oil over onion rings, close with its lid, and cook for 16 minutes until nicely golden and thoroughly cooked, flipping the onion rings halfway through the frying.
7. When the air fryer beeps, open its lid, transfer onion rings onto a serving plate and cook the remaining onion rings in the same manner.
8. Serve straight away.

Nutrition:
Calories: 121.68
Fat: 6.8g
Protein: 7.9g
Carbs: 8g
Sodium: 240.47mg

370. CAULIFLOWER FRITTERS

Preparation Time: 10 minutes
Cooking Time: 14 minutes
Servings: 2
Ingredients:

- 5 cups chopped cauliflower florets
- ½ cup almond flour
- ½ teaspoon baking powder
- ½ teaspoon ground black pepper
- ½ teaspoon salt
- 2 eggs, pastured

Directions:

1. Add chopped cauliflower in a blender or food processor, pulse until minced, and then tip the mixture in a bowl.
2. Add remaining ingredients, stir well and then shape the mixture into ⅓-inch patties, an ice cream scoop of mixture per patty.
3. Switch on the air fryer, insert fryer basket, grease it with olive oil, then shut with its lid, set the fryer at 390°F, and preheat for 5 minutes.
4. Then open the fryer, add cauliflower patties in it in a single layer, spray oil over patties, close with its lid and cook for 14 minutes at 375°F until nicely golden and cooked, flipping the patties halfway through the frying.
5. Serve straight away with the dip.

Nutrition:
Calories: 284
Fat: 17.19g
Protein: 17.4g
Carbs: 21.6g
Sodium: 845mg

371. ZUCCHINI FRITTERS

Preparation Time: 20 minutes
Cooking Time: 12 minutes
Servings: 4
Ingredients:
- 2 medium zucchinis, ends trimmed
- 3 tablespoons almond flour
- 1 tablespoon salt
- 1 teaspoon garlic powder
- ¼ teaspoon paprika
- ¼ teaspoon ground black pepper
- ¼ teaspoon onion powder
- 1 egg

Directions:
1. Wash and pat dry the zucchini, then cut its ends and grate the zucchini.
2. Place grated zucchini in a colander, sprinkle with salt and let it rest for 10 minutes.
3. Then wrap zucchini in a kitchen cloth and squeeze moisture from it as much as possible and place dried zucchini in another bowl.
4. Add remaining ingredients into the zucchini and then stir until mixed.
5. Take fryer basket, line it with parchment paper, grease it with oil, and drop zucchini mixture on it by a spoonful, about 1-inch apart and then spray well with oil.
6. Switch on the air fryer, insert fryer basket, then shut with its lid, set the fryer at 360°F, and cook the fritter for 12 minutes until nicely golden and cooked, flipping the fritters halfway through the frying.
7. Serve straight away.

Nutrition:
Calories: 61.64
Fat: 3.6g
Protein: 3.6 g
Carbs: 4.8g
Sodium: 1767mg

372. AIR-FRIED KALE CHIPS

Preparation Time: 5 minutes
Cooking Time: 7 minutes
Servings: 2
Ingredients:
- 1 large bunch of kale
- ¾ teaspoon red chili powder
- 1 teaspoon salt
- ¾ teaspoon ground black pepper

Directions:

1. Remove the hard spines from the kale leaves, then cut kale into small pieces and place them in a fryer basket.
2. Spray oil over kale, then sprinkle with salt, chili powder, and black pepper and toss until well mixed.
3. Switch on the air fryer, insert fryer basket, then shut with its lid, set the fryer at 375°F, and cook for 7 minutes until kale is crispy, shaking halfway through the frying.
4. When the air fryer beeps, open its lid, transfer kale chips onto a serving plate and serve.

Nutrition:
Calories: 80.46
Fat: 1.59g
Protein: 6.8g
Carbs: 14.5g
Sodium: 1222mg

373. RADISH CHIPS

Preparation Time: 5 minutes
Cooking Time: 20 minutes
Servings: 2
Ingredients:
- 8 ounces radish slices
- ½ teaspoon garlic powder
- 1 teaspoon salt
- ½ teaspoon onion powder
- ½ teaspoon ground black pepper

Directions:
1. Wash the radish slices, pat them dry, place them in a fryer basket, and then spray oil on them until well coated.
2. Sprinkle salt, garlic powder, onion powder, and black pepper over radish slices and then toss until well coated.
3. Switch on the air fryer, insert fryer basket, then shut with its lid, set the fryer at 370°F, and cook for 10 minutes, stirring the slices halfway through.
4. Then spray oil on radish slices, shake the basket and continue frying for 10 minutes, stirring the chips halfway through.
5. Serve straight away.

Nutrition:
Calories: 21
Fat: 1.8 g
Protein: 0.2 g
Carbs: 3.83g
Sodium: 1191mg

374. ZUCCHINI FRIES

Preparation Time: 10 minutes
Cooking Time: 20 minutes
Servings: 4
Ingredients:
- 2 medium zucchinis
- ½ cup almond flour
- ⅛ teaspoon ground black pepper
- ½ teaspoon garlic powder
- ⅛ teaspoon salt
- 1 teaspoon Italian seasoning
- ½ cup grated Parmesan cheese, reduced fat
- 1 egg, beaten

Directions:
1. Switch on the air fryer, insert fryer basket, grease it with olive oil, then shut with its lid, set the fryer at 400°F, and preheat for 10 minutes.
2. Meanwhile, cut each zucchini in half and then cut each zucchini half into 4-inch-long pieces, each about ½ inch thick.
3. Place flour in a shallow dish, add remaining ingredients except for the egg, and stir until mixed.
4. Crack the egg in a bowl and then whisk it until blended.
5. Working on one zucchini piece at a time, first dip it in the egg, then coat it in the almond flour mixture and place it on a wire rack.
6. Open the fryer, add zucchini pieces in it in a single layer, spray oil over zucchini, close with its lid and cook for 10 minutes until nicely golden and crispy, shaking halfway through the frying.
7. Cook remaining zucchini pieces in the same manner and serve.

Nutrition:
Calories: 142
Fat: 9.89g
Protein: 8.74g
Carbs: 6.22g
Sodium: 213.37mg

375. ROASTED PEANUT BUTTER SQUASH

Preparation Time: 5 minutes
Cooking Time: 22 minutes
Servings: 4
Ingredients:
- 1 butternut squash, peeled
- 1 teaspoon cinnamon
- 1 tablespoon olive oil

Directions:

1. Switch on the air fryer, insert fryer basket, grease it with olive oil, then shut with its lid, set the fryer at 220°F, and preheat for 5 minutes.
2. Meanwhile, peel the squash and cut it into 1-inch pieces, and then place them in a bowl.
3. Drizzle oil over squash pieces, sprinkle with cinnamon, and then toss until well coated.
4. Open the fryer, add squash pieces in it, close with its lid and cook for 17 minutes until nicely golden and crispy, shaking every 5 minutes.
5. When the air fryer beeps, open its lid, transfer squash onto a serving plate and serve.

Nutrition:
Calories: 99.92
Fat: 3.7g
Protein: 1.51g
Carbs: 17.88g
Sodium: 6.08mg

376. ROASTED CHICKPEAS

Preparation Time: 35 minutes
Cooking Time: 25 minutes
Servings: 6
Ingredients:
- 15 ounces cooked chickpeas
- 1 teaspoon garlic powder
- 1 tablespoon nutritional yeast
- ⅛ teaspoon cumin
- 1 teaspoon smoked paprika
- ½ teaspoon salt
- 1 tablespoon olive oil

Directions:
1. Take a large baking sheet, line it with paper towels, then spread chickpeas on it, cover the peas with paper towels, and let rest for 30 minutes or until chickpeas are dried.
2. Then switch on the air fryer, insert the fryer basket, grease it with olive oil, then shut with its lid, set the fryer at 355°F, and preheat for 5 minutes.
3. Place dried chickpeas in a bowl, add remaining ingredients and toss until well coated.
4. Open the fryer, add chickpeas in it, close with its lid and cook for 20 minutes until nicely golden and crispy, shaking the chickpeas every 5 minutes.
5. When the air fryer beeps, open its lid, transfer chickpeas onto a serving bowl, and serve.

Nutrition:
Calories: 145.49

Fat: 4.27g
Protein: 7.08g
Carbs: 20.42g
Sodium: 199.13mg

377. BUFFALO CAULIFLOWER WINGS

Preparation Time: 5 minutes
Cooking Time: 30 minutes
Servings: 6
Ingredients:
- 1 tablespoon almond flour
- 1 medium head of cauliflower
- 1 ½ teaspoon salt
- 4 tablespoons hot sauce
- 1 tablespoon olive oil

Directions:
1. Switch on the air fryer, insert fryer basket, grease it with olive oil, then close lid, set the fryer at 400°F, and preheat for 5 minutes.
2. Meanwhile, cut cauliflower into bite-size florets and set aside.
3. Place flour in a large bowl, whisk in salt, oil, and hot sauce until combined, add cauliflower florets and toss until combined.
4. Open the fryer, add cauliflower florets it in a single layer, close lid and cook for 15 minutes until nicely golden and crispy, shaking halfway through the frying.
5. When the air fryer beeps, open its lid, transfer cauliflower florets onto a serving plate and keep warm.
6. Cook the remaining cauliflower florets in the same manner and serve.

Nutrition:
Calories: 38.88
Fat: 3g
Protein: 1.11g
Sodium: 843.09mg
Carbs: 2.57g

378. OKRA

Preparation Time: 10 minutes
Cooking Time: 10 minutes
Servings: 4
Ingredients:
- 1 cup almond flour
- 8 ounces fresh okra
- ½ teaspoon sea salt
- 1 cup milk, reduced fat
- 1 egg,

Directions:

1. Crack the egg in a bowl, pour in the milk, and whisk until blended.
2. Cut the stem from each okra, then cut it into ½-inch pieces, add them into the egg and stir until well coated.
3. Mix flour and salt and add them into a large plastic bag.
4. Working on one okra piece at a time, drain the okra well by letting excess egg drip off, add it to the flour mixture, then seal the bag and shake well until okra is well coated.
5. Place the coated okra on a grease air fryer basket, coat remaining okra pieces in the same manner, and place them into the basket.
6. Switch on the air fryer, insert fryer basket, spray okra with oil, then shut with its lid, set the fryer at 390°F, and cook for 10 minutes until nicely golden and cooked, stirring okra halfway through the frying.
7. Serve straight away.

Nutrition:
Calories: 199
Fat: 13.8g
Protein: 9.66g
Sodium: 282.84mg

379. QUINOA TABBOULEH

Preparation Time: 8 minutes
Cooking Time: 16 minutes
Servings: 6
Ingredients:
- 1 cup quinoa, rinsed
- 1 large English cucumber
- 2 scallions, sliced
- 2 cups cherry tomatoes, halved
- ⅔ cup chopped parsley
- ½ cup chopped mint
- ½ teaspoon minced garlic
- ½ teaspoon salt
- ½ teaspoon ground black pepper
- 2 tablespoons lemon juice
- ½ cup olive oil

Directions:
1. Plug in Instant Pot, insert the inner pot, add quinoa, then pour in water and stir until mixed.
2. Close the Instant Pot lid and turn the pressure knob to seal the pot.
3. Select the manual button, then set the timer to 7 minutes and cook on high pressure.

4. Once the timer stops, select the cancel button and do a natural pressure release for 10 minutes, and then do a quick pressure release until pressure knob drops down.
5. Open the Instant Pot, fluff quinoa with a fork, then spoon it on a rimmed baking sheet, spread quinoa evenly and let cool.
6. Meanwhile, place lime juice in a small bowl, add garlic, and stir until just mixed.
7. Then add salt, black pepper, and olive oil and whisk until combined.
8. Transfer cooled quinoa to a large bowl, add remaining ingredients, then drizzle generously with the prepared lime juice mixture and toss until evenly coated.
9. Taste quinoa to adjust seasoning and then serve.

Nutrition:
Calories: 297.87
Carbohydrates: 24g
Fiber: 3.4g
Sodium: 205.8mg

380. LOW FAT ROASTIES

Preparation Time: 8 minutes
Cooking Time: 25 minutes
Servings: 2
Ingredients:
- 1lb roasting potatoes
- 1 garlic clove
- 1 cup vegetable stock
- 2 tablespoons olive oil

Directions:
1. Position potatoes in the steamer basket and add the stock into the Instant Pot.
2. Steam the potatoes in your Instant Pot for 15 minutes.
3. Depressurize and pour away the remaining stock.
4. Set to sauté and add the oil, garlic, and potatoes. Cook until brown.

Nutrition:
Calories: 260.9
Carbohydrates: 30.46g
Fat: 14.5g
Sodium: 382.65mg

381. ROASTED PARSNIPS

Preparation Time: 9 minutes
Cooking Time: 25 minutes
Servings: 2
Ingredients:

- 1 lb parsnips
- 1 cup vegetable stock
- 2 tablespoons herbs
- 2 tablespoons olive oil

Directions:
1. Put the parsnips in the steamer basket and add the stock into the Instant Pot.
2. Steam the parsnips in your Instant Pot for 15 minutes.
3. Depressurize and pour away the remaining stock.
4. Set to sauté and add the oil, herbs, and parsnips.
5. Cook until golden and crisp.

Nutrition:
Calories: 277.44
Carbohydrates: 35.9g
Protein: 2.7g
Sodium: 372.44mg

382. LOWER CARB HUMMUS

Preparation Time: 9 minutes
Cooking Time: 60 minutes
Servings: 2
Ingredients:
- ½ cup dry chickpeas
- 1 cup vegetable stock
- 1 cup pumpkin puree
- 2 tablespoons smoked paprika
- Salt and pepper to taste

Directions:
1. Soak the chickpeas overnight.
2. Place the chickpeas and stock in the Instant Pot.
3. Cook on Beans for 60 minutes.
4. Depressurize naturally.
5. Blend the chickpeas with the remaining ingredients.

Nutrition:
Calories: 258.88
Carbohydrates:44g
Fat: 10.2g
Sodium: 759.65mg

383. SWEET AND SOUR RED CABBAGE

Preparation Time: 7 minutes
Cooking Time: 10 minutes
Servings: 8
Ingredients:
- 2 cups spiced pear applesauce
- 1 small onion, chopped
- ½ cup apple cider vinegar
- ½ teaspoon kosher salt
- 1 head red cabbage

Directions:
1. In the electric pressure cooker, combine the applesauce, onion, vinegar, salt, and a cup of water. Stir in the cabbage.
2. Seal lid of the pressure cooker.

3. Cook on high pressure for 10 minutes.
4. When the cooking is complete, hit Cancel and quickly release the pressure.
5. Once the pin drops, unlock and remove the lid.
6. Spoon into a bowl or platter and serve.

Nutrition:
Calories: 73.75
Carbohydrates: 17.7g
Fiber: 2.6g
Sodium: 140.93mg

384. PINTO BEANS

Preparation Time: 6 minutes
Cooking Time: 55 minutes
Servings: 10
Ingredients:
- 2 cups pinto beans, dried
- 1 medium white onion
- 1½ teaspoon minced garlic
- ¾ teaspoon salt
- ¼ teaspoon ground black pepper
- 1 teaspoon red chili powder
- ¼ teaspoon cumin
- 1 tablespoon olive oil
- 1 teaspoon chopped cilantro
- 5½ cup vegetable stock

Directions:
1. Plug in Instant Pot, insert the inner pot, press sauté/simmer button, add oil and when hot, add onion and garlic and cook for 3 minutes or until onions begin to soften.
2. Add remaining ingredients, stir well, then press the cancel button, shut the instant pot with its lid, and seal the pot.
3. Click the manual button, then press the timer to set the cooking time to 45 minutes and cook at high pressure.
4. Once done, click the cancel button and do a natural pressure release for 10 minutes until the pressure knob drops down.
5. Open the Instant Pot, spoon beans into plates, and serve.

Nutrition:
Calories: 48.44
Carbohydrates: 6.89g
Fiber: 0.24g
Sodium: 624.28mg

385. STEAMED ASPARAGUS

Preparation Time: 3 minutes
Cooking Time: 2 minutes

Servings: 4
Ingredients:
- 1 lb. fresh asparagus, rinsed and tough ends trimmed
- 1 cup water

Directions:
1. Place the asparagus into a wire steamer rack and set it inside your Instant Pot.
2. Add water to the pot. Close and seal the lid, turning the steam release valve to the "Sealing" position.
3. Select the "Steam" function to cook on high pressure for 2 minutes.
4. Once done, do a quick pressure release of the steam.
5. Lift the wire steamer basket out of the pot and place the asparagus onto a serving plate.
6. Season as desired and serve.

Nutrition:
Calories: 22
Carbohydrates: 4g
Protein: 2g
Sodium: 4.05mg

386. SQUASH MEDLEY

Preparation Time: 10 minutes
Cooking Time: 20 minutes.
Servings: 2
Ingredients:
- 2 lbs. mixed squash
- ½ cup mixed veg
- 1 cup vegetable stock
- 2 tablespoons olive oil
- 2 tablespoons mixed herbs

Directions:
1. Put the squash in the steamer basket and add the stock into the Instant Pot.
2. Steam the squash in your Instant Pot for 10 minutes.
3. Depressurize and pour away the remaining stock.
4. Set to sauté and add the oil and remaining ingredients.
5. Cook until a light crust forms.

Nutrition:
Calories: 270.05
Carbohydrates: 34.32g
Fat: 15g
Sodium: 377.49mg

387. EGGPLANT CURRY

Preparation Time: 15 minutes
Cooking Time: 20 minutes
Servings: 2
Ingredients:
- 3 cups chopped eggplant
- 1 thinly sliced onion

- 1 cup coconut milk
- 3 tablespoons curry paste
- 1 tablespoon oil or ghee

Directions:
1. Set Instant Pot to sauté and put the onion, oil, and curry paste.
2. Once the onion is soft, stir in the remaining ingredients and seal.
3. Cook on Stew for 20 minutes. Release the pressure naturally.

Nutrition:
Calories: 457.7
Carbohydrates: 22.31g
Fat: 42g
Sodium: 546.99mg

388. SPLIT PEA STEW

Preparation Time: 5 minutes
Cooking Time: 35 minutes
Servings: 2
Ingredients:
- 1 cup dry split peas
- 1 lb. chopped vegetables
- 1 cup mushroom soup
- 2 tablespoons Old Bay seasoning

Directions:
1. Add all the ingredients in Instant Pot, cook for 33 minutes.
2. Release the pressure naturally.

Nutrition:
Calories: 555
Carbohydrates: 97g
Fat: 5.6g
Sodium: 1953mg

389. KIDNEY BEAN STEW

Preparation Time: 15 minutes
Cooking Time: 15 minutes
Servings: 2
Ingredients:
- 1 lb. cooked kidney beans
- 1 cup tomato passata
- 1 cup low sodium beef broth
- 3 tablespoons Italian herbs

Directions:
1. Combine all the ingredients in your Instant Pot, cook on Stew for 15 minutes.
2. Release the pressure naturally and serve.

Nutrition:
Calories: 321
Carbohydrates: 55.8g
Fat: 1.47g
Sodium: 246.36mg

390. CHILI SIN CARNE

Preparation Time: 15 minutes
Cooking Time: 35 minutes
Servings: 2
Ingredients:
- 3 cups mixed cooked beans
- 2 cups chopped tomatoes
- 1 tablespoon yeast extract
- 2 squares very dark chocolate
- 1 tablespoon red chili flakes

Directions:
1. Combine all the ingredients in your Instant Pot, cook for 35 minutes.
2. Release the pressure naturally and serve.

Nutrition:
Calories: 284.66
Carbohydrates: 48g
Fat: 3g
Sodium: 274.33mg

391. BRUSSELS SPROUTS

Preparation Time: 5 minutes
Cooking Time: 3 minutes
Servings: 5
Ingredients:
- 1 teaspoon extra-virgin olive oil
- 1 lb. halved Brussels sprouts
- 3 tablespoons apple cider vinegar
- 3 tablespoons gluten-free tamari soy sauce
- 3 tablespoons chopped sun-dried tomatoes

Directions:
1. Select the Sauté function on your Instant Pot, add oil and allow the pot to get hot.
2. Cancel the Sauté function and add the Brussels sprouts.
3. Stir well and allow the sprouts to cook in the residual heat for 2-3 minutes.
4. Add the tamari soy sauce and vinegar, and then stir.
5. Cover the Instant Pot, sealing the pressure valve by pointing it to "Sealing."
6. Select the Manual, High Pressure setting and cook for 3 minutes.
7. Once the cook cycle is done, do a quick pressure release, and then stir in the chopped sun-dried tomatoes.
8. Serve immediately.

Nutrition:
Calories: 58.67
Carbohydrates: 10g
Sodium: 627mg

Fat: 1g

392. GARLIC AND HERB CARROTS

Preparation Time: 2 minutes
Cooking Time: 18 minutes
Servings: 3
Ingredients:
- 2 tablespoons unsalted butter
- 1 lb. baby carrots
- 1 cup water
- 1 teaspoon fresh thyme or oregano
- 1 teaspoon minced garlic
- Black pepper
- Coarse sea salt

Directions:
1. Pour water into the inner pot of the Instant Pot, and then put it in a steamer basket.
2. Layer the carrots into the steamer basket.
3. Close and seal the lid, with the pressure vent in the Sealing position.
4. Select the Steam setting and cook for 2 minutes on high pressure.
5. Quickly release the pressure and then carefully remove the steamer basket with the steamed carrots, discarding the water.
6. Add butter to the inner pot of the Instant Pot and allow it to melt on the Sauté function.
7. Add garlic and sauté for 30 seconds, and then add the carrots. Mix well.
8. Stir in the fresh herbs and cook for 2-3 minutes.
9. Season with salt and black pepper, and then transfer to a serving bowl.
10. Serve warm and enjoy!

Nutrition:
Calories: 122
Carbohydrates: 12g
Sodium: 346.12mg
Fat: 7g

393. CILANTRO LIME DRUMSTICKS

Preparation Time: 5 minutes
Cooking Time: 15 minutes
Servings: 6
Ingredients:
- 1 tablespoon olive oil
- 6 chicken drumsticks
- 4 minced garlic cloves
- ½ cup low-sodium chicken broth
- 1 teaspoon cayenne pepper
- 1 teaspoon crushed red peppers

- 1 teaspoon fine sea salt
- Juice of 1 lime
To Serve:
- 2 tablespoon chopped cilantro
- Extra lime zest

Directions:
1. Pour olive oil into the Instant Pot and set it on the "Sauté" function.
2. Once the oil is hot, add the chicken drumsticks and season them well.
3. Using tongs, reposition the drumsticks and brown them for 2 minutes per side.
4. Add the lime juice, fresh cilantro, and chicken broth to the pot.
5. Lock and seal the lid, turning the pressure valve to "Sealing."
6. Cook the drumsticks on the "Manual, High Pressure" setting for 9 minutes.
7. Once done let the pressure release naturally.
8. Carefully transfer the drumsticks to an aluminum-foiled baking sheet and broil them in the oven for 3-5 minutes until golden brown.
9. Serve warm, garnished with more cilantro and lime zest.

Nutrition:
Calories: 162.74
Carbohydrates: 1.85g
Fat: 10.16g
Sodium: 370.94mg

394. EGGPLANT SPREAD

Preparation Time: 5 minutes
Cooking Time: 18 minutes
Servings: 5
Ingredients:
- 4 tablespoons extra-virgin olive oil
- 2 lbs. eggplant
- 4 skin-on garlic cloves
- ½ cup water
- ¼ cup pitted black olives
- 3 sprigs fresh thyme
- Juice of 1 lemon
- 1 tablespoon tahini
- 1 teaspoon sea salt
- Fresh extra-virgin olive oil

Directions:
1. Peel the eggplant in alternating stripes, leaving some areas with skin and some with no skin.
2. Slice into big chunks and layer at the bottom of your Instant Pot.

3. Add olive oil to the pot, and on the "Sauté" function, fry and caramelize the eggplant on one side, about 5 minutes.
4. Add in the garlic cloves with the skin on.
5. Flip over the eggplant and then add in the remaining uncooked eggplant chunks, salt, and water.
6. Close the lid, ensure the pressure release valve is set to "Sealing."
7. Cook for 5 minutes on the "Manual, High Pressure" setting.
8. Once done, carefully open the pot by quickly releasing the pressure through the steam valve.
9. Discard most of the brown cooking liquid.
10. Remove the garlic cloves and peel them.
11. Add the lemon juice, tahini, cooked and fresh garlic cloves, and pitted black olives to the pot.
12. Using a hand-held immersion blender, process all the ingredients until smooth.
13. Pour out the spread into a serving dish and season with fresh thyme, whole black olives, and some extra-virgin olive oil, prior to serving.

Nutrition:
Calories: 201.14
Carbohydrates: 11.1g
Fat: 17.57g
Sodium: 383mg

395. CARROT HUMMUS

Preparation Time: 15 minutes
Cooking Time: 10 minutes
Servings: 2
Ingredients:
- 1 chopped carrot
- 2 oz. cooked chickpeas
- 1 teaspoon lemon juice
- 1 teaspoon tahini
- 1 teaspoon fresh parsley

Directions:
1. Place the carrot and chickpeas in your Instant Pot.
2. Add a cup of water, seal, cook for 10 minutes on Stew.
3. Depressurize naturally. Blend with the remaining ingredients.

Nutrition:
Calories: 77.45
Carbohydrates: 11.37g
Fat: 2.46g
Sodium: 21.48mg

396. FRENCH BROCCOLI SALAD

Preparation Time: 10 minutes
Cooking Time: 10 minutes
Servings: 10
Ingredients:

- 8 cups broccoli florets
- 3 strips of bacon, cooked and crumbled
- ¼ cup sunflower kernels
- 1 bunch of green onions, sliced
- 3 tablespoons seasoned rice vinegar
- 3 tablespoons canola oil
- ½ cup dried cranberries

Directions:

1. Combine the green onion, cranberries, and broccoli in a bowl.
2. Whisk the vinegar, and oil in another bowl. Blend well.
3. Now drizzle over the broccoli mix.
4. Coat well by tossing.
5. Sprinkle bacon and sunflower kernels before serving.

Nutrition:
Calories: 121
Carbohydrates: 14g
Cholesterol: 2mg
Fiber: 3g
Sugar 1g
Fat: 7g
Protein: 3g
Sodium: 233mg

397. TENDERLOIN GRILLED SALAD

Preparation Time: 10 minutes
Cooking Time: 20 minutes
Servings: 5
Ingredients:

- 1 lb. pork tenderloin
- 10 cups mixed salad greens
- 2 oranges, seedless, cut into bite-sized pieces
- 1 tablespoon orange zest, grated
- 2 tablespoons of cider vinegar
- 2 tablespoons olive oil
- 2 teaspoons Dijon mustard
- ½ cup juice of an orange
- 2 teaspoons honey
- ½ teaspoon ground pepper

Directions:

1. Bring together all the dressing ingredients in a bowl.
2. Grill each side of the pork covered over medium heat for 9 minutes.
3. Slice after 5 minutes.
4. Slice the tenderloin thinly.
5. Keep the greens on your serving plate.

6. Top with the pork and oranges.
7. Sprinkle nuts (optional).

Nutrition:
Calories: 211
Carbohydrates: 13g
Cholesterol: 51mg
Fiber: 3g
Sugar 0.8g
Fat: 9g
Protein: 20g
Sodium: 113mg

398. BARLEY VEGGIE SALAD

Preparation Time: 10 minutes
Cooking Time: 20 minutes
Servings: 6
Ingredients:

- 1 tomato, seeded and chopped
- 2 tablespoons parsley, minced
- 1 yellow pepper, chopped
- 1 tablespoon basil, minced
- ¼ cup almonds, toasted
- 1¼ cups vegetable broth
- 1 cup barley
- 1 tablespoon lemon juice
- 2 tablespoons of white wine vinegar
- 3 tablespoons olive oil
- ¼ teaspoon pepper
- ½ teaspoon salt
- 1 cup of water

Directions:

1. Boil the broth, barley, and water in a saucepan.
2. Reduce heat. Cover and let it simmer for 10 minutes.
3. Take out from the heat.
4. In the meantime, bring together the parsley, yellow pepper, and tomato in a bowl.
5. Stir the barley in.
6. Whisk the vinegar, oil, basil, lemon juice, water, pepper, and salt in a bowl.
7. Pour this over your barley mix. Toss to coat well.
8. Stir the almonds in before serving.

Nutrition:
Calories: 211
Carbohydrates: 27g
Fiber: 7g
Fat: 10g
Protein: 6g
Sodium: 334mg

399. SPINACH SHRIMP SALAD

Preparation Time: 10 minutes
Cooking Time: 10 minutes
Servings: 4
Ingredients:

- 1 lb. uncooked shrimp, peeled and deveined
- 2 tablespoons parsley, minced
- ¾ cup halved cherry tomatoes
- 1 medium lemon
- 4 cups baby spinach
- 2 tablespoons unsalted butter
- 3 minced garlic cloves
- ¼ teaspoon pepper
- ¼ teaspoon salt

Directions:

1. Melt the butter over medium heat in a non-stick skillet.
2. Add the shrimp.
3. Now cook the shrimp for 3 minutes until they become pink.
4. Add the parsley and garlic.
5. Cook for another minute. Remove from the heat.
6. Keep the spinach in your salad bowl.
7. Top with the shrimp mix and tomatoes.
8. Drizzle lemon juice on the salad.
9. Sprinkle pepper and salt.

Nutrition:
Calories: 201
Carbohydrates: 6g
Cholesterol: 153mg
Fiber: 2g
Fat: 10g
Protein: 21g
Sodium: 350mg

400. SWEET POTATO AND ROASTED BEET SALAD

Preparation Time: 10 minutes
Cooking Time: 10 minutes
Servings: 4
Ingredients:

- 2 beets
- 1 sweet potato, peeled and cubed
- 1 garlic clove, minced
- 2 tablespoons walnuts, chopped and toasted
- 1 cup fennel bulb, sliced
- 3 tablespoons balsamic vinegar
- 1 teaspoon Dijon mustard
- 1 tablespoon honey
- 3 tablespoons olive oil
- ¼ teaspoon pepper
- ¼ teaspoon salt
- 3 tablespoons water

Directions:

1. Scrub the beets. Trim the tops to 1 inch.
2. Wrap in foil and keep on a baking sheet.
3. Bake until tender. Take off the foil.

4. Combine water and sweet potato in a bowl.
5. Cover. Microwave for 5 minutes. Drain off.
6. Now peel the beets. Cut into small wedges.
7. Arrange the fennel, sweet potato, and beets on 4 salad plates.
8. Sprinkle nuts.
9. Whisk the honey, mustard, vinegar, water, garlic, pepper, and salt.
10. Whisk in oil gradually.
11. Drizzle over the salad.

Nutrition:
Calories: 270
Carbohydrates: 37g
Fiber: 6g
Sugar 0.3g
Fat: 13g
Protein: 5g
Sodium: 309mg

401. POTATO CALICO SALAD

Preparation Time: 15 minutes
Cooking Time: 5 minutes
Servings: 14
Ingredients:
- 4 red potatoes, peeled and cooked
- 1½ cups kernel corn, cooked
- ½ cup green pepper, diced
- ½ cup red onion, chopped
- 1 cup carrot, shredded
- ½ cup olive oil
- ¼ cup vinegar
- 1½ teaspoons chili powder
- 1 teaspoon salt
- Dash of hot pepper sauce

Directions:
1. Keep all the ingredients together in a jar.
2. Close it and shake well.
3. Cube the potatoes. Combine with the carrot, onion, and corn in your salad bowl.
4. Pour the dressing over.
5. Now toss lightly.

Nutrition:
Calories: 146
Carbohydrates: 17g
Fat: 9g
Protein: 2g
Sodium: 212mg

402. MANGO AND JICAMA SALAD

Preparation Time: 15 minutes
Cooking Time: 5 minutes
Servings: 8
Ingredients:
- 1 jicama, peeled
- 1 mango, peeled
- 1 teaspoon ginger root, minced
- ⅓ cup chives, minced
- ½ cup cilantro, chopped
- ¼ cup canola oil
- ½ cup white wine vinegar
- 2 tablespoons of lime juice
- ¼ cup honey
- ⅛ teaspoon pepper
- ¼ teaspoon salt

Directions:
1. Whisk together the vinegar, honey, canola oil, gingerroot, paper, and salt.
2. Cut the mango and jicama into matchsticks.
3. Keep in a bowl.
4. Now toss with the lime juice.
5. Add the dressing and herbs. Combine well by tossing.

Nutrition:
Calories: 143
Carbohydrates: 20g
Fiber: 3g
Sugar 1.6g
Fat: 7g
Protein: 1g
Sodium: 78mg

SALAD

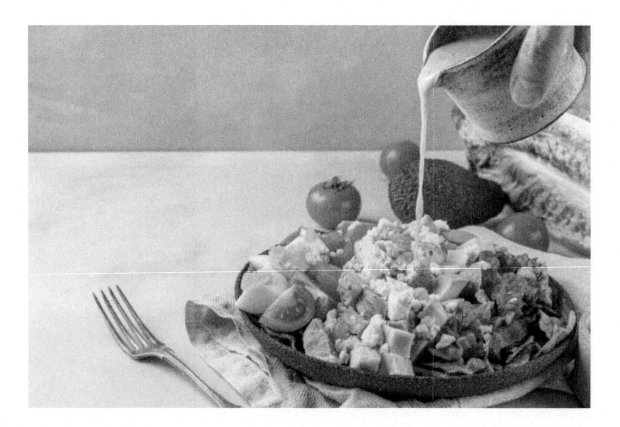

403. SWEET POTATO AND ROASTED BEET SALAD

Preparation Time: 10 minutes
Cooking Time: 10 minutes
Servings: 4
Ingredients:
- 2 beets
- 1 sweet potato, peeled and cubed
- 1 garlic clove, minced
- 2 tablespoons walnuts, chopped and toasted
- 1 cup fennel bulb, sliced
- 3 tablespoons balsamic vinegar
- 1 teaspoon Dijon mustard
- 1 tablespoon honey
- 3 tablespoons olive oil
- ¼ teaspoon pepper
- ¼ teaspoon salt
- 3 tablespoons water

Directions:
1. Scrub the beets. Trim the tops to 1 inch.
2. Wrap in foil and keep on a baking sheet.
3. Bake until tender. Take off the foil. Combine water and sweet potato in a bowl.
4. Cover. Microwave for 5 minutes. Drain off.
5. Now peel the beets. Cut into small wedges.
6. Arrange the fennel, sweet potato, and beets on 4 salad plates.
7. Sprinkle nuts.
8. Whisk the honey, mustard, vinegar, water, garlic, pepper, and salt.
9. Whisk in oil gradually.
10. Drizzle over the salad.

Nutrition:
Calories: 212.16
Fat: 14.26g
Protein: 2.32g
Carbs: 201.g
Sodium: 204.04mg

404. HARVEST SALAD

Preparation Time: 9 minutes
Cooking Time: 25 minutes
Servings: 6
Ingredients:
- 10 oz. kale, deboned and chopped
- 1½ cup blackberries
- ½ butternut squash, cubed
- ¼ cup goat cheese, crumbled
- Maple mustard salad dressing
- 1 cup raw pecans
- ⅓ cup raw pumpkin seeds
- ¼ cup dried cranberries
- 3½ tablespoon olive oil
- 1½ tablespoon sugar-free maple syrup
- 3/8 teaspoon salt, divided
- Pepper, to taste
- Non-stick cooking spray

Directions:

1. Heat oven to 400°F. Spray a baking sheet with cooking spray.
2. Spread squash on the prepared pan, add 1½ tablespoons oil, ⅛ teaspoon salt, and pepper to squash and stir to coat the squash evenly. Bake 20-25 minutes.
3. Place kale in a large bowl. Add 2 tablespoons oil and ½ teaspoon salt and massage it into the kale with your hands for 3-4 minutes.
4. Spray a clean baking sheet with cooking spray. In a medium bowl, stir together pecans, pumpkin seeds, and maple syrup until nuts are coated. Pour onto prepared pan and bake 8-10 minutes, these can be baked at the same time as the squash.
5. To assemble the salad: Place all of the ingredients in a large bowl. Pour dressing over and toss to coat. Serve.

Nutrition:
Calories: 436
Protein: 9g
Carbs: 21.8g
Sodium: 192.67mg
Fat: 37g

405. ASIAN NOODLE SALAD

Preparation Time: 20 minutes
Cooking Time: 15 minutes
 Servings: 4
Ingredients:
- 2 carrots, sliced thin
- 2 radishes, sliced thin
- 1 English cucumber, sliced thin
- 1 mango, julienned
- 1 bell pepper, julienned
- 1 small serrano pepper, seeded and sliced thin
- 1 bag tofu Shirataki fettuccini noodles
- ¼ cup lime juice
- ¼ cup fresh basil, chopped
- ¼ cup fresh cilantro, chopped
- 2 tablespoons fresh mint, chopped
- 2 tablespoons rice vinegar
- 2 tablespoons sweet chili sauce
- 2 tablespoons roasted peanuts finely chopped
- 1 tablespoon Splenda
- ½ teaspoon sesame oil

Directions:
1. Pickle the vegetables: In a large bowl, place radish, cucumbers, and carrots. Add vinegar, coconut sugar, and lime juice and stir to coat the vegetables. Cover and chill 15 – 20 minutes.
2. Prep the noodles: Remove the noodles from the package and rinse them under cold water. Cut into smaller pieces. Pat dry with paper towels.
3. To assemble the salad: Remove the vegetables from the marinade, reserve the marinade, and place them in a large mixing bowl. Add noodles, mango, bell pepper, chili, and herbs.
4. In a small bowl, combine 2 tablespoons marinade with the chili sauce and sesame oil. Pour over salad and toss to coat. Top with peanuts and serve.

Nutrition:
Calories: 129.18
Protein: 3.2g
Fat: 3.55g
Carbs: 25.68g
Sodium: 33mg

406. HEALTHY TACO SALAD

Preparation Time: 20 minutes
Cooking Time: 9 minutes
 Servings: 4
Ingredients:
- 2 whole Romaine hearts, chopped
- 1 lb. lean ground beef
- 1 whole avocado, cubed
- 3 oz. grape tomatoes, halved
- ½ cup cheddar cheese, cubed
- 2 tablespoon sliced red onion
- ½ batch Tangy Mexican Salad Dressing
- 1 teaspoon ground cumin
- Salt and pepper to taste

Directions:
1. Cook ground beef in a skillet over medium heat.
2. Break the beef up into little pieces as it cooks. Add seasonings and stir to combine. Drain grease and let cool for about 5 minutes.
3. To assemble the salad, place all ingredients into a large bowl. Toss to mix then add dressing and toss. Top with reduced-fat sour cream and/or salsa if desired.

Nutrition:
Calories: 449
Protein: 40g
Sodium: 389.45mg
Carbs: 9.63g

Fat: 22g

407. CHICKEN GUACAMOLE SALAD

Preparation Time: 6 minutes
Cooking Time: 25 minutes
 Servings: 6
Ingredients:
- 1 lb. chicken breast, boneless & skinless
- 2 avocados
- 1-2 jalapeño peppers, seeded & diced
- ⅓ cup onion, diced
- 3 tablespoons cilantro, diced
- 2 tablespoons fresh lime juice
- 2 cloves garlic, diced
- 1 tablespoon olive oil
- Salt & pepper, to taste

Directions:
1. Heat oven to 400°F. Line a baking sheet with foil.
2. Season chicken with salt and pepper and place on prepared pan. Bake 20 minutes, or until chicken is cooked through. Let cool completely.
3. Once the chicken has cooled, shred or dice and add to a large bowl. Add remaining ingredients and mix well, mashing the avocado as you mix it in. Taste and season with salt and pepper as desired. Serve immediately.

Nutrition:
Calories: 177.76
Protein: 17.97g
Fat: 9.81g
Carbs: 4.91g
Sodium: 167mg

408. WARM PORTOBELLO SALAD

Preparation Time: 20 minutes
Cooking Time: 9 minutes
 Servings: 4
Ingredients:
- 6 cup mixed salad greens
- 1 cup Portobello mushrooms, sliced
- 1 green onion, sliced
- Walnut or warm bacon vinaigrette
- 1 tablespoon olive oil
- ⅛ teaspoon ground black pepper

Directions:
1. Heat oil in a nonstick skillet over med-high heat. Add mushrooms and cook, stirring occasionally, 10 minutes, or

until they are tender. Stir in onions and reduce heat to low.

2. Place salad greens on serving plates, top with mushrooms, and sprinkle with pepper. Drizzle lightly with your choice of vinaigrette.

Nutrition:
Calories: 76.64
Protein: 2.9g
Fat: 6.28g
Carbs: 3.39g
Sodium: 60mg

409. LAYERED SALAD

Preparation Time: 9 minutes
Cooking Time: 15 minutes
Servings: 10
Ingredients:
- 6 slices bacon, chopped and cooked crisp
- 2 tomatoes, diced
- 2 stalks celery, sliced
- 1 head romaine lettuce, diced
- 1 red bell pepper, diced
- 1 cup frozen peas, thawed
- 1 cup sharp cheddar cheese, grated
- ¼ cup red onion diced fine
- 1 cup fat-free ranch dressing

Directions:
1. Use a 9x13 glass baking dish and layer half the lettuce, pepper, celery, tomatoes, peas, onion, cheese, bacon, and dressing. Repeat. Serve or cover and chill until ready to serve.

Nutrition:
Calories: 177
Protein: 6.49g
Fat: 10.3g
Carbs: 15g
Sodium: 491.58mg

410. BAKED "POTATO" SALAD

Preparation Time: 6 minutes
Cooking Time: 15 minutes
Servings: 8
Ingredients:
- 2 lb. cauliflower, separated into small florets
- 6-8 slices bacon, chopped and fried crisp
- 6 boiled eggs, cooled, peeled, and chopped
- 1 cup sharp cheddar cheese, grated
- ½ cup green onion, sliced
- 1 cup reduced-fat mayonnaise
- 2 teaspoons yellow mustard

- 1½ teaspoons onion powder, divided
- Salt and fresh-ground black pepper to taste

Directions:
1. Place cauliflower in a vegetable steamer, or a pot with a steamer insert, and steam for 5-6 minutes.
2. Drain the cauliflower and set it aside.
3. In a small bowl, whisk together mayonnaise, mustard, 1 teaspoon onion powder, salt, and pepper.
4. Pat cauliflower dry with paper towels and place in a large mixing bowl. Add eggs, salt, pepper, remaining ½ teaspoon onion powder, then dressing. Mix gently to combine ingredients together.
5. Fold in the bacon, cheese, and green onion. Serve warm or cover and chill before serving.

Nutrition:
Calories: 308
Protein: 11g
Fat: 27.48g
Carbs: 4.42g
Sodium: 630.94mg

411. CAPRESE SALAD

Preparation Time: 6 minutes
Cooking Time: 15 minutes
Servings: 4
Ingredients:
- 3 medium tomatoes, cut into 8 slices
- 2 1-oz. slices mozzarella cheese, cut into strips
- ¼ cup fresh basil, sliced thin
- 2 teaspoons extra-virgin olive oil
- ⅛ teaspoon salt
- Pinch black pepper

Directions:
1. Place tomatoes and cheese on serving plates. Sprinkle with salt and pepper. Drizzle oil over and top with basil. Serve.

Nutrition:
Calories: 77
Protein: 5g
Carbs: 3.7g
Sodium: 146mg
Fat: 5g

412. BROCCOLI SALAD

Preparation Time: 10 minutes
Cooking Time: none
Servings: 6

Ingredients:
- 1 medium head broccoli, raw, florets only
- ½ cup red onion, chopped
- 12 oz. turkey bacon, chopped, fried until crisp
- ½ cup cherry tomatoes, halved
- ¼ cup sunflower kernels
- ¾ cup raisins
- ¾ cup mayonnaise
- 2 tablespoon white vinegar

Directions:
1. In a salad bowl combine the broccoli, tomatoes, and onion.
2. Mix mayo with vinegar and sprinkle over the broccoli.
3. Add the sunflower kernels, raisins, and bacon, and toss well.

Nutrition:
Calories: 418.57
Carbohydrates: 19.59g
Protein: 11.57g
Sodium: 748.52mg

413. ASIAN CUCUMBER SALAD

Preparation Time: 10 minutes
Cooking Time: 0 minutes
Servings: 6
Ingredients:
- 1 lb. cucumbers, sliced
- 2 scallions, sliced
- 2 tablespoon sliced pickled ginger, chopped
- ¼ cup cilantro
- ½ red jalapeño, chopped
- 3 tablespoons rice wine vinegar
- 1 tablespoon sesame oil
- 1 tablespoon sesame seeds

Directions:
1. In a salad bowl combine all ingredients and toss together.

Nutrition:
Calories: 44.34
Carbohydrates: 3.4g
Protein: 0.9g
Sodium: 41mg

414. SCALLOP CAESAR SALAD

Preparation Time: 5 minutes
Cooking Time: 2 minutes
Servings: 2
Ingredients:
- 8 sea scallops
- 4 cups romaine lettuce
- 2 teaspoon olive oil
- 3 tablespoon Caesar salad dressing
- 1 teaspoon lemon juice
- Salt and pepper to taste

Directions:

1. In a frying pan, heat olive oil and cook the scallops in one layer no longer than 2 minutes on both sides. Season with salt and pepper to taste.
2. Arrange lettuce on plates and place scallops on top.
3. Pour over the Caesar dressing and lemon juice.

Nutrition:
Calories: 261.67
Carbohydrates: 8g
Protein: 16.14g
Sodium: 1131.89mg

415. CHICKEN SALAD IN CUCUMBER CUPS

Preparation Time: 5 minutes
Cooking Time: 15 minutes
Servings: 4
Ingredients:

- ½ chicken breast, skinless, boiled, and shredded
- 2 long cucumbers, cut into 8 thick rounds each, scooped out (won't use).
- 1 teaspoon ginger, minced
- 1 teaspoon lime zest, grated
- 4 teaspoons olive oil
- 1 teaspoon sesame oil
- 1 teaspoon lime juice
- Salt and pepper to taste

Directions:

1. In a bowl combine lime zest, juice, olive and sesame oils, ginger, and season with salt.
2. Toss the chicken with the dressing and fill the cucumber cups with the salad.

Nutrition:
Calories: 97.76
Carbohydrates: 4g
Protein: 6.7g
Sodium: 207mg
Fat: 6.65g

416. SUNFLOWER SEEDS AND ARUGULA GARDEN SALAD

Preparation Time: 5 minutes
Cooking Time: 10 minutes
Servings: 6
Ingredients:

- ¼ teaspoon black pepper
- ¼ teaspoon salt
- 1 teaspoon fresh thyme, chopped
- 2 tablespoon sunflower seeds, toasted
- 2 cups red grapes, halved
- 7 cups baby arugula, loosely packed

- 1 tablespoon coconut oil
- 2 teaspoon honey
- 3 tablespoon red wine vinegar
- ½ teaspoon stone-ground mustard

Directions:

1. In a small bowl, whisk together mustard, honey, and vinegar. Slowly pour oil as you whisk.
2. In a large salad bowl, mix thyme, seeds, grapes, and arugula.
3. Drizzle with dressing and serve.

Nutrition:
Calories: 86.7g
Protein: 1.6g
Carbs: 13.6g
Sodium: 120.41mg
Fat: 3.1g

417. SUPREME CAESAR SALAD

Preparation Time: 5 minutes
Cooking Time: 10 minutes
Servings: 4
Ingredients:

- ¼ cup olive oil
- ¾ cup mayonnaise
- 1 head romaine lettuce, torn into bite-sized pieces
- 1 tablespoon lemon juice
- 1 teaspoon Dijon mustard
- 1 teaspoon Worcestershire sauce
- 3 cloves garlic, peeled and minced
- 3 cloves garlic, peeled and quartered
- 4 cups day-old bread, cubed
- 5 anchovy filets, minced
- 6 tablespoon grated parmesan cheese, divided
- Ground black pepper to taste
- Salt to taste

Directions:

1. In a small bowl, whisk well lemon juice, mustard, Worcestershire sauce, 2 tablespoons parmesan cheese, anchovies, mayonnaise, and minced garlic. Season with pepper and salt to taste. Set aside in the ref.
2. On medium heat, place a large nonstick saucepan and heat oil.
3. Sauté quartered garlic until browned around a minute or two. Remove and discard.
4. Add bread cubes in the same pan, sauté until lightly browned. Season with pepper and salt. Transfer to a plate.
5. In a large bowl, place lettuce and pour in the dressing. Toss

well to coat. Top with remaining parmesan cheese.
6. Garnish with bread cubes, serve, and enjoy.

Nutrition:
Calories: 443.3g
Fat: 32.1g
Carbs: 36g
Sodium: 978mg
Protein: 11.6g

418. TABBOULEH- ARABIAN SALAD

Preparation Time: 5 minutes
Cooking Time: 10 minutes
Servings: 6
Ingredients:

- ¼ cup chopped fresh mint
- 1⅔ cups boiling water
- 1 cucumber, peeled, seeded, and chopped
- 1 cup bulgur
- 1 cup chopped fresh parsley
- 1 cup chopped green onions
- 1 teaspoon salt
- ⅓ cup lemon juice
- ⅓ cup olive oil
- 3 tomatoes, chopped
- Ground black pepper to taste

Directions:

1. In a large bowl, mix together boiling water and bulgur. Let soak and set aside for an hour while covered.
2. After one hour, toss in cucumber, tomatoes, mint, parsley, onions, lemon juice, and oil. Then season with black pepper and salt to taste. Toss well and refrigerate for another hour while covered before serving.

Nutrition:
Calories: 219.48g
Fat: 13.2g
Protein: 4.27g
Carbs: 24g
Sodium: 405.37mg

419. BACON-BROCCOLI SALAD

Preparation Time: 10 minutes
Cooking Time: 10 minutes
Servings: 10
Ingredients:

- 8 cups broccoli florets
- 3 strips of bacon, cooked and crumbled
- ¼ cup sunflower kernels
- 1 bunch of green onion, sliced
- 3 tablespoons seasoned rice vinegar
- 3 tablespoons canola oil

- ½ cup dried cranberries

Directions:
1. Combine the green onion, cranberries, and broccoli in a bowl.
2. Whisk the vinegar, and oil in another bowl. Blend well.
3. Now drizzle over the broccoli mix.
4. Coat well by tossing.
5. Sprinkle bacon and sunflower kernels before serving.

Nutrition:
Calories: 139
Fat: 9.18g
Protein: 3.45g
Carbs: 13g
Sodium: 136.5mg

420. TENDERLOIN GRILLED SALAD

Preparation Time: 10 minutes
Cooking Time: 20 minutes
Servings: 5
Ingredients:
- 1 lb. pork tenderloin
- 10 cups mixed salad greens
- 2 oranges, seedless, cut into bite-sized pieces
- 1 tablespoon orange zest, grated
- 2 tablespoons of cider vinegar
- 2 tablespoons olive oil
- 2 teaspoons Dijon mustard
- ½ cup juice of an orange
- 2 teaspoons honey
- ½ teaspoon ground pepper

Directions:
1. Bring together all the dressing ingredients in a bowl.
2. Grill each side of the pork covered over medium heat for 9 minutes.
3. Slice after 5 minutes.
4. Slice the tenderloin thinly.
5. Keep the greens on your serving plate.
6. Top with the pork and oranges.
7. Sprinkle nuts (optional).

Nutrition:
Calories: 211
Fat: 9g
Carbs: 11.92g
Sodium: 74.5mg
Protein: 20g

421. BARLEY VEGGIE SALAD

Preparation Time: 10 minutes
Cooking Time: 20 minutes
Servings: 6
Ingredients:
- 1 tomato, seeded and chopped
- 2 tablespoons parsley, minced

- 1 yellow pepper, chopped
- 1 tablespoon basil, minced
- ¼ cup almonds, toasted
- 1¼ cups vegetable broth
- 1 cup barley
- 1 tablespoon lemon juice
- 2 tablespoons of white wine vinegar
- 3 tablespoons olive oil
- ¼ teaspoon pepper
- ½ teaspoon salt
- 1 cup of water

Directions:
1. Boil the broth, barley, and water in a saucepan.
2. Reduce heat. Cover and let it simmer for 10 minutes.
3. Take out from the heat.
4. In the meantime, bring together the parsley, yellow pepper, and tomato in a bowl.
5. Stir the barley in.
6. Whisk the vinegar, oil, basil, lemon juice, water, pepper, and salt in a bowl.
7. Pour this over your barley mix. Toss to coat well.
8. Stir the almonds in before serving.

Nutrition:
Calories: 233.38
Fat: 11.32g
Protein: 5.23g
Carbs: 29.66g
Sodium: 370.39mg

422. SPINACH SHRIMP SALAD

Preparation Time: 10 minutes
Cooking Time: 10 minutes
Servings: 4
Ingredients:
- 1 lb. uncooked shrimp, peeled and deveined
- 2 tablespoons parsley, minced
- ¾ cup halved cherry tomatoes
- 1 medium lemon
- 4 cups baby spinach
- 2 tablespoons unsalted butter
- 3 minced garlic cloves
- ¼ teaspoon pepper
- ¼ teaspoon salt

Directions:
1. Melt the butter over the medium temperature in a nonstick skillet.
2. Add the shrimp.
3. Now cook the shrimp for 3 minutes until they become pink.
4. Add the parsley and garlic.
5. Cook for another minute. Remove from heat.
6. Keep the spinach in your salad bowl.

7. Top with the shrimp mix and tomatoes.
8. Drizzle lemon juice on the salad.
9. Sprinkle pepper and salt.

Nutrition:
Calories: 143.77
Fat: 6.68g
Protein: 17.35g
Carbs: 4g
Sodium: 807.85mg

423. CHOPPED VEGGIE SALAD

Preparation Time: 4 minutes
Cooking Time: 15 minutes
Servings: 4
Ingredients:
- 1 cucumber, chopped
- 1 pint cherry tomatoes, cut in half
- 3 radishes, chopped
- 1 yellow bell pepper chopped
- ½ cup fresh parsley, chopped
- 3 tablespoon lemon juice
- 1 tablespoon olive oil
- Salt to taste

Directions:
1. Place all ingredients in a large bowl and toss to combine. Serve immediately, or cover and chill until ready to serve.

Nutrition:
Calories: 70
Protein: 2g
Fat: 4g
Carbs: 8g
Sodium: 206mg

424. TOFU SALAD SANDWICHES

Preparation Time: 9 minutes
Cooking Time: 16 minutes
Servings: 4
Ingredients:
- 1 pkg. silken firm tofu, pressed
- 4 lettuce leaves
- 2 green onions, diced
- ¼ cup celery, diced
- 8 slices bread
- ¼ cup light mayonnaise
- 2 tablespoons sweet pickle relish
- 1 tablespoon Dijon mustard
- ¼ teaspoon turmeric
- ¼ teaspoon salt
- ⅛ teaspoon cayenne pepper

Directions:
1. Press tofu between layers of paper towels for 15 minutes to remove excess moisture. Cut into small cubes.

2. In a medium bowl, stir together the remaining ingredients. Fold in tofu. Spread over 4 slices of bread. Top with a lettuce leaf and another slice of bread. Serve.

Nutrition:
Calories: 317.23
Protein: 15.83g
Fat: 9.4g
Carbs: 44.7g
Sodium: 728mg

425. LOBSTER ROLL SALAD WITH BACON VINAIGRETTE

Preparation Time: 20 minutes
Cooking Time: 15 minutes
Servings: 6
Ingredients:
- 6 slices bacon
- 2 whole grain ciabatta rolls, halved horizontally
- 3 medium tomatoes, cut into wedges
- 2 8-oz. spiny lobster tails, fresh or frozen (thawed)
- 2 cups fresh baby spinach
- 2 cups romaine lettuce, torn
- 1 cup seeded cucumber, diced
- 1 cup red sweet peppers, diced
- 2 tablespoons shallot, diced fine
- 2 tablespoons fresh chives, diced fine
- 2 cloves garlic, diced fine
- 3 tablespoon white wine vinegar
- 3 tablespoons olive oil, divided

Directions:
1. Heat a grill to medium heat, or medium heat charcoals.
2. Rinse lobster and pat dry. Butterfly lobster tails. Place on the grill, cover, and cook for 25 – 30 minutes, or until meat is opaque.
3. Remove lobster and let cool.
4. In a small bowl, whisk together 2 tablespoons of olive oil and garlic. Brush the cut sides of the rolls with an oil mixture. Place on grill, cut side down, and cook until crisp, about 2 minutes. Transfer to cutting board.
5. While lobster is cooking, chop bacon and cook in a medium skillet until crisp. Transfer to paper towels. Reserve 1 tablespoon bacon grease.
6. To make the vinaigrette: combine reserved bacon grease, vinegar, shallot, remaining 1

tablespoon oil, and chives in a glass jar with an air-tight lid. Screw on the lid and shake to combine.
7. Remove the lobster from the shells and cut it into 1 ½-inch piece. Cut rolls into 1-inch cubes.
8. To assemble salad: In a large bowl, combine spinach, romaine, tomatoes, cucumber, peppers, lobster, and bread cubes. Toss to combine. Transfer to serving platter and drizzle with vinaigrette. Sprinkle bacon over top and serve.

Nutrition:
Calories: 283
Protein: 13.32g
Fat: 18g
Carbs: 18.29g
Sodium: 334mg

426. POMEGRANATE & BRUSSELS SPROUTS SALAD

Preparation Time: 8 minutes
Cooking Time: 12 minutes
Servings: 6
Ingredients:
- 3 slices bacon, cooked crisp & crumbled
- 3 cups Brussels sprouts, shredded
- 3 cup kale, shredded
- 1½ cup pomegranate seeds
- ½ cup almonds, toasted & chopped
- ¼ cup reduced-fat parmesan cheese, grated
- Citrus vinaigrette

Directions:
1. Combine all ingredients in a large bowl.
2. Drizzle vinaigrette over salad and toss to coat well. Serve garnished with more cheese if desired.

Nutrition:
Calories: 223
Protein: 8.98g
Fat: 14.42g
Carbs: 18.58g
Sodium: 182mg

427. STRAWBERRY & AVOCADO SALAD

Preparation Time: 6 minutes
Cooking Time: 9 minutes
Servings: 6
Ingredients:
- 6 oz. baby spinach

- 2 avocados, chopped
- 1 cup strawberries, sliced
- ¼ cup feta cheese, crumbled
- Creamy poppy seed dressing
- ¼ cup almonds, sliced

Directions:
1. Add spinach, berries, avocado, nuts, and cheese to a large bowl and toss to combine.
2. Pour ½ recipe of creamy poppy seed dressing over salad and toss to coat. Add more dressing if desired. Serve.

Nutrition:
Calories: 146.55
Protein: 4g
Fat: 11.89g
Carbs: 8.8g
Sodium: 118.65mg

428. KALE SALAD WITH AVOCADO DRESSING

Preparation Time: 10 minutes
Cooking Time: 0 minutes
Servings: 6
Ingredients:
- 6 cups chopped kale
- 1 cup finely chopped red bell pepper
- 1 bunch scallions, white and green parts, finely chopped
- 1 avocado, pitted and peeled
- ½ cup raw cashews
- 3 garlic cloves, peeled
- Juice of ½ lemon
- ¼ cup extra-virgin olive oil
- Salt
- Freshly ground black pepper

Directions:
1. In a large bowl, toss together the kale, red bell pepper, and scallions.
2. In a high-speed blender or food processor, combine the avocado, cashews, garlic, lemon juice, and olive oil, and process until smooth. Add up to ½ cup of water as needed to create a pourable dressing. Season with salt and pepper. Pour the dressing over the kale, mix well, and serve.

Nutrition:
Calories: 224.3
Total Fat: 18g
Protein: 5.46g
Carbs: 14g
Sodium: 160.32mg

429. ROASTED BEET SALAD

Preparation Time: 20 minutes

Cooking Time: 70 minutes
Servings: 4
Ingredients:
- 6 medium beets, scrubbed, tops removed
- ¼ cup balsamic vinegar
- ¼ cup extra-virgin olive oil
- 1 teaspoon Dijon mustard
- Salt
- Freshly ground black pepper
- ¼ cup walnuts
- 6 ounces baby arugula
- 2 ounces feta cheese, crumbled

Directions:
1. Preheat the oven to 400°F.
2. Wrap each beet tightly in aluminum foil and arrange it on a baking sheet. Roast for 45 to 60 minutes, depending on their size, until tender when pierced with a knife. Remove from the oven, carefully unwrap each beet, and let cool for 10 minutes.
3. Reduce the oven temperature to 350°F.
4. Meanwhile, in a medium bowl, whisk the vinegar, olive oil, and mustard. Season with salt and pepper.
5. On the same baking sheet, spread the walnuts in a single layer. Toast for 5 to 7 minutes, until lightly browned.
6. Using a small knife, peel and slice the beets, and place them in another medium bowl. Add half the vinaigrette and toss to coat.
7. Add the arugula to the remaining vinaigrette and toss to coat.
8. On a serving platter, arrange the arugula and top with the beets. Sprinkle the toasted walnuts and feta cheese over the top and serve.

Nutrition:
Calories: 282.84
Total Fat: 24.44g
Protein: 5.7g
Carbs: 12g
Sodium: 422mg

430. TROPICAL FRUIT SALAD WITH COCONUT MILK

Preparation Time: 10 minutes
Cooking Time: 0 minutes
Servings: 8
Ingredients:
- 2 cups pineapple chunks
- 2 kiwi fruits, peeled and sliced
- 1 mango, peeled and chopped
- ¼ cup canned light coconut milk
- 1 tablespoon freshly squeezed lime juice
- 1 tablespoon honey

Directions:
1. In a medium bowl, toss together the pineapple, kiwi, and mango.
2. In a small bowl, combine the coconut milk, lime juice, and honey, stirring until the honey dissolves. Pour the mixture over the fruits and toss to coat. Serve immediately or refrigerate in an airtight container for up to 3 days.

Nutrition:
Calories: 70.65
Total Fat: 0.72g
Protein: 0.79g
Carbs: 17g
Sodium: 1.97mg

431. CUCUMBER, TOMATO, AND AVOCADO SALAD

Preparation Time: 10 minutes
Cooking Time: 0 minutes
Servings: 4
Ingredients:
- 1 cup cherry tomatoes, halved
- 1 large cucumber, chopped
- 1 small red onion, thinly sliced
- 1 avocado, diced
- 2 tablespoons chopped fresh dill
- 2 tablespoons extra-virgin olive oil
- Juice of 1 lemon
- ¼ teaspoon salt
- ¼ teaspoon freshly ground black pepper

Directions:
1. In a large mixing bowl, combine the tomatoes, cucumber, onion, avocado, and dill.
2. In a small bowl, combine the oil, lemon juice, salt, and pepper, and mix well.
3. Drizzle the dressing over the vegetables and toss to combine. Serve.

Nutrition:
Calories: 131.74
Total Fat: 11.39g
Protein: 1.59g
Carbs: 7.89g
Sodium: 151.44mg

432. CABBAGE SLAW SALAD

Preparation Time: 20 minutes
Cooking Time: 0 minutes
Servings: 6
Ingredients:
- 2 cups finely chopped green cabbage
- 2 cups finely chopped red cabbage
- 2 cups grated carrots
- 3 scallions, both white and green parts, sliced
- 2 tablespoons extra-virgin olive oil
- 2 tablespoons rice vinegar
- 1 teaspoon honey
- 1 garlic clove, minced
- ¼ teaspoon salt

Directions:
1. In a large bowl, toss together the green and red cabbage, carrots, and scallions.
2. In a small bowl, whisk together the oil, vinegar, honey, garlic, and salt.
3. Pour the dressing over the veggies and mix to thoroughly combine.
4. Serve immediately or cover and chill for several hours before serving.

Nutrition:
Calories: 80
Total Fat: 5g
Carbs: 9.07g
Sodium: 138.47mg
Protein: 1.27g

433. GREEN SALAD WITH BLACKBERRIES, GOAT CHEESE, AND SWEET POTATOES

Preparation Time: 20 minutes
Cooking Time: 15 minutes
Servings: 4
Ingredients:
For the vinaigrette:
- 1 pint blackberries
- 2 tablespoons red wine vinegar
- 1 tablespoon honey
- 3 tablespoons extra-virgin olive oil
- ¼ teaspoon salt
- Freshly ground black pepper

For the Salad:
- 1 sweet potato, cubed
- 1 teaspoon extra-virgin olive oil
- 8 cups salad greens (baby spinach, spicy greens, romaine)
- ½ red onion, sliced

- ¼ cup crumbled goat cheese

Directions:
1. To make the vinaigrette: In a blender jar, combine the blackberries, vinegar, honey, oil, salt, and pepper, and process until smooth. Set aside.
2. To make the salad
3. Preheat the oven to 425°F. Line a baking sheet with parchment paper.
4. In a medium mixing bowl, toss the sweet potato with the olive oil. Transfer everything onto the baking sheet and then roast it for 20 minutes, stirring once halfway through, until tender. Remove and cool for a few minutes.
5. In a large bowl, toss the greens with the red onion and cooled sweet potato, and drizzle with the vinaigrette. Serve topped with 1 tablespoon of goat cheese per serving.

Nutrition:
Calories: 253.56
Total Fat: 15.65g
Protein: 5.82g
Carbs: 24.6g
Sodium: 230.87mg

434. 3 BEAN AND BASIL SALAD

Preparation Time: 20 minutes
Cooking Time: 0 minutes
Servings: 8
Ingredients:
- 1 15-ounce can low-sodium chickpeas, drained and rinsed
- 1 15-ounce can low-sodium kidney beans, drained and rinsed
- 1 15-ounce can low-sodium white beans, drained and rinsed
- 1 red bell pepper, seeded and finely chopped
- ¼ cup chopped scallions, both white and green parts
- ¼ cup finely chopped fresh basil
- 3 garlic cloves, minced
- 2 tablespoons extra-virgin olive oil
- 1 tablespoon red wine vinegar
- 1 teaspoon Dijon mustard
- ¼ teaspoon freshly ground black pepper

Directions:
1. In a large mixing bowl, combine the chickpeas, kidney beans, white beans, bell pepper, scallions, basil, and garlic. Toss gently to combine.

2. In a small bowl, combine the olive oil, vinegar, mustard, and pepper. Toss with the salad.
3. Cover and refrigerate for an hour before serving, to allow the flavors to mix.
4. Substitution tip: Feel free to substitute home-cooked beans in place of canned, using about 1½ cups per variety.

Nutrition:
Calories: 158
Total Fat: 6.7g
Protein: 6.6g
Carbs: 18.9g
Sodium: 144.26mg

435. RAINBOW BLACK BEAN SALAD

Preparation Time: 16 minutes
Cooking Time: 0 minutes
Servings: 5
Ingredients:
- 1 15-ounce can low-sodium black beans, drained and rinsed
- 1 avocado, diced
- 1 cup cherry tomatoes, halved
- 1 cup chopped baby spinach
- ½ cup finely chopped red bell pepper
- ¼ cup finely chopped jicama
- ½ cup chopped scallions, both white and green parts
- ¼ cup chopped fresh cilantro
- 2 tablespoons freshly squeezed lime juice
- 1 tablespoon extra-virgin olive oil
- 2 garlic cloves, minced
- 1 teaspoon honey
- ¼ teaspoon salt
- ¼ teaspoon freshly ground black pepper

Directions:
1. In a large bowl, combine the black beans, avocado, tomatoes, spinach, bell pepper, jicama, scallions, and cilantro.
2. In a small bowl, mix the lime juice, oil, garlic, honey, salt, and pepper. Add to the salad and toss.
3. Chill for 1 hour before serving.

Nutrition:
Calories: 169
Total Fat: 7g
Carbs: 19.45g
Sodium: 188mg
Protein: 6g

436. WINTER CHICKEN AND CITRUS SALAD

Preparation Time: 20 minutes
Cooking Time: 0 minutes
Servings: 4
Ingredients:
- 4 cups baby spinach
- 2 tablespoons extra-virgin olive oil
- 1 tablespoon freshly squeezed lemon juice
- ⅛ teaspoon salt
- Freshly ground black pepper
- 2 cups chopped cooked chicken
- 2 mandarin oranges, peeled and sectioned
- ½ peeled grapefruit, sectioned
- ¼ cup sliced almonds

Directions:
1. In a large mixing bowl, toss the spinach with olive oil, lemon juice, salt, and pepper.
2. Add the chicken, oranges, grapefruit, and almonds to the bowl. Toss gently.
3. Arrange on 4 plates and serve.

Nutrition:
Calories: 289
Total Fat: 22g
Protein: 15g
Carbs: 9.54g
Sodium: 141mg

437. FRENCH BROCCOLI SALAD

Preparation Time: 10 minutes
Cooking Time: 10 minutes
Servings: 10
Ingredients:
- 8 cups broccoli florets
- 3 strips of bacon, cooked and crumbled
- ¼ cup sunflower kernels
- 1 bunch of green onion, sliced
- 3 tablespoons seasoned rice vinegar
- 3 tablespoons canola oil
- ½ cup dried cranberries

Directions:
1. Combine the green onion, cranberries, and broccoli in a bowl.
2. Whisk the vinegar, and oil in another bowl. Blend well.
3. Now drizzle over the broccoli mix.
4. Coat well by tossing.
5. Sprinkle bacon and sunflower kernels before serving.

Nutrition:
Calories: 121
Carbohydrates: 14g

Cholesterol 2mg
Fiber: 3g
Sugar 1g
Fat: 7g
Protein: 3g
Sodium: 233mg

438. TENDERLOIN GRILLED SALAD

Preparation Time: 10 minutes
Cooking Time: 20 minutes
Servings: 5
Ingredients:

- 1 lb. pork tenderloin
- 10 cups mixed salad greens
- 2 oranges, seedless, cut into bite-sized pieces
- 1 tablespoon orange zest, grated
- 2 tablespoons of cider vinegar
- 2 tablespoons olive oil
- 2 teaspoons Dijon mustard
- ½ cup juice of an orange
- 2 teaspoons honey
- ½ teaspoon ground pepper

Directions:

1. Bring together all the dressing ingredients in a bowl.
2. Grill each side of the pork covered over medium heat for 9 minutes.
3. Slice after 5 minutes.
4. Slice the tenderloin thinly.
5. Keep the greens on your serving plate.
6. Top with the pork and oranges.
7. Sprinkle nuts (optional).

Nutrition:
Calories: 211
Carbohydrates: 13g
Cholesterol 51mg
Fiber: 3g
Sugar 0.8g
Fat: 9g
Protein: 20g
Sodium: 113mg

439. BARLEY VEGGIE SALAD

Preparation Time: 10 minutes
Cooking Time: 20 minutes
Servings: 6
Ingredients:

- 1 tomato, seeded and chopped
- 2 tablespoons parsley, minced
- 1 yellow pepper, chopped
- 1 tablespoon basil, minced
- ¼ cup almonds, toasted
- 1¼ cups vegetable broth
- 1 cup barley
- 1 tablespoon lemon juice
- 2 tablespoons of white wine vinegar

- 3 tablespoons olive oil
- ¼ teaspoon pepper
- ½ teaspoon salt
- 1 cup of water

Directions:

1. Boil the broth, barley, and water in a saucepan.
2. Reduce heat. Cover and let it simmer for 10 minutes.
3. Take out from the heat.
4. In the meantime, bring together the parsley, yellow pepper, and tomato in a bowl.
5. Stir the barley in.
6. Whisk the vinegar, oil, basil, lemon juice, water, pepper, and salt in a bowl.
7. Pour this over your barley mix. Toss to coat well.
8. Stir the almonds in before serving.

Nutrition:
Calories: 211
Carbohydrates: 27g
Fiber: 7g
Fat: 10g
Protein: 6g
Sodium: 334mg

440. SPINACH SHRIMP SALAD

Preparation Time: 10 minutes
Cooking Time: 10 minutes
Servings: 4
Ingredients:

- 1 lb. uncooked shrimp, peeled and deveined
- 2 tablespoons parsley, minced
- ¾ cup halved cherry tomatoes
- 1 medium lemon
- 4 cups baby spinach
- 2 tablespoons unsalted butter
- 3 minced garlic cloves
- ¼ teaspoon pepper
- ¼ teaspoon salt

Directions:

1. Melt the butter over medium temperature in a nonstick skillet.
2. Add the shrimp.
3. Now cook the shrimp for 3 minutes until your shrimp becomes pink.
4. Add the parsley and garlic.
5. Cook for another minute. Take out from the heat.
6. Keep the spinach in your salad bowl.
7. Top with the shrimp mix and tomatoes.
8. Drizzle lemon juice on the salad.
9. Sprinkle pepper and salt.

Nutrition:

Calories: 201
Carbohydrates: 6g
Cholesterol 153mg
Fiber: 2g
Fat: 10g
Protein: 21g
Sodium: 350mg

441. SWEET POTATO AND ROASTED BEET SALAD

Preparation Time: 10 minutes
Cooking Time: 10 minutes
Servings: 4
Ingredients:

- 2 beets
- 1 sweet potato, peeled and cubed
- 1 garlic clove, minced
- 2 tablespoons walnuts, chopped and toasted
- 1 cup fennel bulb, sliced
- 3 tablespoons balsamic vinegar
- 1 teaspoon Dijon mustard
- 1 tablespoon honey
- 3 tablespoons olive oil
- ¼ teaspoon pepper
- ¼ teaspoon salt
- 3 tablespoons water

Directions:

1. Scrub the beets. Trim the tops to 1 inch.
2. Wrap in foil and keep on a baking sheet.
3. Bake until tender. Take off the foil.
4. Combine water and sweet potato in a bowl.
5. Cover. Microwave for 5 minutes. Drain.
6. Now peel the beets. Cut into small wedges.
7. Arrange the fennel, sweet potato, and beets on 4 salad plates.
8. Sprinkle nuts.
9. Whisk the honey, mustard, vinegar, water, garlic, pepper, and salt. Whisk in oil gradually.
10. Drizzle over the salad.

Nutrition:
Calories: 270
Carbohydrates: 37g
Fiber: 6g
Sugar 0.3g
Fat: 13g
Protein: 5g
Sodium: 309mg

442. POTATO CALICO SALAD

Preparation Time: 15 minutes
Cooking Time: 5 minutes

Servings: 14

Ingredients:

- 4 red potatoes, peeled and cooked
- 1½ cups kernel corn, cooked
- ½ cup green pepper, diced
- ½ cup red onion, chopped
- 1 cup carrots, shredded
- ½ cup olive oil
- ¼ cup vinegar
- 1½ teaspoons chili powder
- 1 teaspoon salt
- Dash of hot pepper sauce

Directions:

1. Keep all the ingredients together in a jar.
2. Close it and shake well.
3. Cube the potatoes. Combine with the carrot, onion, and corn in your salad bowl.
4. Pour the dressing over.
5. Now toss lightly.

Nutrition:
Calories: 146
Carbohydrates: 17g
Fat: 9g
Protein: 2g
Sodium: 212mg

443. MANGO AND JICAMA SALAD

Preparation Time: 15 minutes
Cooking Time: 5 minutes
Servings: 8
Ingredients:

- 1 jicama, peeled
- 1 mango, peeled
- 1 teaspoon ginger root, minced
- ⅓ cup chives, minced
- ½ cup cilantro, chopped
- ¼ cup canola oil
- ½ cup white wine vinegar
- 2 tablespoons of lime juice
- ¼ cup honey
- ⅛ teaspoon pepper
- ¼ teaspoon salt

Directions:

1. Whisk together the vinegar, honey, canola oil, gingerroot, paper, and salt.
2. Cut the mango and jicama into matchsticks.
3. Keep in a bowl.
4. Now toss with the lime juice.
5. Add the dressing and herbs. Combine well by tossing.

Nutrition:
Calories: 143
Carbohydrates: 20g
Fiber: 3g
Sugar 1.6g
Fat: 7g
Protein: 1g
Sodium: 78mg

444. ASIAN CRISPY CHICKEN SALAD

Preparation Time: 10 minutes
Cooking Time: 10 minutes
Servings: 2
Ingredients:

- 2 chicken breasts halved, skinless
- ½ cup panko breadcrumbs
- 4 cups spring mix salad greens
- 4 teaspoons of sesame seeds
- ½ cup mushrooms, sliced
- 1 teaspoon sesame oil
- 2 teaspoons of canola oil
- 2 teaspoons hoisin sauce
- ¼ cup sesame ginger salad dressing

Directions:

1. Flatten the chicken breasts to half-inch thickness.
2. Mix the sesame oil and hoisin sauce. Brush over the chicken.
3. Combine the sesame seeds and panko in a bowl.
4. Now dip the chicken mix in it.
5. Cook each side of the chicken for 5 minutes.
6. In the meantime, divide the salad greens between 2 plates.
7. Top with mushroom.

8. Slice the chicken and keep on top. Drizzle the dressing.

Nutrition:
Calories: 386
Carbohydrates: 29g
Cholesterol: 63mg
Fiber: 6g
Sugar: 1g
Fat: 17g
Protein: 30g
Sodium: 620mg

445. KALE, GRAPE AND BULGUR SALAD

Preparation Time: 10 minutes
Cooking Time: 15 minutes
Servings: 6
Ingredients:

- 1 cup bulgur
- 1 cup pecan, toasted and chopped
- ¼ cup scallions, sliced
- ½ cup parsley, chopped
- 2 cups California grapes, seedless and halved
- 2 tablespoons of extra virgin olive oil
- ¼ cup of juice from a lemon
- Pinch of kosher salt
- Pinch of black pepper
- 2 cups of water

Directions:

1. Boil 2 cups of water in a saucepan
2. Stir the bulgur in and ½ teaspoon of salt.
3. Remove from heat.
4. Keep covered. Drain.
5. Stir in the other ingredients.
6. Season with pepper and salt.

Nutrition:
Calories: 289
Carbohydrates: 33g
Fat: 17g
Protein: 6g
Sodium: 181mg

SOUPS AND STEWS

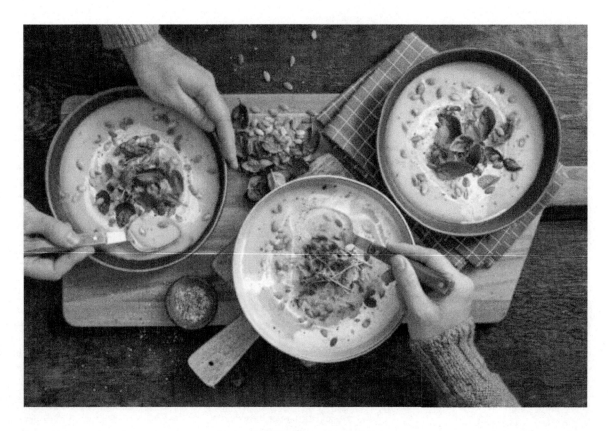

446. DILL CELERY SOUP

Preparation Time: 10 minutes
Cooking Time: 30 minutes
Servings: 4
Ingredients:
- 6 cups celery stalk, chopped
- 2 cups filtered alkaline water
- 1 medium onion, chopped
- ½ teaspoon dill
- 1 cup of coconut milk
- ¼ teaspoon sea salt

Directions:
1. Combine all elements into the direct pot and mix fine.
2. Cover pot with lid and select soup mode it takes 30 minutes.
3. Release pressure using the quick release directions then open the lid carefully.
4. Blend the soup utilizing a submersion blender until smooth.
5. Stir well and serve.

Nutrition:
Calories: 169
Fat: 14.58g
Carbohydrates: 10g
Protein: 2.68g
Sugar: 5g
Sodium: 248.1mg

447. CREAMY AVOCADO-BROCCOLI SOUP

Preparation Time: 10 minutes
Cooking Time: 15 minutes
Servings: 1-2
Ingredients:
- 1 small avocado
- 2-3 broccoli florets
- 1 yellow onion
- 1 green or red pepper
- 1 celery stalk
- 2 cups vegetable broth (yeast-free)
- Celtic Sea Salt to taste

Directions:
1. Warm vegetable stock (don't bubble). Include chopped onion and broccoli, and warm for a few minutes. At that point put in a blender, include the avocado, pepper, and celery, and Blend until the soup is smooth (include some more water whenever wanted). Flavor and serve warm. Delicious!!

Nutrition:
Calories: 124g
Carbohydrates: 14g
Fat: 7.4g
Protein: 2.8g
Sodium: 1073mg

448. FRESH GARDEN VEGETABLE SOUP

Preparation Time: 7 minutes
Cooking Time: 20 minutes
Servings: 1-2
Ingredients:

- 2 large carrots
- 1 small zucchini
- 1 celery stem
- 1 cup of broccoli
- 3 stalks of asparagus
- 1 yellow onion
- 1 quart of water
- 4-5 teaspoons of sans yeast vegetable stock
- 1 teaspoon new basil
- 2 teaspoons sea salt to taste

Directions:

1. Put water in the pot, including the vegetable stock just as the onion, and bring it to a bubble.
2. In the meantime, cleave the zucchini, the broccoli, and the asparagus, and shred the carrots and the celery stem in a food processor.
3. When the water is bubbling, turn off the oven, as we would prefer not to heat up the vegetables. Simply put them all in the high temp water and hold up until the vegetables soften a bit.
4. Let cool and at that point put all fixings into a blender and blend until you get a thick, smooth consistency.

Nutrition:
Calories: 43
Carbohydrates: 16g
Sodium: 1998mg
Fat: 0.56g

449. ALKALINE CARROT SOUP WITH FRESH MUSHROOMS

Preparation Time: 10 minutes
Cooking Time: 20 minutes
Servings: 1-2
Ingredients:

- 4 medium-sized carrots
- 4 medium-sized potatoes
- 10 large new mushrooms (champignons or chanterelles)
- ½ white onion
- 2 tablespoon olive oil (cold squeezed, additional virgin)
- 3 cups vegetable stock
- 2 tablespoon parsley, new and cleaved
- Salt and new white pepper

Directions:

1. Wash and peel carrots and potatoes and dice them.
2. Warm up vegetable stock in a pot on medium heat. Cook carrots and potatoes for around 15 minutes. Meanwhile, finely chop onions and braise them in a container with olive oil for around 3 minutes.
3. Wash mushrooms, slice them to the desired size, and add to the container, cooking approx. an additional 5 minutes, stirring at times. Blend carrots, vegetable stock, and potatoes, and put the blend into the pot.
4. When nearly done, season with parsley, salt, and pepper and serve hot. Appreciate this alkalizing soup!

Nutrition:
Calories: 490
Carbohydrates: 80g
Fat: 15g
Protein: 12.8g
Sodium: 1550mg

450. SWISS CAULIFLOWER-EMMENTAL-SOUP

Preparation Time: 10 minutes
Cooking Time: 15 minutes
Servings: 3-4
Ingredients:

- 2 cups cauliflower pieces
- 1 cup potatoes, cubed
- 2 cups vegetable stock (without yeast)
- 3 tablespoons Swiss Emmental cheddar, cubed
- 2 tablespoons new chives
- 1 tablespoon pumpkin seeds
- 1 touch of nutmeg and cayenne pepper

Directions:

1. Cook cauliflower and potato in vegetable stock until delicate and blend with a blender.
2. Season the soup with nutmeg and cayenne, and possibly somewhat salt and pepper.
3. Add Emmental cheddar and chives and mix a couple of moments until the soup is smooth and prepared to serve. Enhance it with pumpkin seeds.

Nutrition:
Calories: 80
Carbohydrates: 10.8g
Fat: 2.8g
Protein: 3.9g
Sodium: 411.61mg

451. CHILLED AVOCADO TOMATO SOUP

Preparation Time: 7 minutes
Cooking Time: 20 minutes
Servings: 1-2
Ingredients:

- 2 small avocados
- 2 large tomatoes
- 1 stalk of celery
- 1 small onion
- 1 clove of garlic
- Juice of 1 fresh lemon
- 1 cup of water (best: alkaline water)
- A handful of fresh lovage
- Parsley and sea salt to taste

Directions:

1. Scoop the avocados and cut all veggies into little pieces.
2. Add all fixings in a blender and blend until smooth.
3. Serve chilled.

Nutrition:
Calories: 210
Carbohydrates: 20.72g
Fat: 14.6g
Protein: 4.23g
Sodium: 378.32mg

452. PUMPKIN AND WHITE BEAN SOUP WITH SAGE

Preparation Time: 10 minutes
Cooking Time: 40 minutes
Servings: 3-4
Ingredients:

- 1½ pound pumpkin
- ½ pound yams
- ½ pound white beans
- 1 onion
- 2 cloves of garlic
- 1 tablespoon of cold squeezed extra- virgin olive oil
- 1 tablespoon of spices (your top picks)
- 1 tablespoon of sage
- 1½ quart water (best: antacid water)
- A dash of sea salt and pepper

Directions:

1. Cut the pumpkin and potatoes, cut the onion, and cut the garlic, the spices, and the sage into fine pieces.
2. Sauté the onion and garlic in olive oil for around 2 or 3 minutes.
3. Include the potatoes, pumpkin, spices, and sage and fry for an additional 5 minutes.
4. At that point add the water and cook for around 30 minutes

(spread the pot with a top) until vegetables are delicate.

5. Finally, add the beans and some salt and pepper. Cook for an additional 5 minutes and serve right away.

Nutrition:
Calories: 323.66
Carbohydrates: 59g
Sodium: 85.33mg
Fat: 4.5g

453. ALKALINE CARROT SOUP WITH MILLET

Preparation Time: 7 minutes
Cooking Time: 40 minutes
Servings: 3-4
Ingredients:

- 2 cups cauliflower pieces
- 1 cup potatoes, cubed
- 2 cups vegetable stock (without yeast)
- 3 tablespoon Swiss Emmental cheddar, cubed
- 2 tablespoon new chives
- 1 tablespoon pumpkin seeds
- 1 dash of nutmeg and cayenne pepper

Directions:

1. Cook cauliflower and potato in vegetable stock until delicate and blend with a blender.
2. Season the soup with nutmeg and cayenne, salt and pepper.
3. Include Emmental cheddar and chives and mix a couple of moments until the soup is smooth and prepared to serve. Can enhance with pumpkin seeds.

Nutrition:
Calories: 87
Carbohydrates: 12g
Fat: 3g
Protein: 4.4g
Sodium: 419.47mg

454. ALKALINE PUMPKIN TOMATO SOUP

Preparation Time: 15 minutes
Cooking Time: 30 minutes
Servings: 3-4
Ingredients:

- 1 quart of water (if accessible: soluble water)
- 400g new tomatoes, stripped and diced
- 1 medium-sized sweet pumpkin
- 5 yellow onions
- 1 tablespoon cold squeezed extra-virgin olive oil

- 2 teaspoons sea salt or natural salt
- Touch of cayenne pepper
- Your preferred spices
- Bunch of new parsley

Directions:

1. Cut onions in little pieces and sauté with some oil in a large pot.
2. Cut the pumpkin down the middle, at that point remove the stem and scoop out the seeds.
3. Add the pumpking to the pot.
4. Include the tomatoes and the water and cook for around 20 minutes.
5. At that point empty the soup into a food processor and blend well for a couple of moments. Sprinkle with salt pepper and other spices.
6. Fill bowls and trim with new parsley.

Nutrition:
Calories: 250
Carbohydrates: 52g
Fat: 4.5g
Sodium: 971mg
Protein: 8.5g

455. COLD CAULIFLOWER-COCONUT SOUP

Preparation Time: 7 minutes
Cooking Time: 20 minutes
Servings: 3-4
Ingredients:

- 1 pound (450g) new cauliflower
- 1¼ cup (300ml) unsweetened coconut milk
- 1 cup water
- 2 tablespoons new lime juice
- ⅓ cup cold squeezed extra-virgin olive oil
- 1 cup new coriander leaves, chopped
- Dash of salt and cayenne pepper
- Unsweetened coconut chips

Directions:

1. Steam cauliflower for 10 minutes.
2. At that point, combine the cauliflower with coconut milk and water in a food processor and blend until extremely smooth.
3. Add a squeeze of new lime, salt and pepper, The chopped coriander, and the oil and blend for an additional couple of moments.

4. Pour in soup bowls and embellish with coriander and coconut chips.

Nutrition:
Calories: 369.14
Carbohydrates: 7.36g
Fat: 37.21g
Protein: 1.6g
Sodium: 125mg

456. RAW AVOCADO-BROCCOLI SOUP WITH CASHEW NUTS

Preparation Time: 10 minutes
Cooking Time: 30 minutes
Servings: 1-2
Ingredients:

- ½ cup water (if available: alkaline water)
- ½ avocado
- 1 cup chopped broccoli
- ½ cup cashew nuts
- ½ cup alfalfa sprouts
- 1 clove of garlic
- 1 tablespoon cold-pressed extra virgin olive oil
- 1 pinch of sea salt and pepper
- Some parsley to garnish

Directions:

1. Put the cashew nuts in a blender or food processor, include water and puree for a couple of moments.
2. Include the various fixings (with the exception of the avocado) and puree.
3. Pour the soup in a container and warm it up to room temperature. Enhance with salt and pepper. Dice the avocado and chop the parsley.
4. Pour the soup in a container or plate; include the avocado dices and embellish with parsley.

Nutrition:
Calories: 325.76
Carbohydrates: 17.73g
Fat: 27g
Protein: 7.6g
Sodium: 85.24mg

457. KALE CAULIFLOWER SOUP

Preparation Time: 10 minutes
Cooking Time: 25 minutes
Servings: 4
Ingredients:

- 2 cups baby kale
- ½ cup unsweetened coconut milk
- 4 cups of water

- 1 large cauliflower head, chopped
- 3 garlic cloves, peeled
- 2 carrots, peeled and chopped
- 2 onion, chopped
- 3 tablespoon olive oil
- Pepper
- Salt

Directions:
1. Add oil to Instant Pot and set the pot on sauté mode.
2. Add carrot, garlic, and onion to the pot and sauté for 5-7 minutes.
3. Add water and cauliflower and stir well.
4. Cover pot with lid and cook on high pressure for 20 minutes.
5. When finished, release pressure using the quick release then open the lid.
6. Add kale and coconut milk and stir well.
7. Blend the soup utilizing a submersion blender until smooth.
8. Season with pepper and salt.

Nutrition:
Calories: 204.46
Fat: 16.4g
Carbohydrates: 13.27g
Sugar: 5.28g
Protein: 2.6g
Sodium: 258mg

458. HEALTHY BROCCOLI ASPARAGUS SOUP

Preparation Time: 10 minutes
Cooking Time: 20 minutes
Servings: 6
Ingredients:

- 2 cups broccoli florets, chopped
- 15 asparagus spears, ends trimmed and chopped
- 1 teaspoon dried oregano
- 1 tablespoon fresh thyme leaves
- ½ cup unsweetened almond milk
- 3½ cups filtered alkaline water
- 2 cups cauliflower florets, chopped
- 2 teaspoon garlic, chopped
- 1 cup onion, chopped
- 2 tablespoon olive oil
- Pepper
- Salt

Directions:
1. Add oil to the instant pot and set the pot on sauté mode.

2. Add onion to the olive oil and sauté until onion is softened.
3. Add garlic and sauté for 30 seconds.
4. Add all vegetables and water and stir well.
5. Cover pot with lid and cook on manual mode for 3 minutes.
6. When finished, allow to release pressure naturally then open the lid.
7. Blend until smooth.
8. Stir in almond milk, herbs, pepper, and salt.
9. Serve and enjoy.

Nutrition:
Calories: 85
Fat: 5.2g
Sodium: 165.24mg
Carbohydrates: 8.8g
Sugar 3.3g
Protein: 3.3g

459. CREAMY ASPARAGUS SOUP

Preparation Time: 10 minutes
Cooking Time: 30 minutes
Servings: 6
Ingredients:

- 2 lbs. fresh asparagus (cut off woody stems)
- ¼ teaspoon lime zest
- 2 tablespoon lime juice
- 14 oz. coconut milk
- 1 teaspoon dried thyme
- ½ teaspoon oregano
- ½ teaspoon sage
- 1½ cups filtered alkaline water
- 1 cauliflower head, cut into florets
- 1 tablespoon garlic, minced
- 1 leek, sliced
- 3 tablespoons coconut oil
- Pinch of Himalayan salt

Directions:
1. Preheat the oven to 400°F/ 200°C.
2. Line baking tray with parchment paper and set aside.
3. Arrange asparagus spears on a baking tray. Drizzle with 2 tablespoons of coconut oil and sprinkle with salt, thyme, oregano, and sage.
4. Bake in preheated oven for 20-25 minutes.
5. Add remaining oil to the instant pot and set the pot on sauté mode.
6. Put some garlic and leek to the pot and sauté for 2-3 minutes.
7. Add cauliflower florets and water in the pot and stir well.

8. Cover pot with lid and select steam mode and set timer for 4 minutes.
9. When finished, release pressure using the quick release **Directions**.
10. Add roasted asparagus, lime zest, lime juice, and coconut milk and stir well.
11. Blend until smooth.
12. Serve and enjoy.

Nutrition:
Calories: 265
Fat: 22.9g
Sodium: 51.45mg
Carbohydrates: 14.7g
Sugar 6.7g
Protein: 6.1g

460. QUICK BROCCOLI SOUP

Preparation Time: 5 minutes
Cooking Time: 10 minutes
Servings: 6
Ingredients:

- 1 lb. broccoli, chopped
- 6 cups filtered alkaline water
- 1 onion, diced
- 2 tablespoon olive oil
- Pepper
- Salt

Directions:
1. Add oil into the Instant Pot and set the pot on sauté mode.
2. Add the onion in olive oil and sauté until softened.
3. Add broccoli and water and stir well.
4. Cover pot with top and cook on manual high pressure for 3 minutes.
5. When finished, release pressure using the quick release then open the lid.
6. Blend the soup utilizing a submersion blender until smooth.
7. Season soup with pepper and salt.
8. Serve and enjoy.

Nutrition:
Calories: 65
Fat: 4.9g
Carbohydrates: 5g
Protein: 1.5g
Sugar: 1.48g
Sodium: 145.19mg

461. GREEN LENTIL SOUP

Preparation Time: 10 minutes
Cooking Time: 30 minutes
Servings: 4

Ingredients:

- 1½ cups green lentils, rinsed
- 4 cups baby spinach
- 4 cups filtered alkaline water
- 1 teaspoon Italian seasoning
- 2 teaspoons fresh thyme
- 14 oz. tomatoes, diced
- 3 garlic cloves, minced
- 2 celery stalks, chopped
- 1 carrot, chopped
- 1 onion, chopped
- Pepper
- Sea salt

Directions:

1. Add all ingredients except spinach into the pot and mix.
2. Cover pot with top and cook on manual high pressure for 18 minutes.
3. When finished, release pressure using the quick release then open the lid.
4. Add spinach and stir well.
5. Serve and enjoy.

Nutrition:
Calories: 283.65
Fat: 2g
Carbohydrates: 52.7g
Sugar: 6.11g
Protein: 18g
Sodium: 224mg
Cholesterol: 0mg

462. SQUASH SOUP

Preparation Time: 10 minutes
Cooking Time: 40 minutes
Servings: 4
Ingredients:

- 3 lbs. butternut squash, peeled and cubed
- 1 tablespoon curry powder
- ½ cup unsweetened coconut milk
- 3 cups filtered alkaline water
- 2 garlic cloves, minced
- 1 large onion, minced
- 1 teaspoon olive oil

Directions:

1. Add olive oil to the Instant Pot and set the pot on sauté mode.
2. Add onion and cook until tender, about 8 minutes.
3. Add curry powder and garlic and sauté for a minute.
4. Add butternut squash, water, and salt and stir well.
5. Cover pot with lid and cook on soup mode for 30 minutes.
6. When finished, allow to release pressure naturally for 10 minutes then release using quick-release directions then open the lid.

7. Blend the soup until smooth.
8. Add coconut milk and stir well.
9. Serve warm and enjoy.

Nutrition:
Calories: 185
Fat: 6.98g
Carbohydrates: 31.46g
Sugar: 6.79g
Sodium: 24.57mg
Protein: 2.9g

463. TOMATO SOUP

Preparation Time: 5 minutes
Cooking Time: 20 minutes
Servings: 4
Ingredients:

- 6 tomatoes, chopped
- 1 onion, diced
- 14 oz. coconut milk
- 1 teaspoon turmeric
- 1 teaspoon garlic, minced
- ¼ cup cilantro, chopped
- ½ teaspoon cayenne pepper
- 1 teaspoon ginger, minced
- ½ teaspoon sea salt

Directions:

1. Add all ingredients to the pot and mix.
2. Cover the pot with a lid and cook on manual high pressure for 5 minutes.
3. When finished, release pressure naturally for 10 minutes then release using the quick release directions
4. Blend the soup until smooth.
5. Stir well and serve.

Nutrition:
Calories: 273.63
Fat: 24g
Carbohydrates: 15.45g
Sugar: 8.9g
Protein: 4.23g
Sodium: 261.86mg

464. BASIL ZUCCHINI SOUP

Preparation Time: 10 minutes
Cooking Time: 20 minutes
Servings: 4
Ingredients:

- 3 medium zucchinis, peeled and chopped
- ¼ cup basil, chopped
- 1 large leek, chopped
- 3 cups filtered alkaline water
- 1 tablespoon lemon juice
- 3 tablespoon olive oil
- 2 teaspoon sea salt

Directions:

1. Add 2 tablespoons of oil into the pot and set on sauté mode.

2. Add zucchini and sauté for 5 minutes.
3. Add basil and leeks and sauté for 2-3 minutes.
4. Add lemon juice, water, and salt. Stir well.
5. Cover pot with lid and cook on high pressure for 8 minutes.
6. When finished, release pressure naturally then open the lid.
7. Blend the soup until smooth.
8. Top with remaining olive oil and serve.

Nutrition:
Calories: 128.85
Fat: 11.2g
Carbohydrates: 8.9g
Protein: 5.8g
Sodium: 960.99mg
Sugar 4g

465. SUMMER VEGETABLE SOUP

Preparation Time: 5 minutes
Cooking Time: 20 minutes
Servings: 10
Ingredients:

- ½ cup basil, chopped
- 2 bell peppers, seeded and sliced
- 1 cup green beans, trimmed and cut into pieces
- 8 cups filtered alkaline water
- 1 medium summer squash, sliced
- 1 medium zucchini, sliced
- 2 large tomatoes, sliced
- 1 small eggplant, sliced
- 6 garlic cloves, smashed
- 1 medium onion, diced
- Pepper
- Salt

Directions:

1. Combine all ingredients into the direct pot and mix.
2. Cover Instant Pot with lid and cook on soup mode for 10 minutes.
3. Release pressure using quick-release then open the lid.
4. Blend until smooth.
5. Serve and enjoy.

Nutrition:
Calories: 35.16
Fat: 0.35g
Carbohydrates: 7.71g
Protein: 1.68g
Sugar: 4.46g
Sodium: 84.92mg

466. ALMOND-RED BELL PEPPER DIP

Preparation Time: 14 minutes

Cooking Time: 16 minutes
Servings: 3
Ingredients:
- Garlic, 2-3 cloves
- Sea salt, one pinch
- Cayenne pepper, one pinch
- Extra-virgin olive oil (cold-pressed), one tablespoon
- Almonds, 60g
- Red bell pepper, 280g

Directions:
1. Cook garlic and peppers until they are soft.
2. Add all ingredients to a mixer and blend until the mix becomes smooth and creamy.
3. Finally, add pepper and salt to taste.
4. Serve.

Nutrition:
Calories: 180.79
Carbohydrates: 9.61g
Fat: 14.98g
Protein: 5.1g
Sodium: 43.2mg

467. SPICY CARROT SOUP

Preparation Time: 10 minutes
Cooking Time: 20 minutes
Servings: 6
Ingredients:
- 8 large carrots, peeled and chopped
- 1½ cups filtered alkaline water
- 14 oz. coconut milk
- 3 garlic cloves, peeled
- 1 tablespoon red curry paste
- ¼ cup olive oil
- 1 onion, chopped
- Salt

Directions:
1. Combine all ingredients into the Instant pot and mix fine.
2. Cover pot with lid and select manual and set timer for 15 minutes.
3. Release pressure naturally then open the lid.
4. Blend until smooth.
5. Serve and enjoy.

Nutrition:
Calories: 284.39
Fat: 25.6g
Carbohydrates: 14.58g
Protein: 2.8g
Sugar: 7g
Sodium: 282mg
Cholesterol: 0mg

468. ZUCCHINI SOUP

Preparation Time: 10 minutes

Cooking Time: 30 minutes
Servings: 10
Ingredients:
- 10 cups zucchini, chopped
- 32 oz. filtered alkaline water
- 13.5 oz. coconut milk
- 1 tablespoon Thai curry paste

Directions:
1. Combine all ingredients into the Instant Pot and mix.
2. Cover pot with lid and cook on manual high pressure for 10 minutes.
3. Release pressure using quick-release then open the lid.
4. Using a blender, blend the soup until smooth.
5. Serve and enjoy.

Nutrition:
Calories: 112.51
Fat: 9.6g
Carbohydrates: 6.5g
Protein: 2.57g
Sugar: 3.6g
Sodium: 65.33mg

469. KIDNEY BEAN STEW

Preparation Time: 15 minutes
Cooking Time: 15 minutes
Servings: 2
Ingredients:
- 1 lb cooked kidney beans
- 1 cup tomato passata
- 1 cup low sodium beef broth
- 3 tablespoons Italian herbs

Directions:
1. Mix all the ingredients in your Instant Pot.
2. Cook on Stew for 15 minutes.
3. Release the pressure naturally.

Nutrition:
Calories: 321
Carbohydrates: 55.8 g
Sugar: 4.69 g
Fat: 1.47 g
Sodium: 246.36mg
Protein: 22.44 g
GL: 8

470. CABBAGE SOUP

Preparation Time: 15 minutes
Cooking Time: 35 minutes
Servings: 2
Ingredients:
- 1 lb shredded cabbage
- 1 cup low-sodium vegetable broth
- 1 sliced onion
- 2 tablespoons mixed herbs
- 1 tablespoon black pepper

Directions:

1. Mix all the ingredients in your Instant Pot.
2. Cook on Stew for 35 minutes.
3. Release the pressure naturally.

Nutrition:
Calories: 137.6
Carbohydrates: 29.8g
Fat: 1.23g
Sodium: 114.97mg
Protein: 4.7g
GL: 1

471. PUMPKIN SPICE SOUP

Preparation Time: 10 minutes
Cooking Time: 35 minutes
Servings: 2
Ingredients:
- 1 lb cubed pumpkin
- 1 cup low-sodium vegetable broth
- 2 tablespoons mixed spice (cinnamon , cumin, cayenne pepper, salt)

Directions:
1. Mix all the ingredients in your Instant Pot.
2. Cook on "Stew" for 35 minutes.
3. Release the pressure naturally.
4. Blend the soup.

Nutrition:
Calories: 120
Carbohydrates: 24g
Sugar: 7.47g
Fat: 1.45g
Sodium: 81mg
Protein: 3.35g
GL: 1

472. CREAM OF TOMATO SOUP

Preparation Time: 15 minutes
Cooking Time: 15 minutes
Servings: 2
Ingredients:
- 1 lb fresh tomatoes, chopped
- 1½ cups low-sodium tomato puree
- 1 tablespoon black pepper

Directions:
1. Mix all the ingredients in your Instant Pot.
2. Cook on Stew for 15 minutes.
3. Release the pressure naturally.
4. Blend.

Nutrition:
Calories: 118
Carbohydrates: 27.25g
Sugar: 14.6g
Protein: 5.3g
Sodium: 64mg
GL: 1

473. SHIITAKE SOUP

Preparation Time: 15 minutes
Cooking Time: 35 minutes
Servings: 2
Ingredients:
- 1 cup shiitake mushrooms
- 1 cup diced vegetables
- 1 cup low-sodium vegetable broth
- 2 tablespoons Five Spice seasoning

Directions:
1. Mix all the ingredients in your Instant Pot.
2. Cook on Stew for 35 minutes.
3. Release the pressure naturally.

Nutrition:
Calories: 153.8
Carbohydrates: 31.17g
Sugar: 8.6g
Fat: 1.2g
Protein: 6.28g
Sodium: 1439mg
GL: 1

474. SPICY PEPPER SOUP

Preparation Time: 15 minutes
Cooking Time: 15 minutes
Servings: 2
Ingredients:
- 1 lb chopped mixed sweet peppers
- 1 cup low-sodium vegetable broth
- 3 tablespoons chopped chili peppers
- 1 tablespoon black pepper

Directions:
1. Mix all the ingredients in your Instant Pot.
2. Cook on Stew for 15 minutes.
3. Release the pressure naturally. Blend.

Nutrition:
Calories: 132
Carbohydrates: 27g
Sugar: 11.87g
Fat: 1.31g
Sodium: 87.1mg
Protein: 3.87g
GL: 6

475. ZOODLE WON-TON SOUP

Preparation Time: 15 minutes
Cooking Time: 5 minutes
Servings: 2
Ingredients:
- 1 lb spiral zucchini
- 1 pack unfried won tons
- 1 cup low-sodium beef broth
- 2 tablespoons soy sauce

Directions:
1. Mix all the ingredients in your Instant Pot.
2. Cook on Stew for 5 minutes.
3. Release the pressure naturally.

Nutrition:
Calories: 201.15
Carbohydrates: 36.91g
Sugar: 6.09g
Fat: 1.5g
Sodium: 1334.26mg
Protein: 10.96g
GL: 2

476. BROCCOLI STILTON SOUP

Preparation Time: 15 minutes
Cooking Time: 35 minutes
Servings: 4
Ingredients:
- 1 lb chopped broccoli
- ½ lb chopped vegetables
- 1 cup low sodium vegetable broth
- 1 cup Stilton

Directions:
1. Mix all the ingredients in your Instant Pot.
2. Cook on Stew for 35 minutes.
3. Release the pressure naturally.
4. Blend the soup.

Nutrition:
Calories: 209.6
Carbohydrates: 18.97g
Sugar: 4.78g
Fat: 10.36g
Protein: 11.5g
Sodium: 468.79mg
GL: 4

477. LAMB STEW

Preparation Time: 15 minutes
Cooking Time: 35 minutes
Servings: 4
Ingredients:
- 1 lb diced lamb shoulder
- 1 lb chopped winter vegetables
- 1 cup low-sodium vegetable broth
- 1 tablespoon yeast extract
- 1 tablespoon star anise spice mix

Directions:
1. Mix all the ingredients in your Instant Pot.
2. Cook on Stew for 35 minutes.
3. Release the pressure naturally.

Nutrition:
Calories: 365.68
Carbohydrates: 22.1g
Sugar: 5.41g
Fat: 20.7g
Sodium: 403mg
Protein: 21g
GL: 3

478. IRISH STEW

Preparation Time: 15 minutes
Cooking Time: 35 minutes
Servings: 4
Ingredients:
- 1½ lbs. diced lamb shoulder
- 1 lb chopped vegetables
- 1 cup low-sodium beef broth
- 3 minced onions
- 1 tablespoon ghee

Directions:
1. Mix all the ingredients in your Instant Pot.
2. Cook on Stew for 35 minutes.
3. Release the pressure naturally.

Nutrition:
Calories: 508
Carbohydrates: 21.8g
Sugar: 6.7g
Fat: 33.9g
Protein: 28g
Sodium: 225mg
GL: 3

479. SWEET AND SOUR SOUP

Preparation Time: 15 minutes
Cooking Time: 35 minutes
Servings: 5
Ingredients:
- 1 lb cubed chicken breast
- 1 lb chopped vegetables
- 1 cup low-carb sweet and sour sauce
- ½ cup sugar-free marmalade

Directions:
1. Mix all the ingredients in your Instant Pot.
2. Cook on Stew for 35 minutes.
3. Release the pressure naturally.

Nutrition:
Calories: 368.15
Carbohydrates: 33.11g
Sugar: 6.19g
Sodium: 508mg
Fat: 18.27g
Protein: 21.17g

480. MEATBALL STEW

Preparation Time: 15 minutes
Cooking Time: 25 minutes
Servings: 4
Ingredients:
- 1 lb sausage
- 2 cups chopped tomato
- 1 cup chopped vegetables
- 2 tablespoons Italian seasoning
- 1 tablespoon vegetable oil

Directions:

1. Roll the sausage into meatballs.
2. Put the Instant Pot on Sauté and fry the meatballs in the oil until brown.
3. Mix all the ingredients in your Instant Pot.
4. Cook on Stew for 25 minutes.
5. Release the pressure naturally.

Nutrition:
Calories: 410
Carbohydrates: 9.95g
Sugar: 2.6g
Sodium: 979.78mg
Fat: 33.76g

Protein: 15.38g
GL: 2

481. KEBAB STEW

Preparation Time: 15 minutes
Cooking Time: 35 minutes
Servings: 2
Ingredients:

- 1 lb cubed, seasoned kebab meat
- 1 lb cooked chickpeas
- 1 cup low-sodium vegetable broth
- 1 tablespoon black pepper

Directions:

1. Mix all the ingredients in your Instant Pot.
2. Cook on Stew for 35 minutes.
3. Release the pressure naturally.

Nutrition:
Calories: 687.52
Carbohydrates: 116g
Sugar: 44.56g
Fat: 9.07g
Protein: 38.69g
Sodium: 947.85mg
GL: 6

SEAFOOD

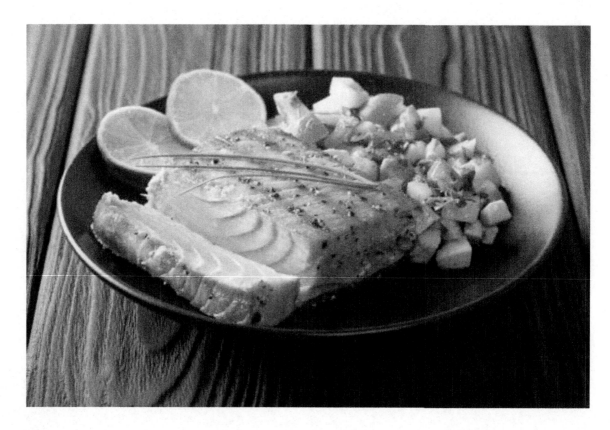

482. TROUT BAKE

Preparation Time: 10 minutes
Cooking Time: 38 minutes
Servings: 2
Ingredients:

- 1 lb trout fillets, boneless
- 1 lb chopped winter vegetables
- 1 cup low-sodium fish broth
- 1 tablespoon mixed herbs
- Sea salt as desired

Directions:

1. Mix all the ingredients except the broth in a foil pouch.
2. Place the pouch in the steamer basket in your Instant Pot.
3. Pour the broth into the Instant Pot.
4. Cook on Steam for 35 minutes.
5. Release the pressure naturally.

Nutrition:
Calories: 504
Fat: 13.6g
Protein: 58.4g

Carbs: 35.8g
Sodium: 1237mg

483. TUNA SWEETCORN CASSEROLE

Preparation Time: 16 minutes
Cooking Time: 35 minutes
Servings: 2
Ingredients:

- 3 small tins of tuna
- ½ lb sweetcorn kernels
- 1 lb chopped vegetables
- 1 cup low-sodium vegetable broth
- 2 tablespoons spicy seasoning

Directions:

1. Mix all the ingredients in your Instant Pot.
2. Cook on Stew for 35 minutes.
3. Release the pressure naturally.

Nutrition:
Calories: 401.43
Fat: 3.6g
Carbs: 33g
Protein: 55g

Sodium: 1865mg

484. SWORDFISH STEAK

Preparation Time: 16 minutes
Cooking Time: 35 minutes
Servings: 2
Ingredients:

- 1 lb swordfish steak, whole
- 1 lb chopped Mediterranean vegetables
- 1 cup low-sodium fish broth
- 2 tablespoons soy sauce

Directions:

1. Mix all the ingredients except the broth in a foil pouch.
2. Place the pouch in the steamer basket for your Instant Pot.
3. Pour the broth into the Instant Pot. Lower the steamer basket into the Instant Pot.
4. Cook on Steam for 35 minutes.
5. Release the pressure naturally.

Nutrition:
Calories: 374.62

Fat: 9g
Protein: 49.6g
Carbs: 13.65g
Sodium: 2474mg

485. SHRIMP COCONUT CURRY

Preparation Time: 14 minutes
Cooking Time: 25 minutes
Servings: 2
Ingredients:
- ½ lb cooked shrimp
- 1 thinly sliced onion
- 1 cup coconut yogurt
- 3 tablespoons curry paste
- 1 tablespoon oil or ghee

Directions:
1. Set the Instant Pot to sauté and add the onion, oil, and curry paste.
2. When the onion is soft, add the remaining ingredients and seal.
3. Cook on Stew for 20 minutes.
4. Release the pressure naturally.

Nutrition:
Calories: 377
Fat: 24g
Protein: 20.71g
Sodium: 697.9mg

486. TUNA AND CHEDDAR

Preparation Time: 20 minutes
Cooking Time: 31 minutes
 Servings: 2
Ingredients:
- 3 small cans of tuna
- 1 lb finely chopped vegetables
- 1 cup low-sodium vegetable broth
- ½ cup shredded cheddar cheese

Directions:
1. Mix all the ingredients in your Instant Pot.
2. Cook on Stew for 35 minutes.
3. Release the pressure naturally.

Nutrition:
Calories: 320
Fat: 11g
Carbs: 42.9g
Sodium: 596mg
Protein: 37g

487. CHILI SHRIMP

Preparation Time: 16 minutes
Cooking Time: 35 minutes
Servings: 2
Ingredients:
- 1.5 lb cooked shrimp
- 1 lb stir fry vegetables
- 1 cup ready-mixed fish sauce
- 2 tablespoons chili flakes

Directions:
1. Mix all the ingredients in your Instant Pot.
2. Cook on Stew for 35 minutes.
3. Release the pressure naturally.

Nutrition:
Calories: 436
Fat: 11.69g
Protein: 58g
Carbs: 22g
Sodium: 1175mg

488. SARDINE CURRY

Preparation Time: 15 minutes
Cooking Time: 35 minutes
Servings: 2
Ingredients:
- 5 tins of sardines in tomato sauce
- 1 lb chopped vegetables
- 1 cup low-sodium fish broth
- 3 tablespoons curry paste

Directions:
1. Mix all the ingredients in your Instant Pot.
2. Cook on Stew for 35 minutes.
3. Release the pressure naturally.

Nutrition:
Calories: 320
Fat: 16g
Protein: 42g
Sodium: 1100mg

489. MUSSELS AND SPAGHETTI SQUASH

Preparation Time: 14 minutes
Cooking Time: 35 minutes
Servings: 2
Ingredients:
- 1 lb cooked, shelled mussels
- ½ spaghetti squash, to fit the Instant Pot
- 1 cup low-sodium fish broth
- 3 tablespoons crushed garlic
- sea salt to taste

Directions:
1. Mix the mussels with garlic and salt.
2. Place the mussels inside the squash.
3. Lower the squash into your Instant Pot.
4. Pour the broth around it.
5. Cook on Stew for 35 minutes.
6. Release the pressure naturally.
7. Shred the squash, mixing the "spaghetti" with the mussels.

Nutrition:
Calories: 265
Fat: 9g
Carbs: 27g
Sodium: 876mg

Protein: 48g

490. COD IN WHITE SAUCE

Preparation Time: 16 minutes
Cooking Time: 5 minutes
Servings: 2
Ingredients:
- 1 lb cod fillets
- 1 lb chopped swede (rutabaga) and carrots
- 2 cups French white sauce
- 1 cup peas
- 3 tablespoons black pepper

Directions:
1. Mix all the ingredients in your Instant Pot.
2. Cook on Stew for 5 minutes.
3. Release the pressure naturally.

Nutrition:
Calories: 582
Fat: 19.97g
Protein: 53.54g
Carbs: 51.77g
Sodium: 699mg

491. LEMON SOLE

Preparation Time: 16 minutes
Cooking Time: 5 minutes
Servings: 2
Ingredients:
- 1 lb sole fillets, boned and skinned
- 1 cup low-sodium fish broth
- 2 diced sweet onions
- Juice of half a lemon
- 2 tablespoons dried cilantro

Directions:
1. Mix all the ingredients in your Instant Pot.
2. Cook on Stew for 5 minutes.
3. Release the pressure naturally.

Nutrition:
Calories: 209.58
Fat: 4.5g
Protein: 30.56g
Carbs: 10.32g
Sodium: 987mg

492. COD IN PARSLEY SAUCE

Preparation Time: 17 minutes
Cooking Time: 5 minutes
Servings: 2
Ingredients:
- 1 lb boneless, skinless cod fillets
- ½ lb green peas
- 1 cup white sauce
- Juice of a lemon
- 2 tablespoons dry parsley

Directions:

1. Mix all the ingredients in your Instant Pot.
2. Cook on Stew for 35 minutes.
3. Release the pressure naturally.

Nutrition:
Calories: 492.2
Fat: 17.8g
Protein: 51.6g
Carbs: 32.7g
Sodium: 732.48mg

493. CRAB CURRY

Preparation Time: 13 minutes
Cooking Time: 25 minutes
Servings: 2
Ingredients:
- ½ lb chopped crab
- 1 thinly sliced red onion
- ½ cup chopped tomato
- 3 tablespoons curry paste
- 1 tablespoon oil or ghee

Directions:
1. Set the Instant Pot to sauté and add the onion, oil, and curry paste.
2. When the onion is soft, add the remaining ingredients and seal.
3. Cook on Stew for 20 minutes.
4. Release the pressure naturally.

Nutrition:
Calories: 177.43
Fat: 13.48g
Protein: 6.98g
Carbs: 7.89g
Sodium: 765.37mg

494. SHRIMP WITH TOMATOES AND FETA

Preparation Time: 10 minutes
Cooking Time: 30 minutes
Servings: 4
Ingredients:
- 3 tomatoes, coarsely chopped
- ½ cup chopped sun-dried tomatoes
- 2 teaspoons minced garlic
- 2 teaspoons extra-virgin olive oil
- 1 teaspoon chopped fresh oregano
- Freshly ground black pepper
- 1½ pounds (16–20 count) shrimp, peeled, deveined, tails removed
- 4 teaspoons freshly squeezed lemon juice
- ½ cup low-sodium feta cheese, crumbled

Directions:
1. Heat the oven to 450°F.
2. In a medium bowl, toss the tomatoes, sun-dried tomatoes,

garlic, oil, and oregano until well combined.
3. Season the mixture lightly with pepper.
4. Transfer the tomato mixture to a 9x13" glass baking dish.
5. Bake until softened, about 15 minutes.
6. Stir the shrimp and lemon juice into the hot tomato mixture and top evenly with the feta.
7. Bake until the shrimp are cooked through, about 15 minutes more.

Nutrition:
Calories: 222.49
Fat: 8.2g
Protein: 28.36g
Carbs: 9.21g
Sodium: 1178mg

495. SEAFOOD STEW

Preparation Time: 20 minutes
Cooking Time: 31 minutes
Servings: 6
Ingredients:
- 1 tablespoon extra-virgin olive oil
- 1 sweet onion, chopped
- 2 teaspoons minced garlic
- 3 celery stalks, chopped
- 2 carrots, peeled and chopped
- 1 28-ounce can sodium-free diced tomatoes, undrained
- 3 cups low-sodium chicken broth
- ½ cup clam juice
- ¼ cup dry white wine
- 2 teaspoons chopped fresh basil
- 2 teaspoons chopped fresh oregano
- 2 4-ounce haddock fillets, cut into 1-inch chunks
- 1 pound mussels, scrubbed, debearded
- 8 ounces (16–20 count) shrimp, peeled, deveined, quartered
- Sea salt
- Freshly ground black pepper
- 2 tablespoons chopped fresh parsley

Directions:
1. Place a large saucepan over medium-high heat and add the olive oil.
2. Sauté the onion and garlic until softened and translucent, about 3 minutes.
3. Stir in the celery and carrots and sauté for 4 minutes.

4. Stir in the tomatoes, chicken broth, clam juice, white wine, basil, and oregano.
5. Bring the sauce to a boil, then reduce the heat to low. Simmer for 15 minutes.
6. Add the fish and mussels, cover, and cook until the mussels open, about 5 minutes.
7. Discard any unopened mussels. Add the shrimp to the pan and cook until the shrimp are opaque about 2 minutes.
8. Season with salt and pepper. Serve garnished with chopped parsley.

Nutrition:
Calories: 174
Fat: 5.25g
Protein: 21g
Carbs: 9.86g
Sodium: 667.68mg

496. SPICY CITRUS SOLE

Preparation Time: 10 minutes
Cooking Time: 12 minutes
Servings: 4
Ingredients:
- 1 teaspoon chili powder
- 1 teaspoon garlic powder
- ½ teaspoon lime zest
- ½ teaspoon lemon zest
- ¼ teaspoon freshly ground black pepper
- ¼ teaspoon smoked paprika
- Pinch sea salt
- 4 6-ounce sole fillets, patted dry
- 1 tablespoon extra-virgin olive oil
- 2 teaspoons freshly squeezed lime juice

Directions:
1. Preheat the oven to 450°F.
2. Line a baking sheet with aluminum foil and set it aside.
3. In a small bowl, stir together the chili powder, garlic powder, lime zest, lemon zest, pepper, paprika, and salt until well mixed.
4. Pat the fish fillets dry with paper towels, place them on the baking sheet and rub them lightly all over with the spice mixture.
5. Drizzle the olive oil and lime juice on the top of the fish.
6. Bake until the fish flakes when pressed lightly with a fork, about 8 minutes. Serve immediately.

Nutrition:

Calories: 156.8
Fat: 6.98g
Protein: 21.39g
Carbs: 1.34g
Sodium: 553.71mg

497. HERB-CRUSTED HALIBUT

Preparation Time: 10 minutes
Cooking Time: 21 minutes
Servings: 4
Ingredients:
- 4 5-ounce halibut fillets
- Extra-virgin olive oil, for brushing
- ½ cup coarsely ground unsalted pistachios
- 1 tablespoon chopped fresh parsley
- 1 teaspoon chopped fresh thyme
- 1 teaspoon chopped fresh basil
- Pinch sea salt
- Pinch freshly ground black pepper

Directions:
1. Preheat the oven to 350°F.
2. Line a baking sheet with parchment paper.
3. Pat the halibut fillets dry with a paper towel and place them on the baking sheet.
4. Brush the halibut generously with olive oil.
5. In a small bowl, stir together the pistachios, parsley, thyme, basil, salt, and pepper.
6. Spoon the nut and herb mixture evenly on the fish, spreading it out so the tops of the fillets are covered.
7. Bake the halibut until it flakes when pressed with a fork, about 20 minutes.
8. Serve immediately.

Nutrition:
Calories: 296.95
Fat: 15.51g
Protein: 36.74g
Carbs: 4.46g
Sodium: 149.57

498. SALMON FLORENTINE

Preparation Time: 10 minutes
Cooking Time: 32 minutes
Servings: 4
Ingredients:
- 1 teaspoon extra-virgin olive oil
- ½ sweet onion, finely chopped
- 1 teaspoon minced garlic
- 3 cups baby spinach

- 1 cup kale, tough stems removed, torn into 3-inch pieces
- Sea salt
- Freshly ground black pepper
- 4 5-ounce salmon fillets
- Lemon wedges, for serving

Directions:
1. Preheat the oven to 350°F.
2. Place a large skillet over medium-high heat and add the oil.
3. Sauté the onion and garlic until softened and translucent, about 3 minutes.
4. Add the spinach and kale and sauté until the greens wilt, about 5 minutes.
5. Remove the skillet from the heat and season the greens with salt and pepper.
6. Place the salmon fillets so they are nestled in the greens and partially covered by them. Bake the salmon until it is opaque, about 20 minutes.
7. Serve immediately with a squeeze of fresh lemon.

Nutrition:
Calories: 294
Fat: 18g
Protein: 29g
Carbs: 3.53g
Sodium: 262mg

499. SALMON CAKES IN AIR FRYER

Preparation Time: 10 minutes
Cooking Time: 10 minutes
Servings: 2
Ingredients:
- 8 oz. fresh salmon fillet
- 1 egg
- ⅛ teaspoon salt
- ¼ teaspoon garlic powder
- 1 sliced lemon

Directions:
1. In a bowl, chop the salmon, add the egg & spices.
2. Form tiny cakes.
3. Let the air fryer preheat to 390°F. On the bottom of the air fryer bowl lay sliced lemons—place cakes on top.
4. Cook them for seven minutes. Eat with your favorite dip.

Nutrition:
Calories: 249.41
Fat: 15.45g
Protein: 25.98g
Carbs: 2.05g
Sodium: 231.59mg

500. COCONUT SHRIMP

Preparation Time: 10 minutes
Cooking Time: 30 minutes
Servings: 4
Ingredients:
- ½ cup pork rinds (crushed)
- 4 cups jumbo shrimp (deveined)
- ½ cup coconut flakes preferably
- 2 eggs
- ½ cup flour of coconut
- Any oil of your choice for frying at least half-inch in pan
- Freshly ground black pepper & kosher salt to taste

For the Dipping sauce (Piña colada flavor):
- 2-3 tablespoons powdered sugar as substitute
- 3 tablespoon mayonnaise
- ½ cup sour cream
- ¼ teaspoon coconut extract or to taste
- 3 tablespoons coconut cream
- ¼ teaspoon pineapple flavoring as much to taste
- 3 tablespoons coconut flakes preferably unsweetened (this is optional).

Directions:
Piña Colada (Sauce)
1. Mix all the ingredients into a tiny bowl for the dipping sauce. Combine well and put in the fridge until ready to serve.

Shrimps
1. Whip all eggs in a deep bowl, and in a small, shallow bowl, add the crushed pork rinds, coconut flour, sea salt, coconut flakes, and freshly ground black pepper.
2. Put the shrimp one by one in the mixed eggs for dipping, then in the coconut flour blend.
3. Place the shrimp, battered, in a single layer in your air fryer basket. Spritz the shrimp with oil and cook for 8-10 minutes at 360°F, flipping them halfway.
4. Enjoy hot with dipping sauce.

Nutrition:
Calories: 517.37
Protein: 36g
Fat: 28.5g
Carbs: 27.11g
Sodium: 1082.4mg

501. CRISPY FISH STICKS IN AIR FRYER

Preparation Time: 10 minutes

Cooking Time: 15 minutes
Servings: 4
Ingredients:

- 1 lb. whitefish such as cod
- ¼ cup mayonnaise
- 2 tablespoon Dijon mustard
- 2 tablespoons water
- 1 ½ cup pork rinds
- ¾ cajun seasoning
- Kosher salt & pepper to taste

Directions:

1. Spray non-stick cooking spray to the air fryer rack.
2. Pat the fish dry & cut into sticks about 1 inch by 2 inches long
3. Stir together the mayo, mustard, and water in a tiny small dish. Mix the pork rinds & cajun seasoning into another small container.
4. Adding kosher salt & pepper to taste (both pork rinds & seasoning can have a decent amount of kosher salt, so you can dip a finger to see how salty it is).
5. Working with one slice of fish at a time, dip to cover in the mayo mix & then tap off the excess. Dip into the mixture of pork rinds, then flip to cover. Place on the rack of an air fryer.
6. Set at 400°F to air fryer & bake for 5 minutes, then turn the fish with tongs and bake for another 5 minutes. Serve.

Nutrition:
Calories: 218
Fat: 16g
Protein: 15.12g
Carbs: 5.91g
Sodium: 5313mg

502. HONEY-GLAZED SALMON

Preparation Time: 10 minutes
Cooking Time: 15 minutes
Servings: 2
Ingredients:

- 6 teaspoons gluten-free soy sauce
- 2 pieces salmon fillets
- 3 teaspoons sweet rice wine
- 1 teaspoon water
- 6 tablespoons honey

Directions:

1. In a bowl, mix sweet rice wine, soy sauce, honey, and water.
2. Set half of it aside.
3. In half of it, marinate the fish and let it rest for 2 hours.
4. Let the air fryer preheat to 350°F (180 C).

5. Cook the fish for 8 minutes, flip halfway through and cook for another five minutes.
6. Baste the salmon with marinade mixture after 3 or 4 minutes.
7. Pour the other half of marinade, into a saucepan, reduce to half, serve with a sauce.

Nutrition:
Calories: 435
Fat: 14g
Protein: 25.6g
Carbs: 53g
Sodium: 956.61mg

503. BASIL-PARMESAN CRUSTED SALMON

Preparation Time: 5 minutes
Cooking Time: 15 minutes
Servings: 4
Ingredients:

- 3 tablespoons grated Parmesan
- 4 skinless salmon fillets
- ¼ teaspoon salt
- Freshly ground black pepper
- 3 tablespoons low-fat mayonnaise
- Basil leaves, chopped
- 1/2 lemon

Directions:

1. Let the air fryer preheat to 400°F. Spray the basket with olive oil.
2. With salt, pepper, and lemon juice, season the salmon.
3. In a bowl, mix 2 tablespoons of Parmesan cheese with mayonnaise and basil leaves.
4. Add this mix and more parmesan on top of salmon and cook for seven minutes or until fully cooked. Serve hot.

Nutrition:
Calories: 248.6
Protein: 25.8g
Fat: 15.35g
Carbs: 1.94g
Sodium: 314.6mg

504. CAJUN SHRIMP IN AIR FRYER

Preparation Time: 10 minutes
Cooking Time: 21 minutes
Servings: 4
Ingredients:

- Peeled, 24 extra-jumbo shrimp
- 2 tablespoon olive oil
- 1 tablespoon cajun seasoning
- 1 zucchini, thick slices (half-moons)
- ¼ cup cooked turkey
- Yellow squash, sliced half-moons

- ¼ teaspoon kosher salt

Directions:

1. In a bowl, mix the shrimp with cajun seasoning.
2. In another bowl, add zucchini, turkey, salt, squash, and coat with oil.
3. Let the air fryer preheat to 400°F
4. Move the shrimp and vegetable mix to the fryer basket and cook for 3 minutes.
5. Serve hot.

Nutrition:
Calories: 108.72
Protein: 6.71g
Fat: 8.14g
Carbs: 2.83g
Sodium: 685.51mg

505. CRISPY AIR FRYER FISH

Preparation Time: 10 minutes
Cooking Time: 17 minutes
Servings: 4
Ingredients:

- 2 teaspoons Old Bay
- 4-6, Whiting fish fillets (cut in half)
- ¾ cup fine cornmeal
- ¼ cup flour
- 1 teaspoon paprika
- ½ teaspoon garlic powder
- 1 ½ teaspoon salt
- ½ teaspoon freshly ground black pepper

Directions:

1. In a Ziploc bag, add all ingredients and coat the fish fillets with it.
2. Spray oil on the basket of the air fryer and put the fish in it.
3. Cook for ten minutes at 400°F. flip fish if necessary and coat with oil spray and cook for another seven minutes.
4. Serve with salad greens.

Nutrition:
Calories: 222.48
Fat: 3.28g
Protein: 21.74g
Carbs: 29.8g
Sodium: 1314.96mg

506. AIR FRYER LEMON COD

Preparation Time: 5 minutes
Cooking Time: 10 minutes
Servings: 1
Ingredients:

- 1 cod fillet
- Dried parsley
- Kosher salt and pepper to taste
- Garlic powder

- 1 lemon

Directions:

1. In a bowl, mix all ingredients and coat the fish fillet with spices.
2. Slice the lemon and lay it at the bottom of the air fryer basket.
3. Put spiced fish on top. Cover the fish with lemon slices.
4. Cook for ten minutes at 375°F, the internal temperature of fish should be 145°F.
5. Serve with a microgreen salad.

Nutrition:
Calories: 137
Protein: 28g
Fat: 1.27g
Carbs: 5.34g
Sodium: 903.43mg

507. AIR FRYER SALMON FILLETS

Preparation Time: 5 minutes
Cooking Time: 15 minutes
Servings: 2
Ingredients:

- ¼ cup low-fat Greek yogurt
- 2 salmon fillets
- 1 tablespoon fresh dill (chopped)
- One lemon and lemon juice
- ½ teaspoon garlic powder
- Kosher salt and pepper

Directions:

1. Cut the lemon into slices and lay at the bottom of the air fryer basket.
2. Season the salmon with kosher salt and pepper. Put salmon on top of lemons.
3. Let it cook at 330°F For 15 minutes.
4. In the meantime, mix garlic powder, lemon juice, salt, pepper with yogurt and dill.
5. Serve the fish with sauce.

Nutrition:
Calories: 260.42
Protein: 28g
Fat: 14.8g
Carbs: 4.87g
Sodium: 457.63mg

508. AIR FRYER FISH & CHIPS

Preparation Time: 10 minutes
Cooking Time: 35 minutes
Servings: 4
Ingredients:

- 4 cups of any fish fillet
- ½ wheat flour
- 1 cup whole wheat breadcrumbs
- One egg

- 2 tablespoon oil
- Potatoes
- 1 teaspoon salt

Directions:

1. Cut the potatoes into fries. Then coat with oil and salt.
2. Cook in the air fryer for 20 minutes at 400°F, toss the fries halfway through.
3. In the meantime, coat fish in flour, then in the whisked egg, and finally in breadcrumbs mix.
4. Place the fish in the air fryer and let it cook at 330°F for 15 minutes.
5. Flip it halfway through, if needed.
6. Serve with tartar sauce and salad green.

Nutrition:
Calories: 488.65
Protein: 37g
Fat: 27g
Carbs: 23.55g
Sodium: 919.08mg

509. GRILLED SALMON WITH LEMON

Preparation Time: 10 minutes
Cooking Time: 21 minutes
Servings: 4
Ingredients:

- 2 tablespoons olive oil
- 2 salmon fillets
- Lemon juice
- ⅓ cup water
- ⅓ cup gluten-free light soy sauce
- ⅓ cup honey
- Scallion slices
- Cherry tomato
- Freshly ground black pepper, garlic powder, kosher salt to taste

Directions:

1. Season salmon with pepper and salt
2. In a bowl, mix honey, soy sauce, lemon juice, water, oil. Add salmon to this marinade and let it rest for at least 2 hours.
3. Let the air fryer preheat at 350°F (180°C)
4. Place fish in the air fryer and cook for 8 minutes.
5. Move to a dish and top with scallion slices.

Nutrition:
Calories: 275.4
Fat: 14.33g
Protein: 14.11g
Carbs: 25.22g
Sodium: 1681mg

510. AIR-FRIED FISH NUGGETS

Preparation Time: 15 minutes
Cooking Time: 10 minutes
Servings: 4
Ingredients:

- 2 cups fish fillets in cubes (skinless)
- 1 egg, beaten
- 5 tablespoon flour
- 5 tablespoons water
- Kosher salt and pepper to taste
- Breadcrumbs mix
- 1 tablespoon smoked paprika
- ¼ cup whole wheat breadcrumbs
- 1 tablespoon garlic powder

Directions:

1. Season the fish cubes with kosher salt and pepper.
2. In a bowl, add flour and gradually add water, mixing as you add.
3. Then mix in the egg.
4. Coat the cubes in batter, then add in the breadcrumb mix. Coat well.
5. Place the cubes in a baking tray and spray with oil.
6. Let the air fryer preheat to 390°F (200°C).
7. Place cubes in the air fryer and cook for 12 minutes or until well cooked and golden brown.
8. Serve with salad greens.

Nutrition:
Calories: 184
Protein:22g
Fat: 3.8g
Carbs: 14.55g
Sodium: 399.42mg

511. GARLIC ROSEMARY GRILLED PRAWNS

Preparation Time: 6 minutes
Cooking Time: 11 minutes
Servings: 2
Ingredients:

- ½ tablespoon melted unsalted butter
- Green capsicum, sliced
- 8 prawns
- Rosemary leaves
- Kosher salt& freshly ground black pepper
- 3-4 cloves of minced garlic

Directions:

1. In a bowl, mix all the ingredients and marinate the prawns in it for at least 60 minutes or more
2. Add 2 prawns and 2 slices of capsicum on each skewer.

3. Let the air fryer preheat to 350°F (180°C).
4. Cook for 5-6 minutes. Then change the temperature to 390°F (200°C) and cook for another minute.
5. Serve with lemon wedges.

Nutrition:
Calories: 65.78
Fat: 3.31g
Carbohydrates: 4.67g
Sodium: 488mg

512. AIR-FRIED CRUMBED FISH

Preparation Time: 10 minutes
Cooking Time: 13 minutes
Servings: 4
Ingredients:
- 4 fish fillets
- 4 tablespoon olive oil
- One egg, beaten
- ¼ cup whole wheat breadcrumbs

Directions:
1. Let the air fryer preheat to 350°F (180 C).
2. In a bowl, mix breadcrumbs with oil. Mix well.
3. First, coat the fish in the egg mix (egg mix with water) then in the breadcrumb mix. Coat well.
4. Place in the air fryer, let it cook for 10-12 minutes.
5. Serve hot with salad greens and lemon.

Nutrition:
Calories: 383.9
Fat: 29g
Protein: 26g
Carbs: 4.9g
Sodium: 158mg

513. PARMESAN GARLIC CRUSTED SALMON

Preparation Time: 5 minutes
Cooking Time: 15 minutes
Servings: 2
Ingredients:
- ¼ cup whole wheat breadcrumbs
- 4 cups of salmon
- 2 tablespoon unsalted butter, melted
- ¼ teaspoon of freshly ground black pepper
- ¼ cup Parmesan cheese (grated)
- 2 teaspoon minced garlic
- ½ teaspoon of Italian seasoning

Directions:

1. Let the air fryer preheat to 400°F, spray the oil over the air fryer basket.
2. Pat dry the salmon. In a bowl, mix Parmesan cheese, Italian seasoning, and breadcrumbs. In another pan, mix melted butter with garlic and add to the breadcrumbs mix. Mix well
3. Add kosher salt and freshly ground black pepper to salmon. On top of every salmon piece, add the crust mix and press gently.
4. Add the salmon to the pre-heated air fryer. Cook until done to your liking.
5. Serve hot with vegetable side dishes.

Nutrition:
Calories: 321.77
Fat: 21.24g
Protein: 27g
Carbs: 5.6g
Sodium: 167mg

514. AIR FRYER SALMON WITH MAPLE SOY GLAZE

Preparation Time: 6 minutes
Cooking Time: 8 minutes
Servings: 4
Ingredients:
- 3 tablespoon pure maple syrup
- 3 tablespoon gluten-free soy sauce
- 1 tablespoon Sriracha hot sauce
- 1 clove of minced garlic
- 4 fillets salmon, skinless

Directions:
1. In a Ziploc bag, mix sriracha, maple syrup, garlic, and soy sauce with salmon.
2. Mix well and let it marinate for at least half an hour.
3. Let the air fryer preheat to 400°F. With oil, spray the basket.
4. Take fish out from the marinade, pat dry.
5. Put the salmon in the air fryer, cook for 7 to 8 minutes, or longer.
6. In the meantime, in a saucepan, add the marinade, let it simmer until reduced to half.
7. Add glaze over salmon and serve.

Nutrition:
Calories: 275
Protein: 25.27g
Carbs: 11.9g
Sodium: 835.26mg

Fat: 14g

515. AIR-FRIED CAJUN SALMON

Preparation Time: 10 minutes
Cooking Time: 21 minutes
Servings: 1
Ingredients:
- 1 piece fresh salmon
- 2 tablespoon cajun seasoning
- Lemon juice

Directions:
1. Let the air fryer preheat to 350°F (180°C).
2. Pat dry the salmon fillet. Rub lemon juice and cajun seasoning over the fish fillet.
3. Place in the air fryer, cook for 7 minutes. Serve with salad greens and lime wedges.

Nutrition:
Calories: 244.54
Fat: 14g
Protein: 25g
Carbs: 5.13g
Sodium: 3272mg

516. AIR FRYER SHRIMP SCAMPI

Preparation Time: 5 minutes
Cooking Time: 11 minutes
Servings: 2
Ingredients:
- 4 cups raw shrimp
- 1 tablespoon lemon juice
- Chopped fresh basil
- 2 teaspoon red pepper flakes
- 2½ tablespoons unsalted butter
- Chopped chives
- 2 tablespoons chicken stock
- 1 tablespoon minced garlic

Directions:
1. Let the air fryer preheat with a metal pan to 330°F.
2. In the hot pan, add garlic, red pepper flakes, and half of the butter. Let it cook for 2 minutes.
3. Add the butter, shrimp, chicken stock, minced garlic, chives, lemon juice, and basil to the pan. Let it cook for five minutes. Bathe the shrimp in melted butter.
4. Take it out from the air fryer and let it rest for one minute.
5. Add fresh basil leaves and chives and serve.

Nutrition:
Calories: 450
Fat: 19g
Protein: 57.48g
Carbs: 7.8g
Sodium: 1408mg

517. SESAME SEED FISH FILLET

Preparation Time: 10 minutes
Cooking Time: 22 minutes
Servings: 2
Ingredients:
- 2 tablespoons whole wheat flour
- One egg, beaten
- 3 frozen fish fillets
For Coating
- 1 tablespoons oil
- ¼ cup sesame seeds
- Rosemary herbs
- ½ cup biscuit crumbs
- Kosher salt & pepper, to taste

Directions:
1. For 2 minutes, sauté the sesame seeds in a pan, without oil. Brown them and set it aside.
2. On a plate, mix all coating ingredients.
3. Place the aluminum foil on the air fryer basket and let it preheat to 390°F (200°C).
4. First, coat the fish in flour. Then in egg, then in the coating mix.
5. Place in the air fryer. If fillets are frozen, cook for ten minutes, then turn the fillet and cook for another 4 minutes.
6. If not frozen, then cook for 8 minutes and 2 minutes.

Nutrition:
Calories: 594
Fat: 34.9g
Protein: 42g
Carbs: 29.9g
Sodium: 2039.69mg

518. LEMON PEPPER SHRIMP IN THE AIR FRYER

Preparation Time: 6 minutes
Cooking Time: 11 minutes
Servings: 2
Ingredients:
- 1½ cup raw shrimp, peeled and deveined
- ½ tablespoon olive oil
- ¼ teaspoon garlic powder
- 1 teaspoon lemon pepper
- ¼ teaspoon paprika
- Juice of one lemon

Directions:
1. Let the air fryer preheat to 400°F
2. In a bowl, mix lemon pepper, olive oil, paprika, garlic powder, and lemon juice. Mix well. Add shrimp and coat well

3. Add shrimp to the air fryer, cook for 8 minutes and top with lemon slices and serve.

Nutrition:
Calories: 102.57
Fat: 4.42g
Protein: 13.56g
Carbs: 2.08g
Sodium: 745.22mg

519. MONKFISH CURRY

Preparation Time: 15 minutes
Cooking Time: 21 minutes
Servings: 2
Ingredients:
- ½ lb monkfish
- 1 thinly sliced sweet yellow onion
- ½ cup chopped tomato
- 3 tablespoons strong curry paste
- 1 tablespoon oil or ghee

Directions:
1. Set the Instant Pot to sauté and add the onion, oil, and curry paste.
2. When the onion is soft, add the remaining ingredients and seal.
3. Cook on "Stew" for 20 minutes.
4. Release the pressure naturally.

Nutrition:
Calories: 220
Fat: 14.5g
Protein: 13.4g
Sodium: 542mg
Carbs: 9.82g

520. SALMON BAKE

Preparation Time: 15 minutes
Cooking Time: 15 minutes
Servings: 2
Ingredients:
- 1 lb salmon
- 1 lb chopped Mediterranean vegetables
- 1 cup low-sodium fish broth
- Juice of half a lemon
- Sea salt as desired

Directions:
1. Mix all the ingredients except the broth in a foil pouch.
2. Place the pouch in the steamer basket in your Instant Pot.
3. Pour the broth into your Instant Pot.
4. Cook on Steam for 15 minutes.
5. Release the pressure naturally.

Nutrition:
Calories: 510.39
Fat: 26.63g
Protein: 50.34g
Carbs: 13.32g

Sodium: 1825mg

521. ROASTED SALMON WITH HONEY-MUSTARD SAUCE

Preparation Time: 6 minutes
Cooking Time: 21 minutes
Servings: 4
Ingredients:
- Non-stick cooking spray
- 2 tablespoons whole grain mustard
- 1 tablespoon honey
- 2 garlic cloves, minced
- ¼ teaspoon salt
- ¼ teaspoon freshly ground black pepper
- 1-pound salmon fillet

Directions:
1. Preheat the oven to 425°F. Spray a baking sheet with non-stick cooking spray.
2. In a small bowl, whisk together the mustard, honey, garlic, salt, and pepper.
3. Place the salmon fillet on the prepared baking sheet, skin-side down. Spoon the sauce onto the salmon and spread evenly.
4. Roast for 15 to 20 minutes, depending on the thickness of the fillet, until the flesh flakes easily.

Nutrition:
Calories: 259
Fat: 15.7g
Protein: 23.81g
Carbs: 5.7g
Sodium: 288mg

522. ROASTED SALMON WITH SALSA VERDE

Preparation Time: 6 minutes
Cooking Time: 25 minutes
Servings: 4
Ingredients:
- Non-stick cooking spray
- 8 ounces tomatillos, husks removed
- ½ onion, quartered
- 1 jalapeño or serrano pepper, seeded
- 1 garlic clove, unpeeled
- 1 teaspoon extra-virgin olive oil
- ½ teaspoon salt, divided
- 4 4-ounce wild-caught salmon fillets
- ¼ teaspoon freshly ground black pepper

- ¼ cup chopped fresh cilantro
- Juice of 1 lime

Directions:
1. Preheat the oven to 425°F. Spray a baking sheet with non-stick cooking spray.
2. In a large bowl, toss the tomatillos, onion, jalapeño, garlic, olive oil, and ¼ teaspoon of salt to coat. Arrange in a single layer on the prepared baking sheet, and roast for about 10 minutes until just softened. Transfer to a dish or plate and set aside.
3. Arrange the salmon fillets skin-side down on the same baking sheet, and season with the remaining ¼ teaspoon of salt and pepper. Bake for 12 to 15 minutes until the fish is firm and flakes easily.
4. Meanwhile, peel the roasted garlic and place it and the roasted vegetables in a blender or food processor. Add a scant ¼ cup of water to the jar, and process until smooth.
5. Add the cilantro and lime juice and process until smooth. Serve the salmon topped with the salsa verde.

Nutrition:
Calories:222.09
Fat: 10.24g
Protein: 25.9g
Carbs:5.9g
Sodium: 343.58mg

523. SHRIMP WITH GREEN BEANS

Preparation Time: 10 minutes
Cooking Time: 2 Minutes
Servings: 4

Ingredients:
- ¾ pound fresh green beans, trimmed
- 1 pound medium frozen shrimp, peeled and deveined
- 2 tablespoons fresh lemon juice
- 2 tablespoons olive oil
- Salt and ground black pepper, as desired

Directions:
1. Arrange a steamer trivet in the Instant Pot and pour in a cup of water.
2. Arrange the green beans on top of the trivet in a single layer and top with shrimp.
3. Drizzle with oil and lemon juice.

4. Sprinkle with salt and black pepper.
5. Close the lid and place the pressure valve in the "Seal" position.
6. Press "Steam" and just use the default time of 2 minutes.
7. Press "Cancel" and allow a natural release.
8. Open the lid and serve.

Nutrition:
Calories: 223
Fat: 1g
Carbohydrates: 7.9g
Sugar: 1.4g
Protein: 27.4g
Sodium: 322mg

524. CRAB CURRY

Preparation Time: 10 minutes
Cooking Time: 20 Minutes
Servings: 2

Ingredients:
- ½ lb chopped crab
- 1 thinly sliced red onion
- ½ cup chopped tomato
- 3 tablespoons curry paste
- 1 tablespoon oil or ghee

Directions:
1. Set the Instant Pot to sauté and add the onion, oil, and curry paste.
2. When the onion is soft, add the remaining ingredients and seal.
3. Cook on "Stew" for 20 minutes.
4. Release the pressure naturally.

Nutrition:
Calories: 2
Carbohydrates: 11g
Sugar: 4g
Fat: 10g
Protein: 24g
GL: 9

525. MIXED CHOWDER

Preparation Time: 10 minutes
Cooking Time: 35 Minutes
Servings: 2

Ingredients:
- 1 lb fish stew mix
- 2 cups white sauce
- 3 tablespoons Old Bay seasoning

Directions:
1. Mix all the ingredients in your Instant Pot.
2. Cook on "Stew" for 35 minutes.
3. Release the pressure naturally.

Nutrition:
Calories: 320
Carbohydrates: 9g
Sugar: 2g

Sodium: 687mg
Fat: 16g
GL: 4

526. MUSSELS IN TOMATO SAUCE

Preparation Time: 10 minutes
Cooking Time: 3 Minutes
Servings: 4

Ingredients:
- 2 tomatoes, seeded and chopped finely
- 2 pounds mussels, scrubbed and de-bearded
- 1 cup low-sodium chicken broth
- 1 tablespoon fresh lemon juice
- 2 garlic cloves, minced

Directions:
1. In the pot of Instant Pot, place tomatoes, garlic, wine, and bay leaf and stir to combine.
2. Arrange the mussels on top.
3. Close the lid and set the pressure valve in the "Seal" position.
4. Press "Manual" and cook under "High Pressure" for about 3 minutes.
5. Press "Cancel" and carefully allow a "Quick" release.
6. Open the lid and serve hot.

Nutrition:
Calories: 213
Fat: 25.2g
Carbohydrates: 11g
Sugar: 1g
Protein: 28.2g
Sodium: 670mg

527. CITRUS SALMON

Preparation Time: 10 minutes
Cooking Time: 7 Minutes
Servings: 4

Ingredients:
- 4 4-ounce salmon fillets
- 1 cup low-sodium chicken broth
- 1 teaspoon fresh ginger, minced
- 2 teaspoons fresh orange zest, grated finely
- 3 tablespoons fresh orange juice
- 1 tablespoon olive oil
- Ground black pepper, as desired

Directions:
1. In an Instant Pot, add all ingredients and mix.

2. Close the lid and set the pressure valve to the "Seal" position.
3. Press "Manual" and cook on "High Pressure" for about 7 minutes.
4. Press "Cancel" and allow a natural release.
5. Open the lid and serve the salmon fillets with a drizzle of the cooking sauce.

Nutrition:
Calories: 190
Fat: 10.5g
Carbohydrates: 1.8g
Sugar: 1g
Protein: 22g
Sodium: 68mg

528. HERBED SALMON

Preparation Time: 10 minutes
Cooking Time: 3 Minutes
Servings: 4
Ingredients:
- 4 4-ounce salmon fillets
- ¼ cup olive oil
- 2 tablespoons fresh lemon juice
- 1 garlic clove, minced
- ¼ teaspoon dried oregano
- Salt and ground black pepper, as desired
- 4 fresh rosemary sprigs
- 4 lemon slices

Directions:
1. For the dressing: In a large bowl, add oil, lemon juice, garlic, oregano, salt, and black pepper and beat until well-combined.
2. Arrange a steamer trivet in the Instant Pot and pour 1½ cups of water in Instant Pot.
3. Place the salmon fillets on top of the trivet in a single layer and top with dressing.
4. Arrange 1 rosemary sprig and 1 lemon slice over each fillet.
5. Close the lid and set the pressure valve to the "Seal" position.
6. Press "Steam" and just use the default time of 3 minutes.
7. Press "Cancel" and carefully allow a quick release.
8. Open the lid and serve hot.

Nutrition:
Calories: 262
Fat: 17g
Carbohydrates: 0.7g
Sugar: 0.2g
Protein: 22.1g
Sodium: 91mg

529. SALMON IN GREEN SAUCE

Preparation Time: 10 minutes
Cooking Time: 12 Minutes
Servings: 4
Ingredients:
- 4 6-ounce salmon fillets
- 1 avocado, peeled, pitted, and chopped
- ½ cup fresh basil, chopped
- 3 garlic cloves, chopped
- 1 tablespoon fresh lemon zest, grated finely

Directions:
1. Grease a large piece of foil.
2. In a large bowl, add all ingredients except salmon and water, and with a fork, mash completely.
3. Place fillets in the center of foil and top with the avocado mixture evenly.
4. Fold the foil around fillets to seal them.
5. Arrange a steamer trivet in the Instant Pot and pour ½ cup of water.
6. Place the foil packet on top of the trivet.
7. Close the lid and place the pressure valve in the "Seal" position.
8. Press "Manual" and cook under "High Pressure" for about minutes.
9. Meanwhile, preheat the oven to the broiler.
10. Press "Cancel" and allow a natural release.
11. Open the lid and transfer the salmon fillets onto a broiler pan.
12. Broil for about 3-4 minutes.
13. Serve warm.

Nutrition:
Calories: 333
Fat: 20.3g
Carbohydrates: 5.5g
Sugar: 0.4g
Protein: 34.2g
Sodium: 79mg

530. BRAISED SHRIMP

Preparation Time: 10 minutes
Cooking Time: 4 Minutes
Servings: 4
Ingredients:
- 1 pound frozen large shrimp, peeled and deveined
- 2 shallots, chopped
- ¾ cup low-sodium chicken broth
- 2 tablespoons fresh lemon juice

- 2 tablespoons olive oil
- 1 tablespoon garlic, crushed
- Ground black pepper, as desired

Directions:
1. In the Instant Pot, place oil and press the Sauté button. Now add the shallots and cook for about 2 minutes.
2. Add the garlic and cook for about 1 minute.
3. Press "Cancel" and stir in the shrimp, broth, lemon juice, and black pepper.
4. Close the lid and place the pressure valve in the "Seal" position.
5. Press "Manual" and cook under "High Pressure" for about 1 minute.
6. Press "Cancel" and carefully allow a quick release.
7. Open the lid and serve hot.

Nutrition:
Calories: 209
Fat: 9g
Carbohydrates: 4.3g
Sugar: 0.2g
Protein: 26.6g
Sodium: 293mg

531. SHRIMP COCONUT CURRY

Preparation Time: 10 minutes
Cooking Time: 20 Minutes
Servings: 2
Ingredients:
- ½ lb cooked shrimp
- 1 thinly sliced onion
- 1 cup coconut yogurt
- 3 tablespoons curry paste
- 1 tablespoon oil or ghee

Directions:
1. Set the Instant Pot to "Sauté" and add the onion, oil, and curry paste.
2. When the onion is soft, add the remaining ingredients and seal.
3. Cook on "Stew" for 20 minutes.
4. Release the pressure naturally.

Nutrition:
Calories: 377
Carbohydrates: 20.7g
Sugar: 13.9g
Fat: 24g
Sodium: 697.9mg
Protein: 20.7g
GL: 14

532. TROUT BAKE

Preparation Time: 10 minutes
Cooking Time: 35 Minutes
Servings: 2

Ingredients:
- 1 lb trout fillets, boneless
- 1 lb chopped winter vegetables
- 1 cup low-sodium fish broth
- 1 tablespoon mixed herbs
- Sea salt, as desired

Directions:
1. Mix all the ingredients except the broth in a foil pouch.
2. Place the pouch in the steamer basket in your Instant Pot.
3. Pour the broth into the Instant Pot.
4. Cook on Steam for 35 minutes.
5. Release the pressure naturally.

Nutrition:
Calories: 310
Carbohydrates: 14g
Sugar: 2g
Fat: 12g
Protein: 40g
Sodium: 856mg
GL: 5

533. SWORDFISH STEAK

Preparation Time: 10 minutes
Cooking Time: 35 Minutes
Servings: 2
Ingredients:
- 1 lb swordfish steak, whole
- 1 lb chopped Mediterranean vegetables
- 1 cup low-sodium fish broth
- 2 tablespoons soy sauce

Directions:
1. Mix all the ingredients except the broth in a foil pouch.
2. Place the pouch in the steamer basket for your Instant Pot.
3. Pour the broth into the Instant Pot. Lower the steamer basket into the Instant Pot.
4. Cook on "Steam" for 35 minutes.
5. Release the pressure naturally.

Nutrition:
Calories: 374
Carbohydrates: 13.65g
Sugar: 7.8g
Fat: 9g
Protein: 48g
GL: 1
Sodium: 2474.8mg

534. LEMON SOLE

Preparation Time: 10 minutes
Cooking Time: 5 Minutes
Servings: 2
Ingredients:
- 1 lb sole fillets, boned and skinned
- 1 cup low-sodium fish broth

- 2 shredded sweet onions
- Juice of half a lemon
- 2 tablespoons dried cilantro

Directions:
1. Mix all the ingredients in your Instant Pot.
2. Cook on "Stew" for 5 minutes.
3. Release the pressure naturally.

Nutrition:
Calories: 209.58
Sugar: 6.5g
Fat: 4.5g
Protein: 30.56g
GL: 1
Sodium: 945.06mg

535. TUNA SWEET CORN CASSEROLE

Preparation Time: 10 minutes
Cooking Time: 35 Minutes
Servings: 2
Ingredients:
- 3 small tins of tuna
- ½ lb sweet corn kernels
- 1 lb chopped vegetables
- 1 cup low-sodium vegetable broth
- 2 tablespoons spicy seasoning

Directions:
1. Mix all the ingredients in your Instant Pot.
2. Cook on "Stew" for 35 minutes.
3. Release the pressure naturally.

Nutrition:
Calories: 300
Carbohydrates: 6g
Sugar: 1g
Fat: 9g
Sodium: 495mg
GL: 2

536. LEMON PEPPER SALMON

Preparation Time: 10 minutes
Cooking Time: 10 Minutes
Servings: 4
Ingredients:
- 3 tablespoons ghee or avocado oil
- 1 lb skin-on salmon filet
- 1 julienned red bell pepper
- 1 julienned green zucchini
- 1 julienned carrot
- ¾ cup water
- A few sprigs of parsley, tarragon, dill, basil, or a combination
- ½ sliced lemon
- ½ teaspoon black pepper
- ¼ teaspoon sea salt

Directions:
1. Add the water and the herbs into the bottom of the Instant

Pot and put in a wire steamer rack making sure the handles extend upwards.
2. Place the salmon filet onto the wire rack, with the skin side facing down.
3. Drizzle the salmon with ghee, season with black pepper and salt, and top with the lemon slices.
4. Close and seal the Instant Pot, making sure the vent is turned to "Sealing".
5. Select the "Steam" setting and cook for 3 minutes.
6. While the salmon cooks, julienne the vegetables and set them aside.
7. Once done, quickly release the pressure, and then press the "Keep Warm/Cancel" button.
8. Uncover and wear oven mitts, carefully remove the steamer rack with the salmon.
9. Remove the herbs and discard them.
10. Add the vegetables to the pot and put the lid back on.
11. Select the "Sauté" function and cook for 1-2 minutes.
12. Serve the vegetables with salmon and add the remaining fat to the pot.
13. Pour a little of the sauce over the fish and vegetables if desired.

Nutrition:
Calories: 296
Carbohydrates 8g
Fat: 15 g
Protein: 31 g
Potassium: 1084 mg
Sodium: 284 mg

537. BAKED SALMON WITH GARLIC PARMESAN TOPPING

Preparation Time: 5 minutes
Cooking Time: 20 minutes
Servings: 4
Ingredients:
- 1 lb wild-caught salmon filets
- 2 tablespoons margarine or unsalted butter
- ¼ cup reduced-fat Parmesan cheese, grated
- ¼ cup light mayonnaise
- 2-3 cloves garlic, diced
- 2 tablespoons parsley
- Salt and pepper

Directions:
1. Heat oven to 350°F and line a baking pan with parchment paper.

2. Place salmon on pan and season with salt and pepper.
3. In a medium skillet, over medium heat, melt butter. Add garlic and cook, stirring 1 minute.
4. Reduce heat to low and add remaining ingredients. Stir until everything is melted and combined.
5. Spread evenly over salmon and bake 15 minutes for thawed fish or 20 for frozen. Salmon is done when it flakes easily with a fork. Serve.

Nutrition:
Calories: 274
Total Carbohydrates: 0.91g
Protein: 26.59g
Fat: 17g
Sugar: 0.03g
Sodium: 519.41mg

538. BLACKENED SHRIMP

Preparation Time: 5 minutes
Cooking Time: 5 minutes
Servings: 4
Ingredients:
- 1½ lb shrimp, peeled & deveined
- 4 lime wedges
- 4 tablespoon cilantro, chopped
- 4 cloves garlic, diced
- 1 tablespoon chili powder
- 1 tablespoon paprika
- 1 tablespoon olive oil
- 2 teaspoon Splenda brown sugar
- 1 teaspoon cumin
- 1 teaspoon oregano
- 1 teaspoon garlic powder
- 1 teaspoon salt
- ½ teaspoon pepper

Directions:
1. In a small bowl combine seasonings and Splenda brown sugar.
2. Heat oil in a skillet over med-high heat. Add shrimp, in a single layer, and cook 1-2 minutes per side.
3. Add seasonings and cook, stirring, 30 seconds. Serve garnished with cilantro and a lime wedge.

Nutrition:
Calories: 176.11
Total Carbohydrates: 7g
Net Carbohydrates: 6g
Protein: 24.89g
Fat: 5.6g
Sugar: 2.41g
Sodium: 1596mg

Fiber: 2.8g

539. CAJUN CATFISH

Preparation Time: 5 minutes
Cooking Time: 15 minutes
Servings: 4
Ingredients:
- 4 8-oz. catfish fillets
- 2 tablespoons olive oil
- 2 teaspoons garlic salt
- 2 teaspoons thyme
- 2 teaspoons paprika
- ½ teaspoon cayenne pepper
- ½ teaspoon red hot sauce
- ¼ teaspoon black pepper
- Non-stick cooking spray

Directions:
1. Heat oven to 450°F. Spray a 9x13" baking dish with cooking spray.
2. In a small bowl whisk together everything but catfish. Brush both sides of fillets, using all the spice mix.
3. Bake 10-13 minutes or until fish flakes easily with a fork. Serve.

Nutrition:
Calories: 263.52
Protein: 32.64g
Fat: 15.8g
Carbs: 1.32g
Sodium: 1309.23mg

540. CAJUN FLOUNDER & TOMATOES

Preparation Time: 10 minutes
Cooking Time: 15 minutes
Servings: 4
Ingredients:
- 4 flounder fillets
- 2½ cups tomatoes, diced
- ¾ cup onion, diced
- ¾ cup green bell pepper, diced
- 2 cloves garlic, diced fine
- 1 tablespoon cajun seasoning
- 1 teaspoon olive oil

Directions:
1. Heat oil in a large skillet over med-high heat. Add onion and garlic and cook 2 minutes, or until soft. Add tomatoes, peppers, and spices, and cook 2-3 minutes until tomatoes soften.
2. Lay fish over top. Cover, reduce heat to medium, and cook, 5-8 minutes, or until fish flakes easily with a fork. Transfer fish to serving plates and top with sauce.

Nutrition:

Calories: 194
Total Carbohydrates: 8g
Net Carbohydrates: 6g
Protein: 32g
Fat: 3g
Sugar: 5g
Sodium: 597.11mg
Fiber: 2g

541. CAJUN SHRIMP & ROASTED VEGETABLES

Preparation Time: 5 minutes
Cooking Time: 15 minutes
Servings: 4
Ingredients:
- 1 lb. large shrimp, peeled and deveined
- 2 zucchinis, sliced
- 2 yellow squash, sliced
- ½ bunch asparagus, cut into thirds
- 2 red bell peppers, cut into chunks
- /2 tablespoon olive oil
- 2 tablespoon Cajun Seasoning
- Salt & pepper, to taste

Directions:
1. Heat oven to 400°F.
2. Combine shrimp and vegetables in a large bowl. Add oil and seasoning and toss to coat.
3. Spread evenly in a large baking sheet and bake 15-20 minutes, or until vegetables are tender. Serve.

Nutrition:
Calories: 162.67
Total Carbohydrates: 11.08g
Sodium: 1650mg
Protein: 19.5g
Fat: 5.35g
Sugar: 7.5g
Fiber: 4.48g

542. CILANTRO LIME GRILLED SHRIMP

Preparation Time: 5 minutes
Cooking Time: 5 minutes
Servings: 6
Ingredients:
- 1 ½ lb. large shrimp raw, peeled, deveined with tails on
- Juice and zest of 1 lime
- 2 tablespoon fresh cilantro chopped

What You'll Need From Store Cupboard:
- ¼ cup olive oil
- 2 cloves garlic, diced fine
- 1 teaspoon smoked paprika
- ¼ teaspoon cumin
- ½ teaspoon salt

- ¼ teaspoon cayenne pepper

Directions:
1. Place the shrimp in a large Ziploc bag.
2. Mix remaining ingredients in a small bowl and pour over shrimp. Let marinate for 20-30 minutes.
3. Heat up the grill. Skewer the shrimp and cook 2-3 minutes, per side, just until they turn pink. Be careful not to overcook them. Serve garnished with cilantro.

Nutrition:
Calories: 166
Total Carbohydrates: 1.6g
Protein: 16g
Fat: 10.5g
Sodium: 829.98mg

543. CRAB FRITTATA

Preparation Time: 10 minutes
Cooking Time: 50 minutes
Servings: 4
Ingredients:
- 4 eggs
- 2 cups lump crabmeat
- 1 cup half-n-half
- 1 cup green onions, diced
- 1 cup reduced-fat parmesan cheese, grated
- 1 teaspoon salt
- 1 teaspoon pepper
- 1 teaspoon smoked paprika
- 1 teaspoon Italian seasoning
- Non-stick cooking spray

Directions:
1. Heat oven to 350°F. Spray an 8-inch springform pan or pie plate with cooking spray.
2. In a large bowl, whisk together the eggs and half-n-half. Add seasonings and parmesan cheese, stir to mix.
3. Stir in the onions and crab meat. Pour into prepared pan and bake 35-40 minutes, or until eggs are set and the top is lightly browned.
4. Let cool for 10 minutes, then slice and serve warm or at room temperature.

Nutrition:
Calories: 276
Total Carbohydrates: 5g
Net Carbohydrates: 4g
Protein: 25g
Fat: 17g
Sugar: 1g
Sodium: 1412.22mg
Fiber: 1g

544. CRUNCHY LEMON SHRIMP

Preparation Time: 5 minutes
Cooking Time: 10 minutes
Servings: 4
Ingredients:
- 1 lb. raw shrimp, peeled and deveined
- 2 tablespoon Italian parsley, roughly chopped
- 2 tablespoons lemon juice, divided
- ⅔ cup panko breadcrumbs
- 2½ tablespoons olive oil, divided
- Salt and pepper, to taste

Directions:
1. Heat oven to 400°F.
2. Sprinkle salt and pepper on top of the shrimp in a baking dish. Drizzle 1 tablespoon lemon juice and 1 tablespoon olive oil over the top. Place aside.
3. Combine the parsley, remaining lemon juice, breadcrumbs, remaining olive oil, and 1/4 tsp salt and pepper in a medium mixing bowl. Arrange the panko mixture on top of the shrimp in an equal layer.
4. Bake 8-10 minutes or until shrimp are cooked through and the panko is golden brown.

Nutrition:
Calories: 192
Total Carbohydrates: 7.78g
Net Carbohydrates: 14g
Protein: 17g
Fat: 9.8g
Sugar: 0.67g
Sodium: 847mg
Fiber: 1g

545. GRILLED TUNA STEAKS

Preparation Time: 5 minutes
Cooking Time: 10 minutes
Servings: 6
Ingredients:
- 6 6-oz. tuna steaks
- 3 tablespoons fresh basil, diced
- 4½ teaspoons olive oil
- ¾ teaspoon salt
- ¼ teaspoon pepper
- Non-stick cooking spray

Directions:
1. Heat grill to medium heat. Spray rack with cooking spray.
2. Drizzle both sides of the tuna with oil. Sprinkle with basil, salt, and pepper.
3. Place on grill and cook 5 minutes per side, tuna should

be slightly pink in the center. Serve.

Nutrition:
Calories: 273
Protein: 40.35g
Fat: 12.34g
Carbs: 0.33g
Sodium: 325.53mg

546. RED CLAM SAUCE & PASTA

Preparation Time: 10 minutes
Cooking Time: 3 hours
Servings: 4
Ingredients:
- 1 onion, diced
- ¼ cup fresh parsley, diced
- 2 6½-oz. cans clams, chopped, undrained
- 14½ oz. tomatoes, diced, undrained
- 6 oz. tomato paste
- 2 cloves garlic, diced
- 1 bay leaf
- 1 tablespoon sunflower oil
- 1 teaspoon Splenda
- 1 teaspoon basil
- ½ teaspoon thyme
- ½ homemade Pasta, cook & drain

Directions:
1. Heat oil in a small skillet over med-high heat. Add onion and cook until tender, add garlic and cook 1 minute more. Transfer to crockpot.
2. Add remaining ingredients, except pasta, cover, and cook on low for 3-4 hours.
3. Discard bay leaf and serve over cooked pasta.

Nutrition:
Calories: 309
Total Carbohydrates: 32g
Net Carbohydrates: 27g
Protein: 22.44g
Fat: 4.23g
Sugar: 7.5g
Fiber: 3.6g
Sodium: 93.45mg

547. SALMON MILANO

Preparation Time: 10 minutes
Cooking Time: 20 minutes
Servings: 6
Ingredients:
- 2½ lb. salmon filet
- 2 tomatoes, sliced
- ½ cup margarine
- ½ cup basil pesto

Directions:

1. Heat the oven to 400°F. Line a 9x15" baking sheet with foil, making sure it covers the sides. Place another large piece of foil onto the baking sheet and place the salmon filet on top of it.
2. Place the pesto and margarine in a blender or food processor and pulse until smooth. Spread evenly over salmon. Place tomato slices on top.
3. Wrap the foil around the salmon, tenting around the top to prevent foil from touching the salmon as much as possible. Bake 15-25 minutes, or salmon flakes easily with a fork. Serve.

Nutrition:
Calories: 570.29
Total Carbohydrates: 3g
Protein: 39.5g
Fat: 44.8g
Sugar: 1.5g
Sodium: 445.15mg

548. SHRIMP & ARTICHOKE SKILLET

Preparation Time: 5 minutes
Cooking Time: 10 minutes
Servings: 4
Ingredients:
- 1½ cups shrimp, peel & devein
- 2 shallots, diced
- 1 tablespoon margarine
- 2 12-oz. jars artichoke hearts, drain & rinse
- 2 cups white wine
- 2 cloves garlic, diced fine

Directions:
1. Melt margarine in a large skillet over med-high heat. Add shallot and garlic and cook until they start to brown, stirring frequently.
2. Add artichokes and cook for 5 minutes. Reduce heat and add wine. Cook 3 minutes, stirring occasionally.
3. Add the shrimp and cook just until they turn pink. Serve.

Nutrition:

Calories: 277
Total Carbohydrates: 26g
Net Carbohydrates: 17g
Protein: 15.9g
Fat: 5g
Sugar: 3.8g
Fiber: 9g
Sodium: 769.93mg

549. TUNA CARBONARA

Preparation Time: 5 minutes
Cooking Time: 25 minutes
Servings: 4
Ingredients:
- ½ lb. tuna fillet, cut into pieces
- 2 eggs
- 4 tablespoons fresh parsley, diced
- ½ cup homemade pasta, cook & drain,
- ½ cup reduced-fat Parmesan cheese
- 2 cloves garlic, peeled
- 2 tablespoons extra-virgin olive oil
- Salt & pepper, to taste

Directions:
1. In a small bowl, beat the eggs, parmesan, and a dash of pepper.
2. Heat the oil in a large skillet over med-high heat. Add garlic and cook until browned. Add the tuna and cook 2-3 minutes, or until the tuna is almost cooked through. Discard the garlic.
3. Add the pasta and reduce heat. Stir in egg mixture and cook, stirring constantly, 2 minutes. If the sauce is too thick, thin with water, a little bit at a time until it has a creamy texture.
4. Salt and pepper to taste and serve garnished with parsley.

Nutrition:
Calories: 248.8
Total Carbohydrates: 9.6g
Protein: 21.8g
Sodium: 460mg
Fat: 12.41g
Sugar: 0.43g

Fiber: 0.58g

550. MEDITERRANEAN FISH FILLETS

Preparation Time: 10 minutes
Cooking Time: 3 minutes
Servings: 4
Ingredients:
- 4 cod fillets
- 1 lb. grape tomatoes, halved
- 1 cup olives, pitted and sliced
- 2 tablespoons capers
- 1 teaspoon dried thyme
- 2 tablespoons olive oil
- 1 teaspoon garlic, minced
- Pepper
- Salt

Directions:
1. Pour 1 cup of water into the Instant Pot then place the steamer rack in the pot.
2. Spray heat-safe baking dish with cooking spray.
3. Add half of the grape tomatoes into the dish and season with pepper and salt.
4. Arrange fish fillets on top of cherry tomatoes. Drizzle with oil and season with garlic, thyme, capers, pepper, and salt.
5. Spread olives and remaining grape tomatoes on top of fish fillets.
6. Place dish on top of steamer rack in the pot.
7. Seal pot with a lid and select manual and cook on high for 3 minutes.
8. Once done, release pressure using quick release. Remove lid.
9. Serve and enjoy.

Nutrition:
Calories: 243
Fat: 12 g
Carbohydrates: 7.4 g
Sugar: 3 g
Protein: 28.4 g
Cholesterol: 0 mg
Sodium: 667.91mg

VEGETABLES

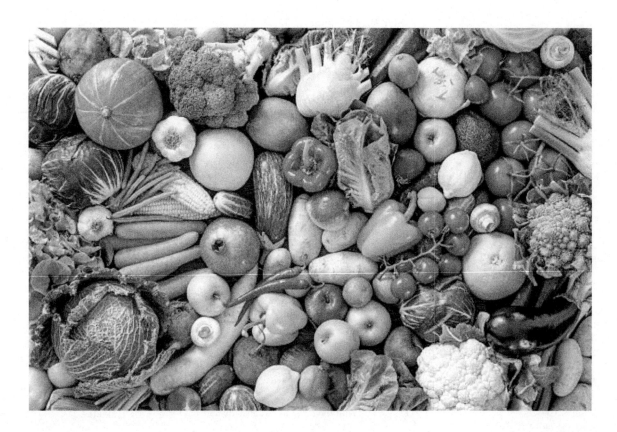

551. EGGPLANT PASTA

Preparation Time: 05 min
Cooking Time: 20 min
Servings: 4
Ingredients:

- 3 tablespoons olive oil, divided
- 1 lemon, ½ zested and juiced, ½ cut into wedges
- ⅛ teaspoon salt plus ¼ teaspoon, divided
- 1 large eggplant (about 1 lb.) sliced into ½-inch-thick rounds
- ¼ cup grated Parmesan cheese
- 2 ounces rotini or penne
- 1 large garlic clove, minced
- 1⅓ cups roasted red peppers
- 3 cups packed baby kale
- 2 tablespoons thinly sliced fresh basil
- 2 tablespoons walnuts, toasted

Directions:

1. Preheat the oven to 450°F. Line a large baking sheet with parchment paper.
2. Mix 2 tablespoons oil, 1½ teaspoons lemon juice, and ⅛ teaspoon salt in a small bowl. Place the eggplant slices on the prepared baking sheet. Brush both sides of the eggplant with the lemon juice mixture. Sprinkle the top with Parmesan. Grill, about 20 to 25 minutes, until the eggplant is golden and tender.
3. In the meantime, bring a large pot of water to a boil. Add the pasta and cook according to package directions for about 8 minutes. Drain.
4. Return the pasta to the pot. Add the lemon zest, garlic, roasted red pepper, spinach, and the remaining tablespoon of oil and ¼ teaspoon salt. Cook over medium heat, about 3 minutes, stirring gently until the spinach is tender.
5. Serve the eggplant with pasta and vegetables. Sprinkle with basil and walnuts. Serve with lemon wedges.

Nutrition:
Calories: 223
Total Fat: 13.8g
Saturated Fat: 1.9g
Cholesterol: 1mg
Sodium: 86mg
Total Carbohydrates: 23.2g
Dietary Fiber: 6g
Total Sugar: 4.4g
Protein: 5.8g

552. GARLIC PARMESAN ASPARAGUS

Preparation Time: 05 min
Cooking Time: 10 min
Servings: 4
Ingredients:

- 3 tablespoons extra-virgin olive oil
- 2 cloves garlic, minced
- ½ teaspoon ground pepper
- ¼ teaspoon salt
- 1½ pounds fresh asparagus, trimmed
- ½ cup finely grated Parmesan cheese
- 3 tablespoons whole wheat panko breadcrumbs
- 3 tablespoons chopped walnuts

Directions:
1. Preheat the oven to 425°F. Line a large baking sheet with aluminum foil or parchment paper. Combine oil, garlic, pepper, and salt in a large bowl; add asparagus and massage to coat evenly. Spread the asparagus evenly on the prepared baking sheet.
2. Combine parmesan, panko, and walnuts in a small bowl, sprinkle over the asparagus. Grill for 12 to 15 minutes until the panko is golden brown and the asparagus is tender. Serve immediately.

Nutrition:
Calories: 166
Total Fat: 14.8g
Saturated Fat: 2.2g
Cholesterol: 3mg
Sodium: 185mg
Total Carbohydrates: 6g
Dietary Fiber: 1.9g
Total Sugar: 1.2g
Protein: 4.2g

553. GREEN BEANS WITH SIZZLED GARLIC

Preparation Time: 10 min
Cooking Time: 15 min
Servings: 4
Ingredients:
- 3 tablespoons coconut oil, divided
- 4 cloves garlic, thinly sliced
- 1 pound green beans, trimmed and cut into 1½-inch pieces
- ¼ teaspoon salt
- ⅓ cup water
- 1 cup grape tomatoes, halved
- ¼ cup chopped fresh basil

Directions:
1. Heat 2 tablespoons oil in a large skillet over medium heat. Add the garlic; cook, stirring occasionally, until golden brown, 2 to 3 minutes. Using a slotted spoon on a small plate, remove the garlic and leave the oil.
2. Add the beans and salt to the pan. Stir to coat. Add water; cover and cook, stirring occasionally until the beans are tender and most of the water has evaporated (about 8 minutes). Add the remaining tablespoon of oil and the tomatoes to the pan. Cook, stirring occasionally, for about 2 minutes until the tomatoes begin to break. Remove from heat.
3. Add the basil and sizzled garlic. Stir to combine.

Nutrition:
Calories: 136
Total Fat: 10.5g
Saturated Fat: 8.9g
Sodium: 157mg
Total Carbohydrates: 10.9g
Dietary Fiber: 4.5g
Total Sugar: 2.8g
Protein: 2.7g

554. GRILLED BROCCOLI STEAKS

Preparation Time: 10 min
Cooking Time: 20 min
Servings: 4
Ingredients:
- 1 large head of broccoli
- 2 cloves garlic, minced
- 3½ tablespoons olive oil, divided
- 1 teaspoon ancho chile powder
- 1 teaspoon ground cumin, divided
- ½ teaspoon salt, divided
- ½ teaspoon ground pepper, divided
- ½ teaspoon lime zest
- 2 tablespoons lime juice
- 1 tablespoon chopped fresh cilantro
- 1 tablespoon maple syrup

Directions:
1. Preheat the grill to medium to high heat. Place a grill basket on the grill while preheating.
2. Remove the tough outer leaves from the broccoli. Cut the stem to get a flat base, leaving the core intact. Place the broccoli upright on a cutting board. Holding the broccoli in place, use a large chef's knife to cut 4 1½-inch-thick leaves from the center, creating 2 large and 2 small florets. Reserve the florets in bulk.
3. Combine the garlic, 1½ teaspoon oil, chili powder, ½ teaspoon cumin, and ¼

teaspoon salt. Place the pepper in a small bowl. Evenly rub the broccoli fillets and florets.
4. Stir in the lime zest, lime juice, cilantro, and the remaining 2 tablespoons oil, ½ teaspoon of cumin, and ¼ teaspoon of salt. Place the pepper in a small bowl. Spoon 2 tablespoons cilantro in a separate small bowl for brushing; reserve the rest to serve.
5. Place the broccoli steaks on the grill and the florets in the grill basket; baste the broccoli with 1 tablespoon of the cilantro mixture. Grill until well-mixed and charred in some spots, 7 to 8 minutes. Flip the steaks and florets and baste with 1 tablespoon cilantro mixture. Grill until the other side is tender and well-marked and charred in some spots, 7 to 8 minutes more.
6. Transfer to a serving dish. Pour the remaining sauce over the roasted broccoli.

Nutrition:
Calories: 114
Total Fat: 10.7g
Saturated Fat: 1.5g
Sodium: 358mg
Total Carbohydrates: 5.7g
Dietary Fiber: 0.9g
Total Sugar: 1.8g
Protein: 1g

555. ROASTED BRUSSELS SPROUTS WITH GOAT CHEESE

Preparation Time: 05 min
Cooking Time: 20 min
Servings: 4
Ingredients:
- 1 pound Brussels sprouts, trimmed and halved
- 1 large shallot, sliced
- 1 tablespoon extra-virgin olive oil
- ¼ teaspoon salt
- ¼ teaspoon ground pepper
- 2-3 teaspoons white balsamic vinegar
- ⅓ cup crumbled goat cheese
- ¼ cup pomegranate seeds

Directions:
1. Preheat oven to 400°F. Combine Brussels sprouts with shallot, oil, salt, and pepper in a medium bowl. Spread out on a large-rimmed baking sheet.
2. Roast Brussels sprouts until tender, 20 to 22 minutes.

Return to the bowl and toss with vinegar to taste. Sprinkle with goat cheese and pomegranate seeds.

Nutrition:
Calories: 103
Total Fat: 4.7g
Saturated Fat: 1.2g
Cholesterol: 2mg
Sodium: 184mg
Total Carbohydrates: 13.9g
Dietary Fiber: 4.3g
Total Sugar: 4.8g
Protein: 4.7g

556. MUSHROOM & TOFU STIR FRY

Preparation Time: 05 min
Cooking Time: 10 min
Servings: 4
Ingredients:
- 4 tablespoons coconut oil, divided
- 1 pound mixed mushrooms, sliced
- 1 medium red bell pepper, diced
- 1 bunch scallions, trimmed and cut into 2-inch pieces
- 1 tablespoon grated fresh ginger
- 1 large clove garlic, grated
- 1 8-ounce container baked tofu or smoked tofu, diced

Directions:
1. Heat 2 tablespoons of oil in a large flat-bottomed wok or cast-iron skillet over high heat. Add mushrooms and bell peppers; cook, stirring occasionally, until smooth, about 4 minutes. Add the scallions, ginger, and garlic; Cook for 30 seconds. Transfer the vegetables to a bowl.
2. Add the remaining 2 tablespoons of oil and tofu to the pan. Flip once, cook 3 to 4 minutes, until browned. Add the vegetables and the oyster sauce. Cook for 1 minute, stirring constantly.

Nutrition:
Calories: 741
Total Fat: 36.5g
Saturated Fat: 13.4g
Sodium: 5908mg
Total Carbohydrates: 55g
Dietary Fiber: 2.9g
Total Sugar: 3.2g
Protein: 33g

557. ROASTED CARROTS

Preparation Time: 05 min
Cooking Time: 20 min
Servings: 4
Ingredients:
- 2 tablespoons balsamic vinegar
- 1 tablespoon pure maple syrup
- 2 tablespoons olive oil, divided
- 1 pound carrots, preferably multicolored, cut into 2-inch pieces
- ¼ teaspoon salt
- 2 tablespoons chopped toasted pine nuts

Directions:
1. Preheat the oven to 400°F.
2. Whisk the vinegar, maple syrup, and 1 tablespoon of oil in a small bowl; put aside.
3. Combine carrots, salt, and the remaining 1 tablespoon of oil in a large bowl; toss to coat. Spread in a layer on a baking sheet.
4. Cook the carrots for 16 to 18 minutes, until they begin to brown and are almost tender but not completely cooked.
5. Pour the balsamic mixture over the carrots and cover completely with a spatula.
6. Continue roasting until carrots are tender and glazed, another 5 minutes. If desired, sprinkle with toasted pine nuts.
7. Serve immediately.

Nutrition:
Calories: 150
Total Fat: 10g
Saturated Fat: 1.2g
Sodium: 226mg
Total Carbohydrates: 15.1g
Dietary Fiber: 3g
Total Sugar: 8.7g
Protein: 1.5g

558. BAKED ZUCCHINI CHIPS

Preparation Time: 05 min
Cooking Time: 20 min
Servings: 2
Ingredients:
- 2 medium zucchini, peeled (about 7 oz. each)
- Cooking spray
- 2 teaspoons lime juice
- ¼ teaspoon chili powder
- ¼ teaspoon salt

Directions:
1. Place the racks in the upper and lower thirds of the oven. Preheat to 225°F. Line 2 large baking sheets with parchment paper.
2. Cut the zucchini into ⅛-inch-thick slices (a mandolin slicer will help you with this). Lay the slices in a layer on the prepared forms and dry them with paper towels. (The slices should not overlap, but it's okay if they are close together.) Brush lightly with cooking spray. Sprinkle with lemon juice, chili powder, and salt.
3. Bake for 1 hour, halving the positions of the shapes. Flip the zucchini slices over and cook for another 45 to 55 minutes, until golden brown and not moist. (Check every 5-10 minutes after the first hour and season the darker slices as soon as they are cooked.) Transfer the zucchini chips to a wire rack to cool.

Nutrition:
Calories: 104
Total Fat: 7.2g
Saturated Fat: 1g
Sodium: 315mg
Total Carbohydrates: 10.5g
Dietary Fiber 2.5g
Total Sugar: 4.2g
Protein: 2.6g

559. BLACK BEAN TORTILLA WRAPS

Preparation Time: 5 min
Cooking Time: 20 min
Servings: 4
Ingredients:
- ½ cup reduced-fat sour cream
- ½ teaspoon ground cumin
- 1 15-ounce can black beans, rinsed and drained
- 1 cup ripe diced peeled avocado
- ½ poblano chile, finely chopped
- ¼ cup finely chopped red onion
- ¼ cup chopped fresh cilantro leaves
- 3 tablespoons fresh lime juice
- ¼ teaspoon salt
- 4 8-inch flour tortillas

Directions:
1. Combine sour cream and cumin seeds in a small bowl; Stir with a whisk.
2. Combine the beans and the next 6 ingredients in a bowl. Place equal amounts of the black bean mixture in the center of each tortilla. Roll it

up, cut it in half, and secure it with wooden toothpicks if necessary. Serve with the sour cream mixture.

Nutrition:
Calories: 578
Total Fat: 15.7g
Saturated Fat: 5.8g
Cholesterol: 13mg
Sodium: 187mg
Total Carbohydrates: 88.2g
Fiber: 21.8g
Total Sugar: 5.5g
Protein: 26.7g

560. ASPARAGUS-TOFU STIR FRY

Preparation Time: 10 min
Cooking Time: 10 min
Servings: 6
Ingredients:
- ¾ pound asparagus spears
- ¾ cup vegetable broth
- ¼ cup low-sodium soy sauce
- 2 teaspoons corn-starch
- 2 tablespoons sesame oil, divided
- 1 8-ounce package tofu thinly sliced
- 4 garlic cloves, minced
- ½ teaspoon crushed red pepper
- 1 6-ounce package sliced shiitake mushrooms

Directions:
1. Remove the tough ends from the asparagus. Cut the spears diagonally into 2-inch pieces. Put aside.
2. Combine vegetable broth, soy sauce, and cornstarch in a small bowl; beat with a whisk until smooth. Put aside.
3. Heat 1 tablespoon of sesame oil in a large nonstick skillet over medium-high heat. Add tofu and sauté for 4 to 5 minutes or until golden brown. Take the tofu out of the pan; put it aside.
4. Heat the remaining tablespoon of sesame oil in the same pan. Add the garlic, red peppers, asparagus, and mushrooms to the pan and sauté for 3 minutes or until the asparagus is crisp and tender. Add the broth; Bring to a boil and cook for 2 to 3 minutes or until thickened. Add tofu and cook 1 minute or until heated through. Serve with brown rice.

Nutrition:
Calories: 215
Total Fat: 12.3g

Saturated Fat: 1.8g
Sodium: 1135mg
Total Carbohydrates: 17.4g
Fiber: 4.1g
Total Sugar: 4.3g
Protein: 13.6g

561. BLACK BEAN-ORANGE CHILI

Preparation Time: 10 min
Cooking Time: 10 min
Servings: 4
Ingredients:
- 2 tablespoons olive oil
- 1 large onion, chopped
- 1 medium green pepper, chopped
- 3 garlic cloves, minced
- 1 teaspoon ground cinnamon
- 1 teaspoon ground cumin
- 1 teaspoon chili powder
- ¼ teaspoon pepper
- 3 cans (14½ ounces each) diced tomatoes, undrained
- 2 cans (15 ounces each) black beans, rinsed and drained
- 1 cup orange juice

Directions:
1. In a Dutch oven, heat the oil over medium-high heat. Add onion and green pepper; cook and stir 8 to 10 minutes or until tender. Add garlic and spices; Cook for 1 more minute.
2. Add remaining ingredients; bring to a boil. Reduce the heat; Simmer, covered, 20-25 minutes to allow flavors to combine, stirring occasionally.

Nutrition:
Calories: 473
Total Fat: 9.1g
Saturated Fat: 1.5g
Sodium: 22mg
Total Carbohydrates: 79g
Fiber: 18.5g
Total Sugar: 13.2g
Protein: 23.6g

562. CUMIN QUINOA PATTIES

Preparation Time: 10 min
Cooking Time: 10 min
Servings: 4
Ingredients:
- 1 cup water
- ½ cup quinoa, rinsed
- 1 medium carrot, cut into 1-inch pieces
- 1 cup canned cannellini beans, rinsed and drained
- ¼ cup panko breadcrumbs
- 3 green onions, chopped

- 3 teaspoons ground cumin
- ¼ teaspoon salt
- ⅛ teaspoon pepper
- 2 tablespoons olive oil

Directions:
1. Bring the water to a boil in a small saucepan. Add the quinoa. Reduce the heat; Cook, covered, over low heat for 12 to 15 minutes until the liquid is absorbed. Remove from heat.
2. In the meantime, put the carrot in the food processor. Mix until coarsely chopped. Add the beans; mix until chopped. Transfer the mixture to a large bowl. Stir in the cooked quinoa, breadcrumbs, onion, and spices. Shape into 8 patties with the mixture.
3. In a large skillet, heat the oil over medium heat. Add the patties. Cook until the thermometer reads 160°, 3-4 minutes per side, turning carefully. Serve with optional garnishes if desired.

Nutrition:
Calories: 352
Total Fat: 10.6g
Saturated Fat: 1.7g
Cholesterol: 47mg
Sodium: 243mg
Total Carbohydrates: 49.3g
Fiber: 14.1g
Total Sugar: 2.6g
Protein: 17g

563. KALE QUESADILLAS

Preparation Time: 05 min
Cooking Time: 10 min
Servings: 4
Ingredients:
- 3 ounces fresh baby kale (about 4 cups)
- 4 green onions, chopped
- 1 small tomato, chopped
- 2 tablespoons lemon juice
- 1 teaspoon ground cumin
- ¼ teaspoon garlic powder
- 1 cup shredded reduced-fat Monterey Jack cheese
- ¼ cup reduced-fat ricotta cheese
- 6 flour tortillas (6 inches)

Directions:
1. In a large non-stick skillet, cook the first 6 ingredients and stir until the kale is tender. Remove from heat; add cheese.

2. The top half of each tortilla with the kale mixture; Fold the other half over the filling. Place on a pan covered with cooking spray. Cook over medium heat for 1 to 2 minutes per side until golden brown. Cut the quesadillas in half; Serve with sour cream if desired.

Nutrition:
Calories: 236
Total Fat: 11.9g
Saturated Fat: 6.7g
Cholesterol: 32mg
Sodium: 212mg
Total Carbohydrates: 21.5g
Fiber: 3.3g
Total Sugar: 2.9g
Protein: 12.2g

564. QUINOA-STUFFED ZUCCHINI

Preparation Time: 10 min
Cooking Time: 20 min
Servings: 8
Ingredients:
- 4 zucchini
- 3 teaspoons olive oil, divided
- ⅛ teaspoon pepper
- 1 teaspoon salt, divided
- 1½ cups vegetable broth
- 1 cup quinoa, rinsed
- 1 can (15 ounces) chickpeas or garbanzo beans, rinsed and drained
- ¼ cup dried cranberries
- 1 green onion, thinly sliced
- 1 teaspoon minced fresh sage
- ½ teaspoon grated lemon zest
- 1 teaspoon lemon juice
- ½ cup crumbled goat cheese

Directions:
1. Preheat the oven to 450°F. Cut each zucchini in half lengthwise; remove and discard the seeds. Lightly brush cut sides with 1 teaspoon of oil. Sprinkle with pepper and ½ teaspoon of salt. Place them face down on a baking sheet. Bake for 15-20 minutes until tender.
2. Combine broth and quinoa in a large saucepan. Bring to a boil. Reduce the heat; Cook, covered, over low heat for 12 to 15 minutes until the liquid is absorbed.
3. Add the chickpeas, cranberries, green onions, sage, lemon zest, lemon juice, and remaining oil and salt; pour into the zucchini. Sprinkle with cheese.

Nutrition:
Calories: 216
Total Fat: 5.6g
Saturated Fat: 1.1g
Cholesterol: 2mg
Sodium: 410mg
Total Carbohydrates: 32.8g
Fiber: 7.2g
Total Sugar: 4.7g
Protein: 10.2g

565. QUINOA WITH VEGETABLE STIR FRY

Preparation Time: 10 min
Cooking Time: 20 min
Servings: 4
Ingredients:
- 1 tablespoon olive oil
- 1 cup quinoa, rinsed and well-drained
- 2 garlic cloves, minced
- 1 medium zucchini, chopped
- 2 cups water
- ¾ cup canned chickpeas, rinsed and drained
- 1 medium tomato, finely chopped
- ½ cup crumbled feta cheese
- 2 tablespoons minced fresh basil
- ¼ teaspoon pepper

Directions:
1. In a large saucepan, heat oil over medium-high heat.
2. Add the quinoa and garlic; cook and stir for 2-3 minutes or until quinoa is lightly browned.
3. Add zucchini and water; bring to a boil. Reduce the heat; Cook, covered, over low heat for 12 to 15 minutes until the liquid is absorbed.
4. Add remaining ingredients; Serve hot.

Nutrition:
Calories: 389
Total Fat: 12.5g
Saturated Fat: 3.9g
Cholesterol: 17mg
Sodium: 231mg
Total Carbohydrates: 54.2g
Fiber: 10.5g
Total Sugar: 6.5g
Protein: 16.9g

566. KALE WITH GARLIC, RAISINS, AND PEANUTS

Preparation Time: 10 min
Cooking Time: 20 min
Servings: 4
Ingredients:
- 1 tablespoon peanut oil

- 2 garlic cloves, thinly sliced
- A pinch of dried hot red pepper flakes
- 1 small red bell pepper, cored, seeded, and cut into thin strips
- 2 pounds fresh baby kale, rinsed and spun
- ¼ cup golden raisins
- ¼ cup unsalted dry-roasted peanuts, chopped
- Salt and freshly ground black pepper

Directions:
1. In a large non-stick skillet, heat oil over medium-high heat. Add the garlic and chili flakes and cook
2. Add the red pepper and cook for another minute, stirring or stirring. Add kale, raisins, and peanuts; with the help of tongs, turn the kale upside down to distribute the mixture and cook evenly.
3. Fry only until wilted and most of the released water has evaporated about 2 minutes. Season with salt and pepper.

Nutrition:
Calories: 104
Total Fat: 4.7g
Saturated Fat: 0.7g
Sodium: 82mg
Total Carbohydrates: 14.9g
Fiber: 2.4g
Total Sugar: 7.5g
Protein: 3.1g

567. ASIAN FRIED EGGPLANT

Preparation Time: 10 minutes
Cooking Time: 40 minutes
Servings: 4
Ingredients:
- 1 large eggplant, sliced into 4ths
- 3 green onions, diced, green tips only
- 1 teaspoon fresh ginger, peeled & diced fine
- ¼ cup + 1 teaspoon cornstarch
- 1½ tablespoons soy sauce
- 1½ tablespoons sesame oil
- 1 tablespoon vegetable oil
- 1 tablespoon fish sauce
- 2 teaspoons Splenda
- ¼ teaspoon salt

Directions:
1. Place eggplant on paper towels and sprinkle both sides with salt. Let rest for 1 hour to remove excess moisture. Pat dry with more paper towels.

2. In a small bowl, whisk together soy sauce, sesame oil, fish sauce, Splenda, and 1 teaspoon cornstarch.
3. Coat both sides of the eggplant with the ¼ cup cornstarch. Use more if needed.
4. Heat oil in a large skillet over med-high heat. Add ½ the ginger and 1 green onion, then lay 2 slices of eggplant on top. Use ½ the sauce mixture to lightly coat both sides of the eggplant. Cook 8-10 minutes per side. Repeat.
5. Serve garnished with remaining green onions.

Nutrition:
Calories: 155
Total Carbohydrates: 18g
Net Carbohydrates: 13g
Protein: 2g
Fat: 9g
Sugar 6g
Sodium: 839mg
Fiber: 5g

568. CUCUMBER DILL SALAD

Preparation Time: 5 minutes
Cooking Time: 0 minutes
Servings: 2
Ingredients:
- 2 Persian cucumbers, peeled and sliced into very thin rounds
- 6 tablespoons nonfat Greek yogurt
- 1 teaspoon seasoned rice vinegar
- ½ teaspoon dill, fresh or dried
- ¼ teaspoon garlic powder

Directions:
1. Combine all of the ingredients in a small bowl.

Nutrition:
Calories: 20
Protein: 2g
Carbohydrates: 3g
Sodium: 35mg

569. BEET AND WALNUT SALAD

Preparation Time: 5 minutes
Cooking Time: 0 minutes
Servings: 4
Ingredients:
- 4 cups salad greens
- 1 cup chopped beets (canned and rinsed, or freshly cooked and cooled)
- 2 tablespoons chopped walnuts
- 2 tablespoons goat cheese
- Maple mustard vinaigrette

Directions:

1. Combine all of the ingredients in a large bowl and toss with the dressing.

Nutrition:
Calories: 65
Protein: 2g
Carbohydrates: 5g
Fat: 3.5g
Saturated Fat: 1g
Cholesterol: 5mg
Sodium: 100mg
Fiber: 2g

570. BROCCOLI SALAD

Preparation Time: 10 minutes
Cooking Time: 0 minutes
Servings: 5
Ingredients:
- ½ cup nonfat Greek yogurt
- ½ cup light mayonnaise
- 2 tablespoons seasoned rice vinegar
- 1 tablespoon sugar
- 5 cups chopped raw broccoli
- ¼ cup raisins, dried currants, or dried cranberries
- ¼ cup chopped nuts, such as cashews, pecans, or almonds

Directions:
1. In a medium bowl, combine the yogurt, mayonnaise, vinegar, and sugar. Stir in the broccoli, dried fruit, and nuts.
2. Mix well until evenly coated with the dressing.

Nutrition:
Calories: 80
Protein: 2g
Carbohydrates: 9g
Fat: 4.5g
Saturated Fat: 0.5g
Sodium: 160mg
Fiber: 2g

571. DRIED FRUIT SQUASH

Preparation Time: 15 minutes
Cooking Time: 40 minutes
Servings: 4
Ingredients:
- ¼ cup water
- 1 medium butternut squash, halved and seeded
- ½ tablespoon olive oil
- ½ tablespoon balsamic vinegar
- Salt and ground black pepper, to taste
- 4 large dates, pitted and chopped
- 4 fresh figs, chopped
- 3 tablespoons pistachios, chopped

- 2 tablespoons pumpkin seeds

Directions:
1. Preheat the oven to 375°F.
2. Place the water in the bottom of a baking dish.
3. Arrange the squash halves in a large baking dish, hollow side up, and drizzle with oil and vinegar.
4. Sprinkle with salt and black pepper.
5. Spread the dates, figs, and pistachios on top.
6. Bake for about 40 minutes, or until squash becomes tender.
7. Serve hot with the garnishing of pumpkin seeds.

Nutrition:
Calories: 227
Total Fat: 5.5g
Saturated Fat: 0.8g
Sodium: 66mg
Total Carbohydrates: 46.4g
Fiber: 7.5g
Sugar 19.6g
Protein: 5g

572. BANANA CURRY

Preparation Time: 15 minutes
Cooking Time: 15 minutes
Servings: 3
Ingredients:
- 2 tablespoons olive oil
- 2 yellow onions, chopped
- 8 garlic cloves, minced
- 2 tablespoons curry powder
- 1 tablespoon ground ginger
- 1 tablespoon ground cumin
- 1 teaspoon ground turmeric
- 1 teaspoon ground cinnamon
- 1 teaspoon red chili powder
- Salt and ground black pepper, to taste
- ⅔ cup soy yogurt
- 1 cup tomato puree
- 2 bananas, peeled and sliced
- 3 tomatoes, chopped finely
- ¼ cup unsweetened coconut flakes

Directions:
1. In a large pan, heat the oil over medium heat and sauté onion for about 4-5 minutes.
2. Add the garlic, curry powder, and spices, and sauté for about 1 minute.
3. Add the soy yogurt and tomato sauce and bring to a gentle boil.
4. Stir in the bananas and simmer for about 3 minutes.
5. Stir in the tomatoes and simmer for about 1–2 minutes.

6. Stir in the coconut flakes and immediately remove them from the heat.
7. Serve hot.

Nutrition:
Calories: 382
Total Fat: 18.2g
Saturated Fat: 6.6g
Sodium: 108mg
Total Carbohydrates: 53.4g
Fiber: 11.3g
Sugar 24.8g
Protein: 9g

573. MUSHROOM CURRY

Preparation Time: 15 minutes
Cooking Time: 20 minutes
Servings: 3
Ingredients:
- 2 cups tomatoes, chopped
- 1 green chili, chopped
- 1 teaspoon fresh ginger, chopped
- ¼ cup cashews
- 2 tablespoons canola oil
- ½ teaspoon cumin seeds
- ¼ teaspoon ground coriander
- ¼ teaspoon ground turmeric
- ¼ teaspoon red chili powder
- 1½ cups fresh shiitake mushrooms, sliced
- 1½ cups fresh button mushrooms, sliced
- 1 cup frozen corn kernels
- 1¼ cups water
- ¼ cup unsweetened coconut milk
- Salt and ground black pepper, to taste

Directions:
1. In a food processor, add the tomatoes, green chili, ginger, and cashews, and pulse until smooth paste forms.
2. In a pan, heat the oil over medium heat and sauté the cumin seeds for about 1 minute.
3. Add the spices and sauté for about 1 minute.
4. Add the tomato paste and cook for about 5 minutes.
5. Stir in the mushrooms, corn, water, and coconut milk, and bring to a boil.
6. Cook for about 10-12 minutes, stirring occasionally.
7. Season with salt and black pepper and remove from the heat.
8. Serve hot.

Nutrition:
Calories: 311
Total Fat: 20.4g

Saturated Fat: 6.1g
Sodium: 244mg
Total Carbohydrates: 32g
Fiber: 5.6g
Sugar: 9g
Protein: 8g

574. VEGGIE COMBO

Preparation Time: 15 minutes
Cooking Time: 25 minutes
Servings: 4
Ingredients:
- 1 tablespoon olive oil
- 1 small yellow onion, chopped
- 1 teaspoon fresh thyme, chopped
- 1 garlic clove, minced
- 8 ounces fresh button mushroom, sliced
- 1 pound Brussels sprouts
- 3 cups fresh spinach
- 4 tablespoons walnuts
- Salt and ground black pepper, to taste

Directions:
1. In a large skillet, heat the oil over medium heat and sauté the onion for about 3-4 minutes.
2. Add the thyme and garlic and sauté for about 1 minute.
3. Add the mushrooms and cook for about 15 minutes, or until caramelized.
4. Add the Brussels sprouts and cook for about 2-3 minutes.
5. Stir in the spinach and cook for about 3-4 minutes.
6. Stir in the walnuts, salt, and black pepper, and remove from the heat.
7. Serve hot.

Nutrition:
Calories: 153
Total Fat: 8.8g
Saturated Fat: 0.9g
Sodium: 94mg
Total Carbohydrates: 15.8g
Fiber: 6.3g
Sugar 4.4g
Protein: 8.5g

575. BEET SOUP

Preparation Time: 10 minutes
Cooking Time: 5 minutes
Servings: 2
Ingredients:
- 2 cups coconut yogurt
- 4 teaspoons fresh lemon juice
- 2 cups beets, trimmed, peeled, and chopped
- 2 tablespoons fresh dill

- Salt, to taste
- 1 tablespoon pumpkin seeds
- 2 tablespoons coconut cream
- 1 tablespoon fresh chives, minced

Directions:
1. In a high-speed blender, add all ingredients and pulse until smooth.
2. Transfer the soup into a pan over medium heat and cook for about 3-5 minutes or until heated through.
3. Serve immediately with the garnishing of chives and coconut cream.

Nutrition:
Calories: 230
Total Fat: 8g
Saturated Fat: 5.8g
Sodium: 218mg
Total Carbohydrates: 33.5g
Fiber: 4.2g
Sugar: 27.5g
Protein: 8g

576. VEGGIE STEW

Preparation Time: 15 minutes
Cooking Time: 30 minutes
Servings: 3
Ingredients:
- 2 tablespoons olive oil
- 1 large onion, chopped
- 2 garlic cloves, minced
- ¼ teaspoon fresh ginger, grated finely
- 1 teaspoon ground cumin
- 1 teaspoon cayenne pepper
- Salt and ground black pepper, to taste
- 2 cups homemade vegetable broth
- 1½ cups small broccoli florets
- 1½ cups small cauliflower florets
- 1 tablespoon fresh lemon juice
- 1 cup cashews
- 1 teaspoon fresh lemon zest, grated finely

Directions:
1. In a large soup pan, heat oil over medium heat and sauté the onion for about 3-4 minutes.
2. Add the garlic, ginger, and spices and sauté for about 1 minute.
3. Add 1 cup of the broth and bring to a boil.
4. Add the vegetables and again bring to a boil.
5. Cover the soup pan and cook for about 15-20 minutes, stirring occasionally.

6. Stir in the lemon juice and remove from the heat.
7. Serve hot with the topping of cashews and lemon zest.

Nutrition:
Calories: 425
Total Fat: 32g
Saturated Fat: 5.9g
Sodium: 601mg
Total Carbohydrates: 27.6g
Fiber: 5.2g
Sugar 7.1g
Protein: 13.4g

577. TOFU WITH BRUSSELS SPROUTS

Preparation Time: 15 minutes
Cooking Time: 15 minutes
Servings: 3
Ingredients:
- 1½ tablespoons olive oil, divided
- 8 ounces extra-firm tofu, drained, pressed, and cut into slices
- 2 garlic cloves, chopped
- ⅓ cup pecans, toasted, and chopped
- 1 tablespoon unsweetened applesauce
- ¼ cup fresh cilantro, chopped
- ½ pound Brussels sprouts, trimmed and cut into wide ribbons
- ¾ pound mixed bell peppers, seeded and sliced

Directions:
1. In a skillet, heat ½ tablespoon of the oil over medium heat and sauté the tofu and for about 6-7 minutes, or until golden brown.
2. Add the garlic and pecans and sauté for about 1 minute.
3. Add the applesauce and cook for about 2 minutes.
4. Stir in the cilantro and remove from heat.
5. Transfer tofu to a plate and set aside
6. In the same skillet, heat the remaining oil over medium-high heat and cook the Brussels sprouts and bell peppers for about 5 minutes.
7. Stir in the tofu and remove from the heat.
8. Serve immediately.

Nutrition:
Calories: 238
Total Fat: 17.8g
Saturated Fat: 2g

Sodium: 26mg
Total Carbohydrates: 13.6g
Fiber: 4.8g
Sugar 4.5g
Protein: 11.8g

578. TOFU WITH PEAS

Preparation Time: 15 minutes
Cooking Time: 20 minutes
Servings: 5
Ingredients:
- 1 tablespoon chili-garlic sauce
- 3 tablespoons low-sodium soy sauce
- 2 tablespoons canola oil, divided
- 1 16-ounce package extra-firm tofu, drained, pressed, and cubed
- 1 cup yellow onion, chopped
- 1 tablespoon fresh ginger, minced
- 2 garlic cloves, minced
- 2 large tomatoes, chopped finely
- 5 cups frozen peas, thawed
- 1 teaspoon white sesame seeds

Directions:
1. For the sauce: in a bowl, add the chili-garlic sauce and soy sauce and mix until well combined.
2. In a large skillet, heat 1 tablespoon of oil over medium-high heat and cook the tofu for about 4-5 minutes or until browned completely, stirring occasionally.
3. Transfer the tofu into a bowl.
4. In the same skillet, heat the remaining oil over medium heat and sauté the onion for about 3-4 minutes.
5. Add the ginger and garlic and sauté for about 1 minute.
6. Add the tomatoes and cook for about 4-5 minutes, crushing with the back of a spoon.
7. Stir in all 3 peas and cook for about 2-3 minutes.
8. Stir in the sauce mixture and tofu and cook for about 1-2 minutes.
9. Serve hot with the garnishing of sesame seeds.

Nutrition:
Calories: 291
Total Fat: 11.9g
Saturated Fat: 1.1g
Sodium: 732mg
Total Carbohydrates: 31.6g
Fiber: 10.8g
Sugar 11.5g

Protein: 19g

579. CARROT SOUP WITH TEMPEH

Preparation Time: 15 minutes
Cooking Time: 45 minutes
Servings: 6
Ingredients:
- ¼ cup olive oil, divided
- 1 large yellow onion, chopped
- Salt, to taste
- 2 pounds carrots, peeled, and cut into ½-inch rounds
- 2 tablespoons fresh dill, chopped
- 4½ cups homemade vegetable broth
- 12 ounces tempeh, cut into ½-inch cubes
- ¼ cup tomato paste
- 1 teaspoon fresh lemon juice

Directions:
1. In a large soup pan, heat 2 tablespoons of the oil over medium heat and cook the onion with salt for about 6-8 minutes, stirring frequently.
2. Add the carrots and stir to combine.
3. Lower the heat to low and cook, covered for about 5 minutes, stirring frequently.
4. Add in the broth and bring to a boil over high heat.
5. Lower the heat to a low and simmer, covered for about 30 minutes.
6. Meanwhile, in a skillet, heat the remaining oil over medium-high heat and cook the tempeh for about 3-5 minutes.
7. Stir in the dill and cook for about 1 minute.
8. Remove from the heat.
9. Remove the pan of soup from heat and stir in tomato paste and lemon juice.
10. With an immersion blender, blend the soup until smooth and creamy.
11. Serve the soup hot with the topping of tempeh.

Nutrition:
Calories: 294
Total Fat: 15.7g
Saturated Fat: 2.8g
Sodium: 723mg
Total Carbohydrates: 25.9g
Fiber: 4.9g
Sugar 10.4g
Protein: 16.4g

580. TEMPEH WITH BELL PEPPERS

Preparation Time: 15 minutes
Cooking Time: 15 minutes
Servings: 3
Ingredients:

- 2 tablespoons balsamic vinegar
- 2 tablespoons low-sodium soy sauce
- 2 tablespoons tomato sauce
- 1 teaspoon maple syrup
- ½ teaspoon garlic powder
- ⅛ teaspoon red pepper flakes, crushed
- 1 tablespoon vegetable oil
- 8 ounces tempeh, cut into cubes
- 1 medium onion, chopped
- 2 large green bell peppers, seeded and chopped

Directions:

1. In a small bowl, add the vinegar, soy sauce, tomato sauce, maple syrup, garlic powder, and red pepper flakes and beat until well combined. Set aside.
2. Heat 1 tablespoon of oil in a large skillet over medium heat and cook the tempeh for about 2-3 minutes per side.
3. Add the onion and bell peppers and heat for about 2-3 minutes.
4. Stir in the sauce mixture and cook for about 3-5 minutes, stirring frequently.
5. Serve hot.

Nutrition:
Calories: 241
Total Fat: 13g
Saturated Fat: 2.6g
Sodium: 65mg
Total Carbohydrates: 19.7g
Fiber: 2.1g
Sugar 8.1g
Protein: 16.1g

581. SQUASH MEDLEY

Preparation Time: 10 minutes.
Cooking Time: 20 minutes.
Servings: 2
Ingredients:

- 2 lbs mixed squash
- ½ cup mixed veg
- 1 cup vegetable stock
- 2 tablespoons olive oil
- 2 tablespoons mixed herbs

Directions:

1. Put the squash in the steamer basket and add the stock into the Instant Pot.
2. Steam the squash in your Instant Pot for 10 minutes.

3. Depressurize and pour away the remaining stock.
4. Set to sauté and add the oil and remaining ingredients.
5. Cook until a light crust forms.

Nutrition:
Calories: 100
Carbohydrates: 10g
Sugar: 3g
Fat: 6g
Sodium: 123mg
Protein: 5g
GL: 20

582. FRIED TOFU HOTPOT

Preparation Time: 15 minutes
Cooking Time: 15 minutes
Servings: 2
Ingredients:

- ½ lb fried tofu
- 1 lb chopped Chinese vegetable mix
- 1 cup low-sodium vegetable broth
- 2 tablespoons 5 spice seasoning
- 1 tablespoon smoked paprika

Directions:

1. Mix all the ingredients in your Instant Pot.
2. Cook on Stew for 15 minutes.
3. Release the pressure naturally.

Nutrition:
Calories: 268.6
Carbohydrates: 30.25g
Sugar: 14g
Fat: 7.8g
Protein: 16.81g
GL: 6
Sodium: 680mg

583. PEA AND MINT SOUP

Preparation Time: 15 minutes
Cooking Time: 35 minutes
Servings: 2
Ingredients:

- 1 lb green peas
- 2 cups low-sodium vegetable broth
- 3 tablespoons mint sauce

Directions:

1. Mix all the ingredients in your Instant Pot.
2. Cook on "Stew" for 35 minutes.
3. Release the pressure naturally.
4. Blend into a rough soup.

Nutrition:
Calories: 390.7
Carbohydrates: 75g
Sugar: 28g
Fat: 2.7g
Protein: 16.87g

GL: 11
Sodium: 470mg

584. LENTIL AND EGGPLANT STEW

Preparation Time: 15 minutes
Cooking Time: 35 minutes
Servings: 5
Ingredients:

- 1 lb eggplant
- 1 lb dry lentils
- 1 cup chopped vegetables
- 1 cup low-sodium vegetable broth

Directions:

1. Mix all the ingredients in your Instant Pot.
2. Cook on "Stew" for 35 minutes.
3. Release the pressure naturally.

Nutrition:
Calories: 385
Carbohydrates: 71.49g
Sugar: 6.9g
Fat: 1.39g
Protein: 24.66g
GL: 16
Sodium: 50.84mg

585. TOFU CURRY

Preparation Time: 15 minutes
Cooking Time: 20 minutes
Servings: 2
Ingredients:

- 2 cups cubed extra firm tofu
- 2 cups mixed stir fry vegetables
- ½ cup soy yogurt
- 3 tablespoons curry paste
- 1 tablespoon oil or ghee

Directions:

1. Set the Instant Pot to sauté and add the oil and curry paste.
2. When the onion is soft, add the remaining ingredients except for the yogurt and seal.
3. Cook on Stew for 20 minutes.
4. Release the pressure naturally and serve with a scoop of soy yogurt.

Nutrition:
Calories: 484
Carbohydrates: 30.74g
Sugar: 9.88g
Fat: 30.7g
Protein: 28.89g
GL: 7
Sodium: 582mg

586. FAKE ON-STEW

Preparation Time: 15 minutes
Cooking Time: 25 minutes

Servings: 2

Ingredients:

- ½ lb soy bacon
- 1 lb chopped vegetables
- 1 cup low-sodium vegetable broth
- 1 tablespoon nutritional yeast

Directions:

1. Mix all the ingredients in your Instant Pot.
2. Cook on "Stew" for 25 minutes.
3. Release the pressure naturally.

Nutrition:

Calories: 695
Carbohydrates: 45g
Sugar: 12g
Fat: 45.9g
Protein: 24g
GL: 5
Sodium: 908mg

587. LENTIL AND CHICKPEA CURRY

Preparation Time: 15 minutes
Cooking Time: 20 minutes
Servings: 2
Ingredients:

- 2 cups dry lentils and chickpeas
- 1 thinly sliced onion
- 1 cup chopped tomato
- 3 tablespoons curry paste
- 1 tablespoon oil or ghee

Directions:

1. Set the Instant Pot to sauté and add the onion, oil, and curry paste.
2. When the onion is soft, add the remaining ingredients and seal.
3. Cook on Stew for 20 minutes.
4. Release the pressure naturally.

Nutrition:

Calories: 360
Carbohydrates: 26g
Sugar: 6g
Fat: 19g
Protein: 23g
Sodium: 560mg
GL: 10

588. SEITAN ROAST

Preparation Time: 15 minutes
Cooking Time: 35 minutes
Servings: 2
Ingredients:

- 1 lb seitan roulade
- 1 lb chopped winter vegetables
- 1 cup low-sodium vegetable broth
- 4 tablespoons roast rub

Directions:

1. Rub the roast rub into your roulade.
2. Place the roulade and vegetables in your Instant Pot.
3. Add the broth. Seal.
4. Cook on "Stew" for 35 minutes.
5. Release the pressure naturally.

Nutrition:

Calories: 260
Carbohydrates: 9g
Sugar: 2g
Fat: 2g
Sodium: 88mg
Protein: 49g
GL: 4

589. ZUCCHINI WITH TOMATOES

Preparation Time: 15 minutes
Cooking Time: 11 minutes
Servings: 8
Ingredients:

- 6 medium zucchinis, chopped roughly
- 1 pound cherry tomatoes
- 2 small onions, chopped roughly
- 2 tablespoons fresh basil, chopped
- 1 cup water
- 1 tablespoon olive oil
- 2 garlic cloves, minced
- Salt and ground black pepper, as desired

Directions:

1. In the Instant Pot, place oil and press "Sauté." Now add the onion, garlic, ginger, and spices and cook for about 3-4 minutes.
2. Add the zucchinis and tomatoes and cook for about 1-2 minutes.
3. Press "Cancel" and stir in the remaining ingredients except for basil.
4. Close the lid and place the pressure valve in the "Seal" position.
5. Press "Manual" and cook under high pressure for about 5 minutes.
6. Press "Cancel" and allow a natural release.
7. Open the lid and transfer the vegetable mixture onto a serving platter.
8. Garnish with basil and serve.

Nutrition:

Calories: 57
Fat: 2.1g
Carbohydrates: 9g
Sugar: 4.8g
Protein: 2.5g

Sodium: 39mg

590. CHICKPEAS ON MIXED GREENS

Preparation Time: 10 minutes
Cooking Time: 0 minutes
Servings: 2
Ingredients:

- 12¾ ounces canned chickpeas, drained, rinsed, coarsely mashed
- 1⅓ ounces celery, chopped
- 1⅓ ounces red pepper, chopped
- 4 tablespoons red onion, chopped
- ⅛ teaspoon ground black pepper
- 2 tablespoons low-fat mayonnaise
- ½ 5-ounce package mixed baby salad greens

Directions:

1. Combine chickpeas, celery, red pepper, onion, pepper, and mayonnaise. Toss to mix.
2. Divide mix green among plates. Top with chickpeas mixture and serve.

Nutrition:

Calories: 206
Carbohydrates: 26g
Protein: 10g
Fat: 3g
Sodium: 55mg

591. TOMATO AND BASIL SALAD

Preparation Time: 10 minutes
Cooking Time: 0 minutes
Servings: 2
Ingredients:

- 4 medium tomatoes, finely diced
- 1 garlic clove, crushed
- 6 basil leaves, rolled tightly and thinly sliced crosswise to form strips (chiffonade)
- 2 tablespoons organic extra-virgin olive oil
- 1 tablespoon balsamic vinegar
- ½ teaspoon black pepper

Directions:

1. In a bowl, combine all the ingredients. Toss to mix. Season with pepper.
2. Divide among plates and serve.

Nutrition:

Calories: 99
Carbohydrates: 3g
Protein: 1g
Fat: 7g
Sodium: 8mg

592. ANNIE'S EVERYDAY SALAD

Preparation Time: 20 minutes
Cooking Time: 0 minutes
Servings: 6
Ingredients:

- 4 blood oranges, skinned, pitted, sliced
- 3 ripe avocados, pitted, halved, cubed to a ½-inch thickness
- 1 teaspoon ground black pepper
- 2 fennel bulbs, outer layer removed, thinly sliced
- Juice of 1 lemon
- 2 tablespoons organic extra-virgin olive oil

Directions:

1. On a large platter, arrange sliced orange in a single layer.
2. Season cubed avocado with black pepper. Arrange on top of sliced oranges.
3. Place fennel in a bowl. Add lemon juice and olive oil. Toss to mix. Transfer fennel onto sliced orange.
4. Drizzle juice and oil mixture onto the salad.
5. Serve salad on a platter.

Nutrition:
Calories: 251
Carbohydrates: 13g
Protein: 4g
Fat: 17g
Sodium: 17mg

593. POTATO HEAD SALAD

Preparation Time: 20 minutes
Cooking Time: 0 minutes
Servings: 10
Ingredients:

- 1½ pounds russet potatoes, peeled, cooked, cubed, warm
- 1 cup celery, sliced
- ½ cup green onions, sliced
- ¼ cup green and red bell pepper, chopped
- ¼ cup sweet pickle relish
- 2 hard-boiled eggs, chopped
- 4 slices bacon, fried, well-drained, crumbled
- 1 cup fat-free mayonnaise
- ½ cup fat-free sour cream
- 2 tablespoons cider vinegar
- 1 tablespoon yellow mustard
- ½ teaspoon celery seeds
- ⅛ teaspoon sea salt
- ⅛ teaspoon pepper

Directions:

1. In a bowl, combine potatoes, celery, green onions, green and red pepper, pickle relish, eggs,

and bacon. Toss and mix well. Add mayonnaise, sour cream, cider vinegar, yellow mustard, and celery seeds. Toss and mix well. Season with sea salt and pepper.

2. Divide among plates and serve.

Nutrition:
Calories: 132
Carbohydrates: 25g
Protein: 4g
Fat: 3g
Sodium: 495mg

594. ITALIAN CRUNCHY SALAD

Preparation Time: 20 minutes
Cooking Time: 0 minutes
Servings: 8
Ingredients:

- 1 ¾-ounce package Good Seasons Italian dressing mix
- 2 tablespoons plus 2 teaspoons lemon juice, freshly squeezed
- 1 cup water
- 1 teaspoon fructose
- 1½ teaspoons instant thickener
- 1½ cups fresh tomato, chunked to 1-inch
- 1½ cups cucumber peeled, chunked to 1-inch
- ¼ cup onion, chopped
- ½ cup black olives, sliced
- ½ cup avocado chunked to 1-inch
- ¼ cup fat-free Italian Dressing

Directions:

1. Prepare the Italian dressing. In a blender, combine all ingredients. Blend till well mixed. Transfer to a bowl and let stand for 10 minutes. Set aside ¼ cup and refrigerate the rest for later use.
2. In a bowl, combine all the ingredients. Toss to mix well.
3. Divide among plates and serve.

Nutrition:
Calories: 39
Carbohydrates: 4g
Protein: 1g
Fat: 3g
Sodium: 145mg

595. GRILLED VEGETABLES SALAD WITH HERB VINAIGRETTE

Preparation Time: 25 minutes
Cooking Time: 0 minutes
Servings: 6
Ingredients:

- 1 tablespoon organic extra virgin olive oil

- 2 teaspoons cider vinegar
- 1 teaspoon fresh parsley, snipped
- ¼ teaspoon fresh thyme snipped
- ¼ teaspoon fresh rosemary snipped
- ⅛ teaspoon sea salt
- ⅛ teaspoon ground black pepper
- 1 medium eggplant, cut crosswise into ½-inch slices
- 1 medium onion, cut into ½-inch wedges
- 2 green or red sweet peppers, halved, stemmed, seeded, membranes removed
- 3 Roma tomatoes, halved lengthwise
- 6 large cremini mushrooms, stemmed
- 3 tablespoons organic extra virgin olive oil
- 1 tablespoon cider vinegar

Directions:

1. Prepare the herb vinaigrette. In a small bowl, combine all ingredients. Mix well and set aside.
2. In a very large bowl, combine eggplant, onion, sweet peppers, tomatoes, and mushrooms. Drizzle oil and vinegar over vegetables. Toss to coat.
3. Preheat the grill over medium heat. Uncover and grill vegetables till tender turning once midway through the grilling (about 6 minutes). Remove and cool for 5 minutes.
4. Cut halved sweet pepper to strips. Divide grilled vegetables among plates. Drizzle with herb vinaigrette and serve warm.

Nutrition:
Calories: 126
Carbohydrates: 11g
Protein: 2g
Fat: 9g
Sodium: 55mg

596. FRUITS AND BEANS SALAD

Preparation Time: 25 minutes
Cooking Time: 0 minutes
Servings: 8
Ingredients:

- 2 tablespoons organic extra virgin olive oil
- 2 tablespoons water
- 1 tablespoon raw honey
- 1 tablespoon tarragon wine vinegar

- 1 tablespoon lime zest, grated
- 3 teaspoons lime juice
- ½ teaspoon dried mint leaves
- ⅛ teaspoon of sea salt
- 4 large ripe mangoes, peeled, pitted, cubed
- 1 cup pineapple, cubed
- ½ medium cucumber, seeded, sliced
- ¼ cup red bell pepper, finely chopped
- ¼ cup green onions, sliced
- 1 15-ounce can black beans, rinsed, drained
- ⅓ cup honey-lime dressing
- 1 teaspoon mint sprigs

Directions:

1. Prepare the honey-lime dressing. In a bowl, combine all the ingredients. Stir to mix and set aside ⅓ cup.
2. In a salad bowl, combine all the ingredients (excluding mint). Toss to mix.
3. To serve, transfer to plates and top with mint sprigs.

Nutrition:
Calories: 164
Carbohydrates: 33g
Protein: 5g
Fat: 4g
Sodium: 169mg

597. TOMATO CUCUMBER MINT SALAD

Preparation Time: 25 minutes
Cooking Time: 0 minutes
Servings: 6
Ingredients:

- 2 cucumbers, cut to ½-inch wide pieces
- ⅓ cup red wine vinegar
- 1 teaspoon sugar
- ½ teaspoon sea salt
- 2 cups tomatoes, chopped
- ⅔ Cup red onion, chopped
- ¼ cup fresh mint, chopped
- 2 tablespoons organic extra virgin olive oil

Directions:

1. In a medium bowl, combine cucumbers, vinegar, sugar, and sea salt. Mix well and let stand at room temperature for 15 minutes.
2. Add tomatoes, red onion, mint, and olive oil. Toss to mix.
3. Divide and transfer salad to plates and serve.

Nutrition:
Calories: 68
Carbohydrates: 7g
Protein: 1g
Fat: 5g

Sodium: 202mg

598. ASPARAGUS MASHED EGGS SALAD

Preparation Time: 30 minutes
Cooking Time: 10 minutes
Servings: 4

Ingredients:

- 5 hard-boiled eggs, shell removed
- ¼ cup red onion, minced
- 2 tablespoons full-fat mayonnaise
- 1 rib celery, finely diced
- 1 tablespoon lemon juice, freshly squeezed
- 1 tablespoon fresh parsley, chopped
- 2 teaspoons Dijon mustard
- 1 teaspoon of water
- 20 large asparagus spears (about 1 pound), peeled, ends trimmed

Directions:

1. Prepare the salad dressing. Halve eggs and separate the whites and yolks. In 2 separate bowls, mash all the egg whites and 2 egg yolks. Set aside. (Save the remaining 3 egg yolks for other uses.)
2. In a bowl, combine the onion, mayonnaise, celery, lemon juice, parsley, mustard, and water. Mix till blended. Add egg white mixture and stir to mix.
3. Bring a medium saucepan half-filled with water to a boil over high heat. In a large bowl, half fill with ice water.
4. Cook asparagus to al dente (about 8 minutes). Remove and soak in ice water to retain color. Pat dry cooled asparagus with paper towels.
5. Divide the asparagus spears among 4 plates. Spoon salad dressing over asparagus spears and top with minced egg yolks.

Nutrition:
Calories: 105
Carbohydrates: 8g
Protein: 8g
Fat: 5g
Sodium: 199mg

599. GREEN BEAN, TOMATO AND ONION SALAD

Preparation Time: 30 minutes

Cooking Time: 5 minutes
Servings: 6
Ingredients:

- ½ teaspoon sea salt
- 1 pound young green beans, trimmed
- 8 small plum tomatoes (about 1 pound), halved lengthwise
- 2 green onions, sliced

For the Dressing:

- ¼ cup organic extra virgin olive oil
- 4 teaspoon red wine vinegar
- 1 tablespoon grainy mustard
- 1 clove garlic, minced
- ½ teaspoon granulated sugar
- ¼ teaspoon sea salt
- ¼ teaspoon ground black pepper
- ¼ cup fresh parsley, chopped

Directions:

1. Half fill a medium saucepan with water. Add sea salt and bring to a boil. Add beans and cook till crispy and tender (about 3 minutes). Remove from heat. Drain and cool bean in chill water. Drain and pat dry with paper towels.
2. With a small metal spoon, scoop out the center of plum tomatoes and discard. Halve each plum tomato again. Combine beans, tomatoes, and green onions in a large bowl. Set aside.
3. Next, prepare the dressing. In a small bowl combine oil, vinegar, mustard, garlic, sugar, sea salt, and pepper. Mix well. Add parsley and stir briefly. Pour dressing over salad and toss well.
4. Divide salad among plates and serve.

Nutrition:
Calories: 128
Carbohydrates: 10g
Protein: 2g
Fat: 10g
Sodium: 150mg

600. NUTRITIONAL BERRIES-PECAN WITH SPINACH SALAD

Preparation Time: 45 minutes
Cooking Time: 20 minutes
Servings: 6
Ingredients:
For the Oil-Free Raspberry Dressing:

- 3 ¾-ounce packages Good Seasons Italian dressing mix

- ½ cup plus 1 tablespoon lemon juice, fresh squeezed
- 2 cups water
- 6 tablespoons raspberry-white grape juice frozen concentrate
- ⅓ cup instant food thickener
- 15 cloves garlic, peeled
- ¼ cup pecans, chopped
- ⅓ cup oil-free raspberry dressing
- 12½ cups packed baby leaf spinach
- ½ cup red onion, thinly sliced
- 1½ cups mixed berries, sliced
- Non-stick cooking spray

Directions:
1. Preheat oven to 275°F.
2. Prepare raspberry dressing. Combine all ingredients in a blender. Blend till smooth (about 30 seconds). Set aside ⅓ cup and refrigerate the rest for a maximum of 10 days.
3. Spread out pecans on a baking sheet. Bake till slightly browned (about 10 minutes). Remove from oven and let cool for 15 minutes.
4. Meanwhile, increase oven to 300°F. Keep garlic in a foil pouch. Lightly coat with a layer of nonstick cooking spray. Seal pouch and bake for 10 minutes. Remove from oven.
5. Combine all ingredients in a large bowl. Toss and mix well.
6. Divide among plates and serve.

Nutrition:
Calories: 76
Carbohydrates: 10g
Protein: 3g
Fat: 4g
Sodium: 181 mg

601. VEGETABLE KABOB SALAD

Preparation Time: 50 minutes
Cooking Time: 15 minutes
Servings: 4
For the Dressing:
- 2 tablespoons organic extra virgin olive oil
- 1 tablespoon red wine vinegar
- 1 tablespoon balsamic vinegar
- 1 teaspoon Dijon mustard
- 1 large clove garlic, minced
- 1 tablespoon fresh parsley, finely chopped
- 2 teaspoons fresh rosemary, finely chopped
- ½ teaspoon sea salt
- ½ teaspoon ground black pepper

Ingredients:

- 1 Vidalia onion, sliced into 4 rounds
- 1 red bell pepper, quartered, ribbed, seeded
- 1 yellow bell pepper, quartered, ribbed, seeded
- 3 small zucchini, halved crosswise then lengthwise
- Non-stick cooking spray

Directions:
1. Prepare the dressing. Combine oil, vinegar, mustard, garlic, parsley, rosemary, sea salt, and pepper in a bowl. Mix well. Brush vegetables with dressing. Set vegetables aside to marinate for at least 30 minutes.
2. Preheat grill at medium-high heat after lightly coated with nonstick cooking spray.
3. Insert bamboo skewers through sliced onions. Arrange all vegetables on a baking sheet.
4. Place a baking sheet over the grill and cook till vegetables are crispy and tender (about 12 minutes). Turn occasionally.
5. Divide vegetables among plates and serve warm.

Nutrition:
Calories: 72
Carbohydrates: 10g
Protein: 1g
Fat: 1g
Sodium: 165mg

602. FENNEL GARLIC SALAD

Preparation Time: 70 minutes
Cooking Time: 0 minutes
Servings: 4
Ingredients:
- 1½ fennel bulbs (about 18 ounces total), very thinly sliced with a mandoline
- 5 large cloves garlic, very thinly sliced
- ¼ cup organic extra virgin olive oil
- Juice of ½ large lemon
- ⅛ teaspoon of coarse sea salt
- ⅛ teaspoon of ground black pepper
- 1 teaspoon fresh chives, minced
- 1 teaspoon fresh parsley leaves, minced

Directions:
1. In a stainless steel bowl, combine fennel and garlic. Chill for 1 hour.

2. In another steel bowl, combine oil, lemon juice, sea salt, and pepper. Mix well.
3. Remove fennel and garlic from the fridge. Pour dressing over fennel and garlic. Toss well. Add chives and parsley. Toss to mix.
4. Divide and transfer salad to 4 plates and serve.

Nutrition:
Calories: 173
Carbohydrates: 11g
Protein: 2g
Fat: 14g
Sodium: 97mg

603. GRANDMA WENDY'S MULTI-LAYER SALAD

Preparation Time: 70 minutes
Cooking Time: 0 minutes
Servings: 8
Ingredients:
For the Dressing:
- ¼ cup organic extra virgin olive oil
- 2 tablespoon lime juice, freshly squeezed
- 1 tablespoon raw honey
- 2 teaspoon Dijon mustard
- ¾ teaspoon ground cumin
- 1 clove garlic, minced
- ½ teaspoon sea salt
- ½ teaspoon pepper

Ingredients:
- 1 10-ounce package fresh baby spinach, stemmed, coarsely chopped
- 1½ cups mushrooms, sliced
- 2 cups carrots, peeled, shredded
- 1½ cups seedless cucumber, halved lengthwise, sliced
- 1 small red onion, thinly sliced
- ⅓ cup dark raisins

Directions:
1. Prepare the dressing. In a bowl, combine oil, lime juice, honey, mustard, cumin, garlic, sea salt, and pepper. Cover and chill.
2. Divide spinach into 3 portions. In a large bowl, layer 1 portion of spinach with mushrooms, another portion of spinach with carrots, then the final portion with spinach only. Top with cucumbers, onion, and raisins. Cover and refrigerate for 1 hour.
3. Remove salad and dressing from the refrigerator. Divide

salad among plates. Drizzle dressing over salad and serve.

Nutrition:
Calories: 122
Carbohydrates: 14g
Protein: 2g
Fat: 7g
Sodium: 220mg

604. BEAN AND CHICKPEA SALAD WITH MUSTARD-HERB DRESSING

Preparation Time: 80 minutes
Cooking Time: 3 minutes
Servings: 6
Ingredients:
- ½ teaspoon sea salt
- 1 pound green beans, ends trimmed, cut to 1-inch length
- 1 19-ounce can chickpeas, drained, rinsed
- ⅓ cup red onions, chopped

For the Dressing:
- 2 tablespoons organic extra virgin olive oil
- 2 tablespoons red wine vinegar
- 1 tablespoon granulated sugar
- 1 tablespoon Dijon mustard
- ¼ teaspoon freshly ground black pepper
- ¼ teaspoon sea salt
- 2 tablespoons fresh dill, finely chopped

Directions:
1. Half fill a medium saucepan with water. Add sea salt and bring to a boil. Add beans and cook till crispy and tender (about 3 minutes). Remove from heat. Drain and cool bean in chill water. Drain and pat dry with paper towels
2. In a bowl, combine green beans, chickpeas, and onions. Set aside.
3. Next, prepare the dressing. In a small bowl, combine oil, vinegar, sugar, mustard, pepper, and sea salt. Mix until smooth. Stir in dill. Drizzle over salad and toss well. Let chill for 1 hour.
4. Divide salad among plates and serve.

Nutrition:
Calories: 161
Carbohydrates: 23g
Protein: 6g
Fat: 6g
Sodium: 325mg

605. MOST IRRESISTIBLE POTATO SALAD

Preparation Time: 105 minutes
Cooking Time: 20 minutes
Servings: 8
Ingredients:
- 6 medium potatoes, rinsed
- ¾ teaspoon sea salt, divided
- ¾ cup frozen peas, thawed
- 2 tablespoon red wine vinegar
- 1 tablespoon Dijon mustard
- 1 clove garlic, minced
- 4 green onions, sliced
- 2 stalks celery, diced
- ¼ cup fresh parsley, chopped
- 3 hard-boiled eggs, chopped
- ½ cup light mayonnaise
- ¼ cup plain low-fat yogurt
- ¼ teaspoon ground black pepper

Directions:
1. Half fill a medium saucepan with water. Add sea salt and bring water to a boil. Cook potatoes till tender (about 20 minutes). Remove from heat. Drain and let cool for 10 minutes. Peel skin and cut to ½-inch cubes. Place in a large bowl and set aside.
2. Rinse peas with boiling water. Drain well.
3. Combine vinegar, mustard, and garlic in a small bowl. Mix well. Add potatoes. Toss gently to mix. Add onions, celery, parsley, eggs, and peas. Mix well.
4. In a separate large bowl, combine mayonnaise, yogurt, ¼ teaspoon sea salt, and pepper. Mix well. Fold in potato mixture till evenly coated. Chill for at least 1 hour.
5. To serve, divide salad among plates.

Nutrition:
Calories: 162
Carbohydrates: 20g
Protein: 5g
Fat: 7g
Sodium: 395mg

606. SALAD ON THE ROCK

Preparation Time: 130 minutes
Cooking Time: 0 minutes
Servings: 8
Ingredients:
- 2 cups cauliflower, finely chopped
- 1 cup broccoli florets, finely chopped
- ½ cup red apple, diced

- 2 tablespoons raw sunflower seeds
- 2 tablespoons dried cranberries
- ¼ cup mayonnaise spread
- 1½ teaspoons lemon juice, freshly squeezed
- ⅛ teaspoon sea salt
- 2 tablespoons frozen apple juice concentrate, thawed
- ⅛ teaspoon cayenne pepper

Directions:
1. In a medium bowl, combine all ingredients. Toss well. Cover and chill for at least 2 hours.
2. Remove from refrigerator. Transfer to plates and serve.

Nutrition:
Calories: 58
Carbohydrates: 7g
Protein: 2g
Fat: 3g
Sodium: 87mg

607. FRESH TOMATO WITH MINTY LENTIL SALAD

Preparation Time: 160 minutes
Cooking Time: 15 minutes
Servings: 6
Ingredients:
- 1 cup dry lentils
- 2 cups water
- ½ cup onion, chopped
- 2 teaspoons garlic, minced
- ¼ cup celery, chopped
- ½ cup green pepper, chopped
- ½ cup parsley, finely chopped
- 2 tablespoons fresh mint, finely chopped
- ¼ cup lemon juice
- ¼ cup extra-virgin olive oil
- ½ teaspoon sea salt
- 1 cup fresh tomato, diced

Directions:
1. In a medium saucepan, combine lentils and water and bring to a boil. Reduce heat till simmering, cover, and let simmer till lentils are tender (about 15 minutes). Remove from heat, drain and transfer to a medium bowl.
2. Add onion, garlic, celery, green pepper, parsley, and mint. Mix well.
3. In a small bowl, combine lemon juice, olive oil, and sea salt. Mix well. Drizzle over lentils mixture and toss to mix. Cover and refrigerate for 2 hours or more.

4. To serve, remove salad from refrigerator, mix in tomatoes and divide salad among plates.

Nutrition:
Calories: 136
Carbohydrates: 11g
Protein: 4g
Fat: 9g
Sodium: 211mg

608. DELICIOUS CARIBBEAN POTATO SALAD

Preparation Time: 3 hours 10 minutes
Cooking Time: 0 minutes
Servings: 8
Ingredients:
- 1½ pounds sweet potatoes, peeled, cooked, ¾-inch cubed
- 1½ pounds russet potatoes, peeled, cooked, ¾-inch cubed
- ¼ cup small pimiento-stuffed olives
- ¾ cup fat-free mayonnaise
- ½ cup fat-free milk
- 2 teaspoons lime juice
- 2 green onions, sliced
- 1 teaspoon ground cumin
- ⅛ teaspoon red cayenne pepper
- ⅛ teaspoon sea salt

Directions:
1. In a bowl, combine potatoes and olives. Add mayonnaise, milk, lime juice, green onions, cumin, and pepper. Toss and mix well. Season with sea salt.
2. Chill for 3 hours.
3. Remove from fridge. Divide among plates and serve.

Nutrition:
Calories: 167
Carbohydrates: 37g
Protein: 3g
Fat: 1g
Sodium: 416mg

609. TEN VEGETABLE SALAD

Preparation Time: 10 minutes +8 hours refrigerate
Cooking Time: 0 minutes
Servings: 8
Ingredients:
For the Herbed Sour Cream Dressing:
- ¾ cup fat-free mayonnaise
- ¾ cup sour cream
- 2 cloves garlic, minced
- ½ teaspoon dried basil
- ½ teaspoon tarragon leaves
- ¼ teaspoon sea salt
- ¼ teaspoon pepper

Ingredients:
- 2 cups romaine lettuce, thinly sliced
- 1 cup red cabbage, sliced
- 1 cup mushrooms, sliced
- 1 cup carrots, sliced
- 1 cup green bell pepper, sliced
- 1 cup cherry tomatoes, halved
- 1 cup small broccoli
- ½ cup cucumber, sliced
- ½ cup red onion, sliced
- 1½ cup sour cream dressing
- 4 teaspoons parsley, finely chopped

Directions:
1. Prepare the herbed sour cream dressing. Combine all ingredients in a bowl. Mix well.
2. In a 1½-quart bowl, arrange lettuce at the bottom. Arrange and layer the remaining vegetables on top of the lecture. Top with sour cream dressing and garnish with parsley.
3. Cover and refrigerate for 8 hours.
4. Remove from fridge. Toss to mix. Transfer to plates and serve.

Nutrition:
Calories: 68
Carbohydrates: 15g
Protein: 3g
Sodium: 380mg

610. BUTTER BEANS

Preparation Time: 5 minutes
Cooking Time: 12 minutes
Servings: 4
Ingredients:
- 2 garlic cloves, minced
- Red pepper flakes to taste
- Salt to taste
- 2 tablespoons clarified butter
- 4 cups green beans, trimmed

Directions:
1. Bring a pot of salted water to boil
2. Once the water starts to boil, add beans and cook for 3 minutes
3. Take a bowl of ice water and drain beans, plunge them in the ice water
4. Once cooled, keep them on the side
5. Take a medium skillet and place it over medium heat, add ghee, and melt
6. Add red pepper, salt, garlic
7. Cook for 1 minute
8. Add beans and toss until coated well, cook for 3 minutes
9. Serve and enjoy!

Nutrition:
Calories: 93
Fat: 8g
Sodium: 200mg
Carbohydrates: 4g
Protein: 2g

611. WALNUTS AND ASPARAGUS

Preparation Time: 5 minutes
Cooking Time: 5 minutes
Servings: 4
Ingredients:
- 1½ tablespoon olive oil
- ¾ pound asparagus, trimmed
- ¼ cup walnuts, chopped
- Salt and pepper to taste

Directions:
1. Heat olive oil in a skillet over medium heat.
2. Add asparagus, sauté for 5 minutes until browned
3. Season with salt and pepper
4. Remove heat
5. Add walnuts and toss
6. Serve warm!

Nutrition:
Calories: 124
Fat: 12g
Carbohydrates: 4g
Sodium: 196mg
Protein: 3g

612. ROASTED CAULIFLOWER

Preparation Time: 5 minutes
Cooking Time: 30 minutes
Servings: 8
Ingredients:
- 1 large cauliflower head
- 2 tablespoons melted coconut oil
- 2 tablespoons fresh thyme
- 1 teaspoon Celtic sea salt
- 1 teaspoon fresh ground pepper
- 1 head roasted garlic
- 8 ounces burrata cheese, for garnish
- 2 tablespoons fresh thyme for garnish

Directions:
1. Preheat your oven to 425°F
2. Rinse cauliflower and trim, core and sliced
3. Lay cauliflower evenly on a rimmed baking tray
4. Drizzle coconut oil evenly over cauliflower, sprinkle thyme leaves
5. Season with a pinch of salt and pepper
6. Squeeze roasted garlic
7. Roast cauliflower until it slightly caramelizes for about

30 minutes, making sure to turn once
8. Garnish with fresh thyme leaves and burrata
9. Enjoy!

Nutrition:
Calories: 129
Fat: 11g
Carbohydrates: 6g
Protein: 7g

613. COOL BRUSSELS PLATTER

Preparation Time: 5 minutes
Cooking Time: 10-15 minutes
Servings: 2
Ingredients:
- ¼ cup Parmesan cheese, grated
- ¼ cup hazelnuts, whole and skinless
- 1 tablespoon olive oil
- 1 pound Brussels sprouts
- Salt to taste

Directions:
1. Preheat your oven to 350°F
2. Line a baking sheet with parchment paper and trim the bottom of the Brussels
3. Put leaves in a medium-sized bowl, making sure that they are broken
4. Toss leaves with olive oil and season with salt
5. Spread leaves on baking sheet
6. Roast for 10-15 minutes until crispy
7. Divide between bowls and toss with remaining ingredients
8. Serve and enjoy!

Nutrition:
Calories: 287
Fat: 19g
Carbohydrates: 13g
Protein: 14g
Sodium: 558mg

614. TANGY PINEAPPLE COLESLAW

Preparation Time: 10 minutes
Cooking Time: 0 minutes
Servings: 6
Ingredients:
- ¼ cup nonfat Greek yogurt
- ¼ cup light mayonnaise
- ¼ cup finely chopped canned pineapple (packed in its own juice)
- 2 tablespoons pineapple juice (from the canned pineapple)
- 2½ cups shredded cabbage
- ½ cup shredded carrots

Directions:
1. In a medium bowl, combine the yogurt, mayonnaise, pineapple, and pineapple juice. Put in the cabbage and carrots and mix well until evenly covered with the dressing.

Nutrition:
Calories: 60
Protein: 1g
Carbohydrates: 6g
Fat: 3.5g
Saturated Fat: 0.5g
Sodium: 85mg
Fiber: 1g

615. VEGETARIAN ANTIPASTO SALAD

Preparation Time: 10 minutes
Cooking Time: 0 minutes
Servings: 8
Ingredients:
- 1 cup halved marinated mushrooms
- 1 cup chopped canned artichokes
- 1 cup chopped roasted red peppers
- ½ cup sliced black olives
- 1 cup cubed light mozzarella cheese
- ½ cup chopped fresh basil
- 4 cups chopped romaine lettuce

Directions:
1. Dressing of your choice
2. Toss all of the ingredients in a large bowl and serve.
3. To keep calories low, try to find the veggies packed/marinated in water or vinegar. If you select the ones packed in oil, simply rinse them before using them.

Nutrition:
Calories: 80
Protein: 5g
Carbohydrates: 9g
Fat: 3.5g
Saturated Fat: 1g
Cholesterol: 5mg
Sodium: 480mg
Fiber: 3g

616. WATERMELON AND FETA SALAD

Preparation Time: 10 minutes
Cooking Time: 0 minutes
Servings: 4
Ingredients:
- 4 cups ½"-cubed watermelon

- 2 tablespoons fresh chopped basil
- 4 tablespoons white balsamic vinegar
- 2 tablespoons water
- 2 teaspoons honey
- A squeeze of fresh lemon juice
- ¼ cup reduced-fat feta cheese

Directions:
1. Put the watermelon into a medium bowl.
2. In a smaller bowl, whisk together the basil, vinegar, water, honey, and lemon. Pour over the watermelon. Mix well to evenly coat. Sprinkle with cheese and lightly stir.

Nutrition:
Calories: 80
Protein: 2g
Carbohydrates: 19g
Fat: 1g
Saturated Fat: 1g
Cholesterol: 5mg
Sodium: 125mg
Fiber: 1g

617. GENEROUS FIERY TOMATO SALAD

Preparation Time: 10 minutes
Cooking Time: 25 minutes
Servings: 4
Ingredients:
- ½ cup scallions, chopped
- 1 pound cherry tomatoes
- 3 teaspoons olive oil
- Sea salt and freshly ground black pepper, to taste
- 1 tablespoon red wine vinegar

Directions:
1. Season tomatoes with spices and oil
2. Heat your oven to 450°F
3. Take a baking sheet and spread the tomatoes
4. Bake for 15 minutes
5. Stir and turn the tomatoes
6. Then again, bake for 10 minutes
7. Take a bowl and mix the roasted tomatoes with all the remaining ingredients
8. Serve and enjoy!

Nutrition:
Calories: 57.23
Fat: 3.82g
Carbohydrates: 5.4g
Protein: 1.2g
Sodium: 177mg

SNACKS

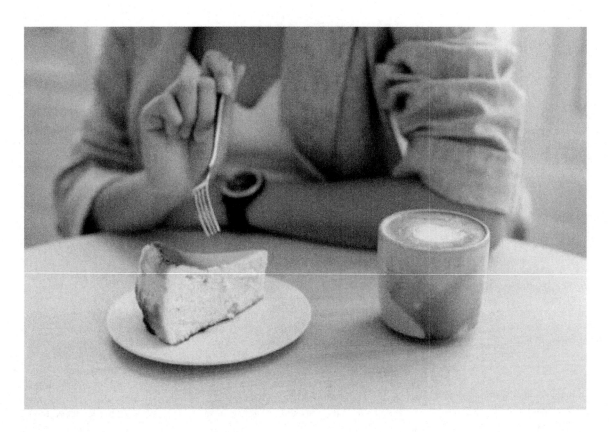

618. ALMOND CHEESECAKE BITES

Preparation Time: 5 minutes
Cooking Time: 0 minutes
Servings: 6
Ingredients:
- ½ cup reduced-fat cream cheese, soft
- ½ cup almonds, ground fine
- ¼ cup almond butter
- 2 drops liquid Stevia

Directions:
1. In a large bowl, beat cream cheese, almond butter, and Stevia on high speed until the mixture is smooth and creamy. Cover and chill for 30 minutes.
2. Use your hands to shape the mixture into 12 balls.
3. Place the ground almonds on a shallow plate. Roll the balls in the nuts completely covering all sides. Store in an airtight container in the refrigerator.

Nutrition:
Calories: 186
Protein: 6.7g
Fat: 16g
Carbs: 6.3g
Sodium: 87.23mg

619. ALMOND COCONUT BISCOTTI

Preparation Time: 5 minutes
Cooking Time: 51 minutes
Servings: 16
Ingredients:

- 1 egg, room temperature
- 1 egg white, room temperature
- ½ cup margarine, melted
- 2½ cup flour
- 1⅓ cup unsweetened coconut, grated
- ¾ cup almonds, sliced
- ⅔ cup Splenda
- 2 teaspoons baking powder
- 1 teaspoon vanilla
- ½ teaspoon salt

Directions:
1. Heat oven to 350°F. Line a baking sheet with parchment paper.
2. In a large bowl, combine dry ingredients.
3. In a separate mixing bowl, beat other Ingredients together. Add to dry ingredients and mix until thoroughly combined.
4. Divide dough in half. Shape each half into a loaf measuring 8x2¾ inches. Place loaves on pan 3 inches apart.
5. Bake 25-30 minutes or until set and golden brown. Cool on a wire rack for 10 minutes.
6. With a serrated knife, cut loaf diagonally into ½-inch slices. Place the cookies, cut side down, back on the pan, and bake another 20 minutes, or until firm and nicely browned.

Store in an airtight container. The serving size is 2 cookies.

Nutrition:
Calories: 274.17
Protein: 5g
Fat: 18g
Carbs: 27.18g
Sodium: 196.88mg

620. CHEESY TACO BITES

Preparation Time: 5 minutes
Cooking Time: 10 minutes
Servings: 12
Ingredients:
- 2 cups of packaged shredded cheddar cheese
- 2 tablespoon of chili powder
- 1 teaspoon of salt
- 2 tablespoons of cumin
- For garnishing, use pico de gallo
- 8 teaspoons of coconut cream for garnishing

Directions:
1. Preheat your oven to 350°F.
2. Place 1 tablespoon piles of cheese on a baking sheet lined with parchment paper, leaving 2 inches between each.
3. Bake for 5 minutes with the baking sheet in the oven.
4. Remove from the oven and allow the cheese to cool for 1 minute before gently lifting and pressing each into the cups of a tiny muffin tray.
5. Make careful to push the cheese's edges to make the shape of little muffins.
6. Allow the cheese to cool completely before removing it.
7. While you're baking the cheese and making your cups.
8. Fill the cheese cups halfway with coconut cream and top with Pico de Gallo.

Nutrition:
Calories:96.19
Carbohydrates:3.58g
Protein: 4.7g
Sodium: 369.58mg

621. ALMOND FLOUR CRACKERS

Preparation Time: 5 minutes
Cooking Time: 15 minutes
Servings: 8
Ingredients:
- ½ cup coconut oil, melted
- 1½ cups almond flour
- ¼ cup Stevia

Directions:

1. Heat oven to 350°F. Line a cookie sheet with parchment paper.
2. In a mixing bowl, combine all ingredients and mix well.
3. Spread dough onto prepared cookie sheet, ¼-inch thick. Use a paring knife to score into 24 crackers.
4. Bake 10-15 minutes or until golden brown.
5. Separate and store in an airtight container.

Nutrition:
Calories: 224.28
Protein: 3.89g
Fat: 23g
Carbs: 9g
Sodium: 0mg

622. CRACKERS

Preparation Time: 7 minutes
Cooking Time: 12 minutes
Servings: 15
Ingredients:
- 2 cups of blanched almond flour
- ½ teaspoon of sea salt
- 1 beaten large egg

Directions:
1. Preheat your oven to 350°F.
2. With parchment paper, line a baking sheet, then combine the almond flour and the salt in a large bowl. Crack in the egg and mix very well until you form a large ball of dough.
3. Place your dough between 2 large pieces of prepared parchment paper, then use a rolling pin to roll the dough into a rectangular shape.
4. Slice the dough into rectangles, prick with a fork, and place on a baking sheet that has been prepared and lined.
5. Bake the crackers for 8 to 12 minutes.
6. Allow the crackers to cool for 10 minutes.
7. Serve the crackers immediately or store them in a jar.

Nutrition:
Calories: 79.39
Fat: 6.7g
Protein: 3.18g
Carbs: 2.79g
Sodium: 67.83mg

623. ASIAN CHICKEN WINGS

Preparation Time: 5 minutes
Cooking Time: 30 minutes

Servings: 12
Ingredients:
- 24 chicken wings
- 6 tablespoons soy sauce
- 6 tablespoon Chinese Five Spice
- Salt & pepper
- Non-stick cooking spray

Directions:
1. Heat oven to 350°F. Spray a baking sheet with cooking spray.
2. Combine the soy sauce, Five Spice, salt, and pepper in a large bowl. Add the wings and toss to coat.
3. Pour the wings onto the prepared pan. Bake 15 minutes. Turn the chicken over and cook another 15 minutes until the chicken is cooked through.
4. Serve with your favorite low-carb dipping sauce.

Nutrition:
Calories: 232
Protein: 20.44g
Fat: 15g
Carbs: 2.76g
Sodium: 858.71mg

624. BANANA NUT COOKIES

Preparation Time: 10 minutes
Cooking Time: 15 minutes
Servings: 18
Ingredients:
- 1½ cup banana, mashed
- 2 cups oats
- 1 cup raisins
- 1 cup walnuts
- ⅓ cup sunflower oil
- 1 teaspoon vanilla
- ½ teaspoon salt

Directions:
1. Heat oven to 350°F.
2. In a large bowl, combine oats, raisins, walnuts, and salt.
3. In a medium bowl, mix banana, oil, and vanilla. Stir into oat mixture until combined. Let rest 15 minutes.
4. Drop by rounded tablespoonful onto 2 ungreased cookie sheets. Bake 15 minutes, or until a light golden brown. Cool and store in an airtight container. The serving size is 2 cookies.

Nutrition:
Calories: 199.6
Protein: 4.69g
Fat: 11.29g
Carbs: 22g
Sodium: 66.19mg

625. BLT STUFFED CUCUMBERS

Preparation Time: 15 minutes
Cooking Time: 15 minutes
 Servings: 4
Ingredients:

- 3 slices bacon, cooked crisp and crumbled
- 1 large cucumber
- ½ cup lettuce, diced fine
- ½ cup baby spinach, diced fine
- ¼ cup tomato, diced fine
- 1 tablespoon + ½ teaspoon fat-free mayonnaise
- ¼ teaspoon black pepper
- ⅛ teaspoon salt

Directions:

1. Peel the cucumber and slice it in half lengthwise. Use a spoon to remove the seeds.
2. In a medium bowl, combine the remaining ingredients and stir well.
3. Spoon the bacon mixture into the cucumber halves. Cut into 2-inch pieces and serve.

Nutrition:
Calories: 95
Protein: 6g
Carbs: 3.95g
Sodium: 233mg
Fat: 6g

626. BUFFALO BITES

Preparation Time: 6 minutes
Cooking Time: 11 minutes
 Servings: 4
Ingredients:

- 1 egg
- ½ head of cauliflower, separated into florets
- 1 cup panko breadcrumbs
- 1 cup low-fat ranch dressing
- ½ cup hot sauce
- ½ teaspoon salt
- ½ teaspoon garlic powder
- Black pepper
- Non-stick cooking spray

Directions:

1. Heat oven to 400°F. Spray a baking sheet with cooking spray.
2. Place the egg in a medium bowl and mix in the salt, pepper, and garlic. Place the panko crumbs into a small bowl.
3. Dip the florets first in the egg then into the panko crumbs. Place in a single layer on prepared pan.
4. Bake 8-10 minutes, stirring halfway through until

cauliflower is golden brown and crisp on the outside.
5. In a small bowl stir the dressing and hot sauce together. Use for dipping.

Nutrition:
Calories: 212.32
Protein: 4.5g
Fat: 10g
Carbs: 26g
Sodium: 1760mg

627. SALTED MACADAMIA KETO BOMBS

Preparation Time: 35 minutes
Cooking Time: 0 minutes
Servings: 12
Ingredients:

- 10 tablespoons of coconut oil
- 5 tablespoons of unsweetened cocoa powder
- 1 tablespoon of granulated Stevia
- 1 pinch coarse sea salt to taste
- 3 tablespoons of coarsely chopped macadamia nuts

Directions:

1. Melt the coconut oil over the stove.
2. Add in the chocolate powder and granulated Stevia.
3. Mix your ingredients and remove them from the heat.
4. Spoon the mixture into silicone candy molds until the mound is about ¾ full.
5. Refrigerate the molds for about 5 minutes.
6. Fill each silicone mold with macadamia nuts and push down; then return the molds to the refrigerator and let cool for about 30 minutes.
7. Sprinkle macadamia nuts into each well. Press down to distribute the nuts.
8. Remove the chocolates from the refrigerator after they have cooled and set; then let them sit at room temperature and sprinkle with coarse salt.
9. Serve your macadamia salted balls and enjoy!

Nutrition:
Calories: 119.18
Fat: 13g
Protein: 0.5g
Carbs: 2.59g
Sodium: 10.98mg

628. ALMOND BUTTER CINNAMON BARS

Preparation Time: 35 minutes
Cooking Time: 0 minutes

Servings: 15
Ingredients:

- ½ cup of creamed coconut, chopped into chunks
- ⅛ teaspoon of ground cinnamon

For the First Icing:

- 1 tablespoon of almond butter
- 1 tablespoon extra virgin coconut oil, non-melted

For the Second Icing:

- ½ teaspoon of ground cinnamon
- 1 tablespoon of extra virgin almond butter

Directions:

1. To begin, line a muffin pan with muffin liners.
2. Combine the coconut cream and cinnamon in a large mixing basin with both hands and well mix.
3. Fill two mini loaf pieces with the mixture after patting it into the dish.
4. Then, make the first frosting by whisking together the coconut oil and almond butter and spreading it over the creamed coconut.
5. Place the bars in the freezer for 6 minutes.
6. Meanwhile, make the second frosting by whisking together the icing almond butter and cinnamon and spreading it over the bars.
7. Place the bars in the refrigerator for 30 minutes or the freezer for 8 minutes.
8. Using a knife, cut the frozen batter into bars.
9. Serve and enjoy your delicious bars!

Nutrition:
Calories: 77.6
Fat: 8.24g
Protein: 0.81g
Carbs: 0.95g
Sodium: 2.38mg

629. PISTACHIO AND COCOA SQUARES

Preparation Time: 25 minutes
Cooking Time: 5 minutes
Servings: 13
Ingredients:

- ½ cup of finely chopped and cacao butter
- 1 cup of roasted almond butter
- 1 cup of creamy coconut butter
- 1 cup of firm coconut oil
- ½ cup of full-fat coconut milk, chilled for an overnight

- ¼ cup of ghee
- 1 tablespoon of pure vanilla extract
- 2 teaspoons of chai spice
- ¼ teaspoon of pure almond extract
- ¼ teaspoon of Himalayan salt
- ¼ cup of chopped raw pistachios shelled

Directions:
1. Grease a 9" square baking pan and line it with parchment paper, leaving a little amount hanging on both sides to help you unmold easily; put aside.
2. Reserve the cacao butter once it has melted in the oven for around 30 seconds.
3. In a large mixing bowl, combine the roasted almonds, coconut butter, coconut oil, coconut milk, ghee, vanilla extract, spice, almond extract, salt, and chopped pistachios. Mix thoroughly on low speed, then raise the speed and mix until the mixture becomes airy.
4. Pour the combined and melted cacao butter into the almond butter and continue to mix on high speed until you have an integrated batter.
5. Transfer the batter to the preheated pan, then sprinkle with the chopped pistachios.
6. Refrigerate the batter for 4 hours or overnight.
7. Cut into 36 squares before serving and enjoying!

Nutrition:
Calories: 538
Fat: 54g
Protein: 6g
Carbs: 10.43g
Sodium: 97.92mg

630. PEPPERMINT AND CHOCOLATE KETO SQUARES

Preparation Time: 10 minutes
Cooking Time: 0 minutes
Servings: 10
Ingredients:
For the Peppermint Filling:
- ½ cup of coconut butter
- 1 tablespoon of melted coconut oil
- 1 teaspoon of peppermint extract
- 2 tablespoons of Stevia

For the Chocolate Layer:
- 2 tablespoons of melted coconut oil
- 4 oz. of 100% dark chocolate

Directions:
1. In a large bowl, add all of the ingredients, including the coconut butter, melted coconut oil, peppermint extract, and stevia, and thoroughly incorporate.
2. Pour a tiny amount of the peppermint mixture into silicone muffin tins to produce a 1/3-inch-thick layer.
3. Freeze for 1 hour, then melt the dark chocolate with the coconut oil and combine.
4. Remove the cups' hard peppermint contents.
5. Pour a tiny amount of the chocolate mixture into each cup, covering the base, and then top with additional chocolate.
6. Then, using the remaining cups, repeat the process.
7. Allow the patties to cool for approximately 2 hours or until firm, then defrost for about 10 minutes.
8. Serve and enjoy your patties!

Nutrition:
Calories: 189
Fat: 16.7g
Protein: 1.4g
Carbs: 11g
Sodium: 5mg

631. GINGER PATTIES

Preparation Time: 10 minutes
Cooking Time: 0 minutes
Servings: 15
Ingredients:
- 1 cup of coconut butter, softened
- 1 cup of coconut oil, softened
- ½ cup of shredded coconut; unsweetened
- 1 teaspoon of Stevia
- 1 teaspoon of ginger powder

Directions:
1. Mix the melted coconut butter, coconut oil, Stevia, shredded coconut, and ginger powder until all of the ingredients are completely dissolved.
2. Pour the batter into the silicone molds and refrigerate for about 10 minutes.
3. Serve and enjoy your ginger patties.

Nutrition:
Calories: 271.43
Fat: 27.71g
Protein: 1.34g
Carbs: 5.65g
Sodium: 6.63mg

632. BLUEBERRY FAT BOMBS

Preparation Time: 5 minutes
Cooking Time: 0 minutes
Servings: 30
Ingredients:
- 4 oz. of soft goat's cheese
- ½ cup of fresh blueberries
- 1 cup of almond flour
- 1 teaspoon of vanilla extract
- ½ cup of pecans
- ½ teaspoon of stevia
- ¼ cup of unsweetened shredded coconut

Directions:
1. In a food processor, combine the goat cheese, fresh blueberries, almond flour, vanilla extract, pecans, stevia, and unsweetened shredded coconut and process until smooth.
2. Roll the mixture into 30 little fat bombs.
3. Pour the coconut flakes into a bowl and lightly roll each of the fat bombs into the shredded coconut
4. Serve and enjoy your delicious fat bombs!

Nutrition:
Calories: 49
Fat: 5g
Protein: 2.3g
Carbs: 1.6g
Sodium: 17.72mg

633. ALMOND "OREO" COOKIES

Preparation Time: 15 minutes
Cooking Time: 12 minutes
Servings: 25
Ingredients:
- 3 tablespoons of coconut flour
- 2¼ cups of hazelnut or almond flour
- 4 tablespoons of cocoa powder
- 1 teaspoon of baking powder
- ½ teaspoon of xanthan gum
- ¼ teaspoon of salt
- ½ cup of softened unsalted butter
- 1 large egg
- ½ cup of Stevia
- 1 teaspoon of vanilla extract

For the Cream Filling:
- 2 tablespoons of almond butter
- 4 oz of softened cream cheese
- ½ teaspoons of pure vanilla extract
- ½ cup of powdered of Swerve

Directions:
1. Preheat your oven to 350°F

2. In a large mixing bowl, combine the almond flour or hazelnut flour with the baking powder, cocoa powder, xanthan gum, Stevia, salt, egg, and vanilla extract.
3. Add the almond butter and mix again.
4. In a separate medium bowl, cream all with the Swerve and the butter until it becomes light and extremely fluffy for 2 to 3 minutes.
5. Mix in the egg and vanilla extract until everything is well mixed.
6. Mix in the previously prepared dry ingredients until thoroughly blended.
7. Roll out the obtained dough between 2 rectangular waxed paper sheets; make sure the thickness is about ⅛.
8. Place the dough on a cookie sheet that has been lined with parchment paper.
9. Continue rolling the cookie dough until it reaches the finish.
10. Bake the cookies for about 12 minutes, then set aside to cool fully before filling.

To Make the Filling:
1. Whip the cream cheese and butter together, then add the vanilla essence.
2. Gradually add in the powdered swerve.
3. Fill the "Oreo" cookies with the cream.
4. Serve and enjoy your delicious cookies!

Nutrition:
Calories: 120.5
Fat: 11.69g
Protein: 2.45g
Carbs: 9.33g
Sodium: 65.38mg

634. BROWNIE COOKIES

Preparation Time: 20 minutes
Cooking Time: 10 minutes
Servings: 11
Ingredients:
- 2 tablespoons of softened almond butter
- 1 large egg
- 1 ablespoon of Truvia
- ¼ cup of Splenda
- ⅛ teaspoon of blackstrap molasses
- 1 tablespoon of VitaFiber syrup
- 1 teaspoon of vanilla extract

- 6 tablespoons of sugar-free chocolate chips
- 1 teaspoon of almond butter
- 6 tablespoons of almond flour
- 1 tablespoon of cocoa powder
- ⅛ teaspoon of baking powder
- ⅛ teaspoon of salt
- ¼ teaspoon of xanthan gum
- ¼ cup of chopped pecans
- 1 tablespoon of sugar-free chocolate chips

Directions:
1. In a medium bowl, using hand mixer, mix all together 2 tablespoons of almond butter with the egg, the sweeteners, the VitaFiber, and the vanilla and combine for about 2 minutes.
2. Microwave the chocolate chips and 1 tablespoon almond butter in a separate medium dish for 30 seconds.
3. Mix the chocolate into the egg and butter mixture until it forms a homogeneous batter.
4. Incorporate the remaining almond flour, cocoa powder, baking powder, salt, xanthan gum, chopped nuts, and chocolate chips.
5. Place the batter in the freezer for 7 to 8 minutes to firm up before preheating the oven to 350°F.
6. Spray a large baking sheet with cooking spray and form the cookies with your hands.
7. Place the cookies on a baking sheet and lightly flatten each one with your hand or the back of an oiled spoon.
8. Bake your cookies for 8 to 10 minutes.
9. Allow the cookies to cool for about 10 minutes.
10. Serve and enjoy your delicious cookies!

Nutrition:
Calories: 112
Fat: 8.25g
Protein: 2.7g
Carbs: 11.35g
Sodium: 47.75mg

635. MACADAMIA COOKIES

Preparation Time: 20 minutes
Cooking Time: 10 minutes
Servings: 11
Ingredients:
- ½ cup coconut oil, melted
- 2 tablespoons almond butter
- 1 egg

- 1½ cup almond flour
- 2 tablespoons unsweetened cocoa powder
- ½ cup granulated erythritol sweetener
- 1 teaspoon vanilla extract
- ½ teaspoon baking soda
- ¼ cup chopped macadamia nuts
- 1 pinch of salt

Directions:
1. Begin by pre-heating your oven to 350°F.
2. In a large mixing bowl, combine the almond butter, coconut oil, almond flour, cocoa powder, Swerve, vanilla extract, baking soda, chopped macadamia nuts, and salt.
3. Set aside after thoroughly mixing your ingredients with a fork or a spoon.
4. Line a cookie sheet with parchment paper or lightly oil it.
5. Drop little 1½" balls onto the baking sheet, then gently flatten the cookies with your hands.
6. Bake your cookies for around 15 minutes, then take them from the oven and cool for about 10 minutes.
7. Serve and enjoy your cookies!

Nutrition:
Calories: 210
Fat: 20.59g
Protein: 4.8g
Carbs: 13.16g
Sodium: 26mg

636. CAULIFLOWER HUMMUS

Preparation Time: 6 minutes
Cooking Time: 15 minutes
Servings: 6
Ingredients:
- 3 cups cauliflower florets
- 3 tablespoons fresh lemon juice
- 5 cloves garlic, divided
- 5 tablespoon olive oil, divided
- 2 tablespoons water
- 1½ tablespoons tahini paste
- 1¼ teaspoons salt, divided
- Smoked paprika & extra olive oil for serving

Directions:
1. In a microwave-safe bowl, combine cauliflower, water, 2 tablespoons oil, ½ teaspoon salt, and 3 whole cloves garlic. Microwave on high for 15

minutes, or until cauliflower is soft and darkened.

2. Transfer mixture to a food processor or blender and process until almost smooth. Add tahini paste, lemon juice, remaining garlic cloves, remaining oil, and salt. Blend until almost smooth.
3. Place the hummus in a bowl and drizzle lightly with olive oil and a sprinkle or 2 of paprika. Serve with your favorite raw vegetables.

Nutrition:
Calories: 177
Protein: 2.4 g
Fat: 16.9g
Carbs: 5.67g
Sodium: 501.9mg

637. CHEESE CRISP CRACKERS

Preparation Time: 6 minutes
Cooking Time: 11 minutes
Servings: 4
Ingredients:
- 4 slices pepper jack cheese, quartered
- 4 slices colby jack cheese, quartered
- 4 slices cheddar cheese, quartered

Directions:
1. Heat oven to 400°F. Line a cooking sheet with parchment paper.
2. Place cheese in a single layer on a prepared pan and bake for 10 minutes, or until cheese gets firm.
3. Transfer to paper towel line surface to absorb excess oil. Let cool, cheese will crisp up more as it cools.
4. Store in an airtight container, or Ziploc bag. Serve with your favorite dip or salsa.

Nutrition:
Calories: 306
Protein: 17.6g
Fat: 25g
Carbs: 1.6g
Sodium: 490.35mg

638. CHEESY ONION DIP

Preparation Time: 6 minutes
Cooking Time: 5 minutes
Servings: 8
Ingredients:
- 8 oz. low-fat cream cheese, soft
- 1 cup onions, grated

- 1 cup low-fat Swiss cheese, grated
- 1 cup light mayonnaise

Directions:
1. Heat oven to broil.
2. Combine all ingredients in a small casserole dish. Microwave on high, stirring every 30 seconds until cheese is melted, and ingredients are combined.
3. Place under the broiler for 1-2 minutes until the top is nicely browned. Serve warm with vegetables for dipping.

Nutrition:
Calories: 164.5
Protein: 6.9g
Fat: 12.6g
Carbs: 3.99g
Sodium: 410mg

639. CHEESY PITA CRISPS

Preparation Time: 6 minutes
Cooking Time: 15 minutes
Servings: 8
Ingredients:
- ½ cup mozzarella cheese
- ¼ cup margarine, melted
- 4 whole wheat pita pocket halves
- 3 tablespoons reduced-fat Parmesan
- ½ teaspoon garlic powder
- ½ teaspoon onion powder
- ¼ teaspoon salt
- ¼ teaspoon pepper
- Non-stick cooking spray

Directions:
1. Heat oven to 400°F. Spray a baking sheet with cooking spray.
2. Cut each pita pocket in half. Cut each half into 2 triangles. Place, rough side up, on prepared pan.
3. In a small bowl, whisk together margarine, Parmesan, and seasonings. Spread each triangle with margarine mixture. Sprinkle mozzarella over top.
4. Bake 12-15 minutes or until golden brown.

Nutrition:
Calories: 131
Protein: 4g
Fat: 7g
Carbs: 10.52g
Sodium: 299.98mg

640. CHEESY TACO CHIPS

Preparation Time: 16 minutes
Cooking Time: 41 minutes
Servings: 6
Ingredients:
- 1 cup Mexican blend cheese, grated
- 2 large egg whites
- 1½ cups crushed pork rinds
- 1 tablespoon taco seasoning
- ¼ teaspoon salt

Directions:
1. Heat oven to 300°F. Line a large baking sheet with parchment paper.
2. In a large bowl, whisk egg whites and salt until frothy. Stir in pork rinds, cheese, and seasoning and stir until thoroughly combined.
3. Turn out onto the prepared pan. Place another sheet of parchment paper on top and roll out very thin, about 12x12 inches. Remove the top sheet of parchment paper, and using a pizza cutter, score dough in 2-inch squares, then score each square in half diagonally.
4. Bake for 20 minutes until they start to brown. Turn off the oven and let them sit inside the oven until they are firm to the touch, about 10-20 minutes.
5. Take from the oven and cool completely before breaking apart. Eat them as is or with your favorite dip.

Nutrition:
Calories: 115.4
Protein: 10g
Fat: 7.8g
Carbs: 1.7g
Sodium: 414mg

641. CHEWY GRANOLA BARS

Preparation Time: 11 minutes
Cooking Time: 35 minutes
Servings: 36
Ingredients:
- 1 egg, beaten
- ⅔ cup margarine, melted
- 3½ cups quick oats
- 1 cup almonds, chopped
- ½ cup honey
- ½ cup sunflower kernels
- ½ cup coconut, unsweetened
- ½ cup dried apples
- ½ cup dried cranberries
- ½ cup Splenda brown sugar
- 1 teaspoon vanilla
- ½ teaspoon cinnamon

- Non-stick cooking spray

Directions:
1. Heat oven to 350°F. Coat baking dish with nonstick cooking spray.
2. Spread oats and almonds on a prepared pan. Bake 12-15 minutes until toasted, stirring every few minutes.
3. In a large bowl, combine egg, margarine, honey, and vanilla. Stir in the remaining ingredients.
4. Stir in oat mixture. Press into baking sheet and bake 13-18 minutes, or until edges are light brown.
5. Cool on a wire rack. Cut into bars and store in an airtight container.

Nutrition:
Calories: 140
Protein: 2.46g
Fat: 7.9g
Carbs: 16.7g
Sodium: 36.64mg

642. CHILI LIME TORTILLA CHIPS

Preparation Time: 6 minutes
Cooking Time: 15 minutes
Servings: 10
Ingredients:
- 12 6-inch corn tortillas, cut into 8 triangles
- 3 tablespoon lime juice
- 1 teaspoon cumin
- 1 teaspoon chili powder

Directions:
1. Heat oven to 350°F.
2. Place tortilla triangles in a single layer on a large baking sheet.
3. In a small bowl stir together spices.
4. Sprinkle half the lime juice over tortillas, followed by ½ the spice mixture. Bake 7 minutes.
5. Remove from oven and turn tortillas over. Sprinkle with remaining lime juice and spices. Bake another 8 minutes or until crisp, but not brown. Serve with your favorite salsa, the serving size is 10 chips.

Nutrition:
Calories: 81
Protein: 2g
Fat: 1g
Carbs: 16.22g
Sodium: 18mg

643. CHOCOLATE CHIP BLONDIES

Preparation Time: 6 minutes
Cooking Time: 21 minutes
Servings: 12
Ingredients:
- 1 egg
- ½ cup semi-sweet chocolate chips
- ⅓ cup flour
- ⅓ cup whole wheat flour
- ¼ cup Splenda brown sugar
- ¼ cup sunflower oil
- 2 tablespoons honey
- 1 teaspoon vanilla
- ½ teaspoon baking powder
- ¼ teaspoon salt
- Non-stick cooking spray

Directions:
1. Heat oven to 350°F. Coat an 8-inch square baking dish with non-stick cooking spray.
2. In a small bowl, combine dry ingredients.
3. In a large bowl, whisk together egg, oil, honey, and vanilla. Stir in dry ingredients just until combined. Stir in chocolate chips.
4. Spread batter in prepared dish. Bake 20-22 minutes or until they pass the toothpick test. Cool on a wire rack then cut into bars.

Nutrition:
Calories: 136
Protein: 2g
Fat: 6g
Carbs: 16.7g
Sodium: 76.47mg

644. CINNAMON APPLE CHIPS

Preparation Time: 6 minutes
Cooking Time: 11 minutes
Servings: 2
Ingredients:
- 1 medium apple, sliced thin
- ¼ teaspoon cinnamon
- ¼ teaspoon nutmeg
- Nonstick cooking spray

Directions:
1. Heat oven to 375°F. Spray a baking sheet with cooking spray.
2. Place apples in a mixing bowl and add spices. Toss to coat.
3. Arrange apples, in a single layer, on the prepared pan. Bake 4 minutes, turn apples over, and bake 4 minutes more.
4. Serve immediately or store in an airtight container.

Nutrition:

Calories: 70
Protein: 0.2g
Fat: 3g
Carbs: 11.41g
Sodium: 2.22mg

645. CINNAMON APPLE POPCORN

Preparation Time: 31 minutes
Cooking Time: 50 minutes
Servings: 11
Ingredients:
- 4 tablespoons margarine, melted
- 10 cup plain popcorn
- 2 cups dried apple rings, unsweetened and chopped
- ½ cup walnuts, chopped
- 2 tablespoons Splenda brown sugar
- 1 teaspoon cinnamon
- ½ teaspoon vanilla

Directions:
1. Heat oven to 250°F.
2. Place chopped apples in a 9x13" baking dish and bake for 20 minutes. Remove from oven and stir in popcorn and nuts.
3. In a small bowl, whisk together margarine, vanilla, Splenda, and cinnamon. Drizzle evenly over popcorn and toss to coat.
4. Bake 30 minutes, stirring quickly every 10 minutes. If apples start to turn a dark brown, remove immediately.
5. Pour onto waxed paper to cool for at least 30 minutes. Store in an airtight container.

Nutrition:
Calories: 171
Protein: 1.7g
Fat: 9.9g
Carbs: 22g
Sodium: 122mg

646. CRAB & SPINACH DIP

Preparation Time: 9 minutes
Cooking Time: 2 hours
Servings: 10
Ingredients:
- 1 pkg. frozen chopped spinach, squeezed nearly dry and thawed
- 8 oz. reduced-fat cream cheese
- 6½ oz. can crab meat, drained and shredded
- 6-oz. jar marinated artichoke hearts, drained and diced fine
- ¼ teaspoon hot pepper sauce
- Melba toast or whole grain crackers (optional)

Directions:

1. Remove any shells or cartilage from the crab.
2. Place all ingredients in a small crockpot. Cover and cook on high 1½-2 hours, or until heated through and cream cheese is melted. Stir after 1 hour.
3. Serve with Melba toast or whole-grain crackers. The serving size is ¼ cup.

Nutrition:
Calories: 81
Protein: 5g
Fat: 4.9g
Carbs: 3g
Sodium: 337mg

647. CRANBERRY & ALMOND GRANOLA BARS

Preparation Time: 14 minutes
Cooking Time: 21 minutes
Servings: 12
Ingredients:
- 1 egg
- 1 egg white
- 2 cups low-fat granola
- ¼ cup dried cranberries, sweetened
- ¼ cup almonds, chopped
- 2 tablespoons Splenda
- 1 teaspoon almond extract
- ½ teaspoon cinnamon

Directions:
1. Heat oven to 350°F. Line the bottom and sides of an 8-inch baking dish with parchment paper.
2. In a large bowl, combine dry Ingredients including the cranberries.
3. In a small bowl, whisk together egg, egg white, and extract. Pour over dry ingredients and mix until combined.
4. Press mixture into the prepared pan. Bake 20 minutes or until light brown.
5. Cool in the pan for 5 minutes. Then carefully lift the bars from the pan onto a cutting board. Use a sharp knife to cut into 12 bars. Cool completely and store in an airtight container.

Nutrition:
Calories: 113.29
Protein: 3g
Fat: 3g
Carbs: 20g
Sodium: 16mg

648. PISTACHIO MUFFINS

Preparation Time: 10 minutes
Cooking Time: 30 minutes
Servings: 12

Ingredients:
- ½ cup of almond butter, unsalted
- 4 large eggs, better to use brown eggs
- ¼ cup of confectioners Swerve
- 1 teaspoon of pistachio extract
- ¼ cup of organic Stevia blend by Pyure
- ½ cup of almond milk, unsweetened
- 1 teaspoon of vanilla extract
- ½ cup of organic coconut flour
- 1 cup of blanched almond flour
- 2 teaspoons of baking powder
- ½ teaspoon of xanthan gum
- ½ cup of crushed pistachio nuts
- 1 teaspoon of Himalayan pink salt

Directions:
1. Preheat the oven to about 325°F.
2. Using a large mixing bowl, beat the eggs thoroughly.
3. Melt the almond butter in a separate dish until it is soft.
4. Combine the butter, sugars, extracts, and almond milk in a mixing bowl.
5. Blend your components until they are completely combined.
6. Mix in the pistachio extract, vanilla extract, almond flour, coconut flour, baking powder, xanthan gum, and salt.
7. Whisk the items together until well combined.
8. In a large mixing bowl, combine all of the dry ingredients and well combine.
9. Fold in the crushed pistachios until well combined.
10. Grease a muffin tray with 12 cup liners.
11. Pour the batter into each muffin cup in an even layer.
12. Bake for 25 to 30 minutes, depending on the size of the muffins.
13. Allow your muffins to cool for 5 minutes.
14. Serve your muffins and enjoy!

Nutrition:
Calories: 189
Fat: 15g
Protein: 7.8g
Carbs: 15g
Sodium: 310mg

649. TACO CHEESE BITES

Preparation Time: 5 minutes
Cooking Time: 10minutes
Servings: 12
Ingredients:
- 2 Cups of packaged shredded cheddar cheese
- 2 tablespoons of cumin
- 2 tablespoon of chili powder
- 1 teaspoon of salt
- 8 teaspoons of coconut cream for garnishing
- For garnishing use pico de gallo

Directions:
1. Preheat your oven to 350°F.
2. Place 1 tablespoon piles of cheese on a baking sheet lined with parchment paper, leaving 2 inches between each.
3. Bake for 5 minutes with the baking sheet in the oven.
4. Remove from the oven and allow the cheese to cool for 1 minute before gently lifting and pressing each into the cups of a muffin tray.
5. Be careful to push the cheese's edges to make the shape of little muffins.
6. Allow the cheese to cool completely before removing it.
7. Fill the cheese cups with coconut cream, then top with the pico de gallo.
8. Serve and enjoy your delicious snack!

Nutrition:
Calories: 96
Fat: 7.25g
Protein: 4.7g
Carbs: 3.58g
Sodium:369mg

650. GARLIC KALE CHIPS

Preparation Time: 5 minutes
Cooking Time: 15 minutes
Servings: 2
Ingredients:
- 1 16-oz. bunch kale, trimmed and cut into 2-inch pieces
- 2 tablespoons extra-virgin olive oil
- 1 teaspoon sea salt
- ½ teaspoon garlic powder
- Pinch cayenne (optional, to taste)

Directions:
1. Preheat the oven to 350°F. Line 2 baking sheets with parchment paper.

2. Wash the kale and pat it completely dry.
3. In a large bowl, toss the kale with the olive oil, sea salt, garlic powder, and cayenne, if using.
4. Spread the kale in a single layer on the prepared baking sheets.
5. Bake until crisp, 12 to 15 minutes, rotating the sheets once.

Nutrition:
Calories: 211
Fat: 15g
Protein: 7g
Carbs: 15g
Sodium: 1011mg

651. CAPRESE SKEWERS

Preparation Time: 5 minutes
Cooking Time: 0 minutes
Servings: 6
Ingredients:
- 12 cherry tomatoes
- 12 basil leaves
- 8 1-inch pieces mozzarella cheese
- ¼ cup Italian vinaigrette (optional, for serving)

Directions:
1. On each of the 4 wooden skewers, thread the following: 1 tomato, 1 basil leaf, 1 piece of cheese, 1 tomato, 1 basil leaf, 1 piece of cheese, 1 basil leaf, 1 tomato.
2. Serve with the vinaigrette, if desired, for dipping.

Nutrition:
Calories: 506.69
Fat: 37g
Protein: 37g
Carbs: 5g
Sodium: 1046mg

652. TURKEY ROLL-UPS WITH VEGGIE CREAM CHEESE

Preparation Time: 10 minutes
Cooking Time: 0 minutes
Servings: 2
Ingredients:
- ¼ cup cream cheese, at room temperature
- 2 tablespoons finely chopped red onion
- 2 tablespoons finely chopped red bell pepper
- 1 tablespoon chopped fresh chives
- 1 teaspoon Dijon mustard
- 1 garlic clove, minced

- ¼ teaspoon sea salt
- 6 slices deli turkey

Directions:
1. The cream cheese, red onion, bell pepper, chives, mustard, garlic, and salt are mixed in a small bowl.
2. Spread the mixture on the turkey slices and roll up.

Nutrition:
Calories: 204.5
Fat: 16.38g
Protein: 14.45g
Carbs: 6.41g
Sodium: 1100mg

653. BAKED PARMESAN CRISPS

Preparation Time: 5 minutes
Cooking Time: 5 minutes
Servings: 2
Ingredients:
- 1 cup grated Parmesan cheese

Directions:
1. Preheat the oven to 400°F. A rimmed baking sheet is lined with parchment paper.
2. Spread the Parmesan on the prepared baking sheet into 4 mounds, spreading each mound out so it is flat but not touching the others.
3. Bake until brown and crisp, 3 to 5 minutes.
4. Cool for 5 minutes. Use a spatula to remove to a plate to continue cooling.

Nutrition:
Calories: 156
Fat: 9.9g
Protein: 14.29g
Carbs: 1.29g
Sodium: 469mg

654. GARLICKY HUMMUS

Preparation Time: 5 minutes
Cooking Time: 10 minutes
Servings: 2
Ingredients:
- 1½ cups canned chickpeas, rinsed and drained
- ¼ cup tahini
- 2 teaspoons minced garlic
- 1 teaspoon ground cumin
- ½ teaspoon ground coriander
- ¼ cup freshly squeezed lemon juice
- 2 tablespoons olive oil
- Sea salt

Directions:

1. Put the chickpeas, tahini, garlic, cumin, coriander, and lemon juice in a food processor, and blend until smooth, scraping down the sides of the processor at least once.
2. Incorporate the olive oil and process until blended. Season with sea salt.
3. Store the hummus in a sealed container in the refrigerator for up to 1 week.

Nutrition:
Calories: 530
Protein: 16g
Fat: 38g
Carbs: 39g
Sodium: 628mg

655. PESTO VEGGIE PIZZA

Preparation Time: 20 minutes
Cooking Time: 15 minutes
Servings: 2
Ingredients:
- Olive oil, for greasing the parchment paper
- ¼ head cauliflower, cut into florets
- 3 tablespoons almond flour
- ½ teaspoons olive oil
- 1 egg, beaten
- Minced garlic
- Pinch sea salt
- ¼ cup simple tomato sauce
- ¼ zucchini, thinly sliced
- ¼ cup baby spinach leaves
- 2½ asparagus spears, woody ends trimmed, cut into 3-inch pieces
- Basil pesto

Directions:
1. Preheat the oven to 450°F. Put a baking sheet without a rim in the oven.
2. Prepare a piece of parchment paper by lightly brushing with olive oil and set aside.
3. Put a large saucepan filled halfway with water over high heat and bring it to a boil.
4. Put the cauliflower in a food processor, and pulse until very finely chopped, almost flour consistency.
5. Transfer the ground cauliflower to a fine-mesh sieve and put it over the boiling water for about 1 minute, until the cauliflower is cooked.
6. Wring out all the water from the cauliflower using a kitchen towel. Transfer the cauliflower to a large bowl.

7. Stir in the almond flour, oil, egg, garlic, and salt, and mix to create a thick dough. Use your hands to press the ingredients together and transfer the cauliflower mixture to the parchment paper.
8. Press the mixture out into a flat circle, about ½ inch thick. Slide the parchment paper onto the baking sheet in the oven.
9. Bake the crust for about 10 minutes, until it is crisp and turns golden brown.
10. Remove the crust from the oven and spread the sauce evenly to the edges of the crust.
11. Arrange the zucchini, spinach, and asparagus on the pizza.
12. Drizzle the pizza with basil pesto and put it back in the oven for about 2 minutes, until the vegetables are tender. Serve.

Nutrition:
Calories: 242
Protein: 7.58g
Fat: 20.7g
Carbs: 8.8g
Sodium: 283mg

656. APPLE LEATHER

Preparation Time: 10 minutes
Cooking Time: 8 to 10 hours
Servings: 24 strips
Ingredients:
- 5 apples, peeled, cored, and sliced
- ¼ cup water
- 1 teaspoon pure vanilla extract
- ¼ teaspoon ground ginger
- ¼ teaspoon ground cloves

Directions:
1. Put the apples, water, vanilla, ginger, and cloves in a large saucepan over medium heat.
2. Bring the mixture to a boil, reduce to low heat, and simmer for about 20 minutes, until the apples are very tender.
3. Transfer the apple mixture to a food processor, and purée until very smooth.
4. Set the oven on the lowest possible setting.
5. Line a baking sheet with parchment paper.
6. Pour the puréed apple mixture onto the baking sheet and spread it out very thinly and evenly.
7. Place the baking sheet in the oven, and bake for 8 to 10

hours, until the leather is smooth and no longer sticky.
8. Cut the apple leather with a pizza cutter into 24 strips, and store this treat in a sealed container in a cool, dark place for up to 2 weeks.

Nutrition:
Calories: 41
Protein: 0.1g
Fat: 0.3g
Carbs: 4.3g
Sodium: 0.13mg

657. SIMPLE APPETIZER MEATBALLS

Preparation Time: 25 minutes
Cooking Time: 25 minutes
Servings: 24 pieces
Ingredients:
- ½ pound lean ground beef
- ½ pound lean ground pork
- ½ cup sodium-free chicken broth
- ¼ cup almond flour
- 1 tablespoon low-sodium tamari sauce
- ½ teaspoon ground cumin
- ¼ teaspoon freshly ground black pepper

Directions:
1. Preheat the oven to 375°F.
2. Combine all the ingredients together until completely incorporated in a large bowl.
3. Roll the mixture into ¾-inch balls and place them on a parchment-lined baking sheet.
4. Bake the meatballs for 25 to 30 minutes, until they are cooked through and golden brown.
5. Serve.

Nutrition:
Calories: 45
Protein: 4g
Fat: 3g
Carbs: 0.34g
Sodium: 45mg

658. FRENCH BREAD PIZZA

Preparation Time: 5 minutes
Cooking Time: 2-3 hours
Servings: 2
Ingredients:
- ½ cup asparagus (diced)
- ½ cup Roma tomatoes (diced)
- ½ cup red bell pepper (diced)
- ½ tablespoon minced garlic
- ½ loaf French bread
- ½ cup pizza sauce
- ½ cup low-fat shredded mozzarella cheese

Directions:
1. Heat the oven to 400°F. Coat the baking sheet lightly with a cooking spray.
2. Add the asparagus, tomatoes, and pepper to a little dish. Add the garlic and stir gently to coat uniformly.
3. Adjust the French bread to the baking sheet. Apply ¼ cup of the pizza sauce and ¼ of the vegetable paste to each portion of the mixture. Sprinkle with ¼ cup of mozzarella cheese.
4. Bake until the cheese is finely browned, and the vegetables are tender for 8 to 10 minutes. Serve straight away.

Nutrition:
Calories: 421.61
Fat: 8.48g
Protein: 20.9g
Carbs: 68g
Sodium: 920mg

659. BEAN SALAD WITH BALSAMIC VINAIGRETTE

Preparation Time: 5 minutes
Cooking Time: 0 hours
Servings: 2
Ingredients:
For the Vinaigrette:
- 2 tablespoons balsamic vinegar
- ⅓ cup fresh parsley, chopped
- 4 garlic cloves, finely chopped
- Ground black pepper, to taste
- ¼ cup extra-virgin olive oil
For the Salad:
- ⅓ can 15 oz. low-sodium garbanzo beans, rinsed and drained
- ⅓ can 15 oz. low-sodium black beans, rinsed and drained
- 1 small red onion, diced
- 2 lettuce leaves
- Celery, finely chopped

Directions:
1. In a small pan, mix the balsamic vinegar, parsley, garlic, and pepper to prepare the vinaigrette. Slowly add the olive oil when whisking.
2. In a large pan, combine the beans and the onion.
3. Pour the vinaigrette over the mixture and stir softly, blend thoroughly and coat equally. Cover and refrigerate until ready to serve.
4. Put one lettuce leaf on each plate to serve. Divide the salad between the individual plates

and garnish with the minced celery. Serve straight away.

Nutrition:
Calories: 436
Fat: 30.29g
Protein: 11.9g
Carbs: 33.2g
Sodium: 225mg

660. EASY CAULIFLOWER HUSH PUPPIES

Preparation Time: 15 minutes
Cooking Time: 10 minutes
Servings: 8 hush puppies
Ingredients:
- 1 whole cauliflower, including stalks and florets, roughly chopped
- ¾ cup buttermilk
- ¾ cup low-fat milk
- 1 medium onion, chopped
- 2 medium eggs
- 2 cups yellow cornmeal
- 1½ teaspoons baking powder
- ½ teaspoon salt

Directions:
1. In a blender, combine the cauliflower, buttermilk, milk, and onion, and purée. Transfer to a large mixing bowl.
2. Crack the eggs into the purée, and gently fold until mixed.
3. In a medium bowl, whisk the cornmeal, baking powder, and salt together.
4. Gently add the dry ingredients to the wet ingredients and mix until just combined, taking care not to overmix.
5. Working in batches, place ⅓-cup portions of the batter into the basket of an air fryer.
6. Set the air fryer to 390°F (199°C), close, and cook for 10 minutes. Transfer the hush puppies to a plate. Repeat until no batter remains.
7. Serve warm with greens.

Nutrition:
Calories: 196.8
Fat: 2.87g
Protein: 5.77g
Carbs: 36.6g
Sodium: 296mg

661. KETO CHOCOLATE BOMBS

Preparation Time: 30 minutes
Cooking Time: 0 minutes
Servings: 12
Ingredients:
- 2 cups of smooth peanut butter
- ¾ cup coconut of flour
- ½ cup of sticky sweetener

- 2 cups of sugar-free chocolate chips

Directions:
1. Start by lining a large tray with parchment paper and setting it aside.
2. In a large mixing basin, add all of the ingredients except the chocolate chips, and mix thoroughly until everything is mixed.
3. If your mixture is excessively thick or crumbly, add a tiny amount of milk or water.
4. Form tiny balls of batter with both hands and place them on the already prepared lined tray. Freeze for about 10 minutes.
5. While the peanut butter balls are chilling, melt the sugar-free chocolate chips in the microwave for 30 seconds to 1 minute.
6. Remove the peanut butter from the freezer, and then dip each of the balls into the melted chocolate, one at a time.
7. Repeat until all of the chocolate balls are coated in chocolate and put on a dish.
8. After you've finished coating all of the balls, store them in the refrigerated for approximately 20 minutes, or until the chocolate has firmed up.
9. Enjoy your delectable chocolate balls!

Nutrition:
Calories: 443.94
Fat: 33.5g
Protein: 12.2g
Carbs: 37.25g
Sodium: 188.15mg

662. COCONUT KETO BOMBS

Preparation Time: 15 minutes
Cooking Time: 0 minutes
Servings: 14
Ingredients:
- ½ cup of shredded coconut
- 1½ cups of walnuts or any type of nuts of your choice
- ¼ cup coconut butter + 1 tablespoon extra coconut butter
- 2 tablespoons of chia seeds
- 2 tablespoons of almond butter
- 2 tablespoons of flax meal
- 1 teaspoon of cinnamon
- 2 tablespoons of hemp seeds
- ½ teaspoon of vanilla bean powder
- ¼ teaspoon of kosher salt

- 2 tablespoons of cacao nibs

For the Chocolate Drizzle:
- 1 oz. of unsweetened chocolate, chopped
- ½ teaspoon of coconut oil

Directions:
1. In a food processor, blend the walnuts, coconut butter, almond butter, chia seeds, flax meal, hemp seeds, cinnamon, vanilla bean powder, shredded coconut, and diced; then drizzle with coconut oil.
2. Pulse your ingredients for 1-2 minutes, or until the mixture begins to break down.
3. Continue to process the mixture until it begins to stay together, but be cautious not to overmix.
4. Add the cacao nibs and pulse until the ingredients are combined.
5. Divide the mixture into equal-sized pieces using a tiny cookie scoop or a tablespoon.
6. Use both your hands to roll the mixture into balls; then arrange it over a platter.
7. Place the balls in an airtight container or freeze them for about 15 minutes.
8. Serve and enjoy your delicious balls!

Nutrition:
Calories: 238
Fat: 22g
Protein: 5.17g
Carbs: 8g
Sodium: 43.6mg

663. RASPBERRY AND CASHEW BALLS

Preparation Time: 15 minutes
Cooking Time: 0 minutes
Servings: 14
Ingredients:
- ¼ cup of cashew or almond butter
- 1⅓ cup of raw cashews or almonds
- 2 tablespoons of coconut oil
- ½ teaspoon of vanilla extract
- 2 pitted Medjool dates, pre-soaked into hot water for about 10 minutes
- ¼ teaspoon of kosher salt
- ⅓ cup of chopped dark chocolate
- ½ cup of freeze-dried and lightly crushed raspberries

Directions:
1. In a high-powered blender or Vitamix, add the cashews or

almonds, butter, coconut oil, Medjool dates, vanilla essence, and salt and process for 1 to 2 minutes, or until the batter begins to stick together.

2. Pulse in the dried raspberries and dark chocolate until you get a thick mixture.
3. Divide the mixture into equal-sized balls using a tablespoon or a tiny cookie scoop.
4. Refrigerate the balls in a container or zip-top bag for around 2 weeks, or just serve and enjoy your wonderful cashew balls!

Nutrition:
Calories: 155.51
Fat: 11.89g
Protein: 3.17g
Carbs: 10.86g
Sodium: 36.51mg

664. COCOA BALLS

Preparation Time: 90 minutes
Cooking Time: 0 minutes
Servings: 9
Ingredients:

- 1 cup of coconut oil, at room temperature
- 1 cup of almond butter
- ½ cup of unsweetened cocoa powder
- ⅓ cup of coconut flour
- ¼ teaspoon of powdered Stevia
- 1/16 teaspoon of pink Himalayan salt

Directions:
1. In a small pot and over medium-high heat, melt the almond butter and combine it with the coconut oil.
2. After adding stir in the coconut flour, cocoa powder, and Himalayan salt.
3. Mix in the stevia, then set aside to chill.
4. Pour the mixture into a large bowl and transfer it to the freezer to solidify for about 60 to 90 minutes.
5. Removing the bowl from the freezer when it has frozen allows you to roll it into balls.
6. Form the batter into balls and place them on a pan lined with parchment paper.
7. Refrigerate the balls for about 15 minutes.
8. Serve and enjoy!

Nutrition:
Calories: 411
Fat: 40.64g
Protein: 7.28g

Carbs: 10.48g
Sodium: 83mg

665. BALANCED TURKEY MEATBALLS

Preparation Time: 12 minutes
Cooking Time: 26 minutes
Servings: 8
Ingredients:

- 20 oz. ground of turkey
- 3½ oz. of fresh or frozen spinach
- ¼ cup of oats
- 2 egg whites
- Celery sticks
- 3 cloves garlic
- ½ green bell peppers
- ½ red onion
- ½ cup parsley
- ½ teaspoon cumin
- 1 teaspoon mustard powder
- 1 teaspoon thyme
- ½ teaspoon turmeric
- ½ teaspoon chipotle pepper
- 1 teaspoon salt
- A pinch of pepper

Directions:
1. First preheat the oven to 350°F (175°C).
2. Chop the onion, garlic, and celery very finely (or use a food processor) and add to a large mixing cup.
3. In the dish, add the ham, egg whites, oats, and spices and combine well. Make sure the mix contains no pockets of spices or oats.
4. Spinach, green peppers (stalked and seeded), and parsley are chopped. The bits need to be about a dime 's size.
5. To a large mixing bowl, add the vegetables and mix them until well-combined.
6. Line the parchment paper with a baking sheet.
7. Roll the turkey mixture into 15 balls (about the size of golf balls) and put them on the baking sheet.
8. Bake for 25 minutes, until fully baked.

Nutrition:
Calories: 187.17
Fat: 13.25g
Carbohydrate: 6.14g
Sodium: 370mg

666. CURRIED CHICKEN WITH APPLES

Preparation Time: 12 minutes
Cooking Time: 13 minutes

Servings: 3
Ingredients:

- 1 lbs of cooked, diced chicken breast
- 1 granny Smith diced apple
- 2 celery stalks, (diced)
- 2 green onions, (diced)
- ½ cup of sliced cashew
- 1 cup of plain Greek yogurt
- 1 tablespoon of tahini
- 4 teaspoon of curry powder
- 1 teaspoon of ground cinnamon

Directions:
1. In a big mixing cup, add the milk, tahini, curry powder, and cinnamon.
2. Add the chicken, apple, celery, cashews, and green onions. Stir to blend.
3. To offer it ever something of a tropical feel, this salad can be eaten on its own, as a snack, or in a hollowed-out papaya.

Nutrition:
Calories: 486.87
Fat: 22.84g
Carbohydrate: 22.8g
Sodium: 128mg

667. HOMEMADE CHICKEN NUGGETS

Preparation Time: 15 minutes
Cooking Time: 23 minutes
Servings: 2
Ingredients:

- ½ cup almond flour
- 1 tablespoon of Italian seasoning
- 2 tablespoons of extra-virgin olive oil
- ½ teaspoon of salt
- ½ teaspoon of pepper

Directions:
1. Preheat the furnace to 200°C (400°F). Use parchment paper to arrange a large baking dish.
2. Whisk the Italian seasoning, almond flour, pepper, and salt together in a dish.
3. Start cutting and remove any fat from the chicken breasts, after which slice into 1-inch-thick bits.
4. Sprinkle the extra virgin olive oil to the chicken.
5. Place each chicken piece in the flour bowl and toss until thoroughly covered, then move the chicken to the baking sheet that has been prepared.
6. For 20 minutes, roast.
7. To get exterior crispy, toggle the broiler on and put the

chicken nuggets underneath the broiler for 3-4 minutes.

Nutrition:
Calories: 267.33
Fat: 26.36g
Carbohydrate: 5.56g
Sodium: 581.77mg

668. TORTILLAS IN GREEN MANGO SALSA

Preparation Time: 30 minutes
Cooking Time: 10 minutes
Servings: 4
Ingredients:
For the Tortillas:
- 4 corn tortillas
- 1 tablespoon of olive oil
- 1/16 teaspoon of sea salt

For the Green Mango Salsa:
- 1 green/unripe mango, minced
- 1 red/ripe Roma tomato, preferably minced
- 1 shallot, peeled, minced
- 1 fresh jalapeño pepper, minced
- ¼ red bell pepper, minced
- 4 tablespoons of fresh cilantro, minced
- ¼ cup of lime juice, freshly squeezed
- 1/16 teaspoon of salt

Directions:
1. Preheat the air fryer to 400°F.
2. Mix lime juice and salt in a bowl. Stir until solids dissolve. Add in the remaining salsa ingredients. Chill in the fridge for at least 30 minutes. Stir again just before using.
3. Lightly brush oil on both sides of tortillas. Cut these into large triangles.
4. Place a generous handful of sliced tortillas in the Air Fryer basket. Fry these for 10 minutes or until bread blisters and turns golden brown. Shake contents of the basket once midway through.
5. Place cooked pieces on a plate. Repeat step for remaining tortillas. Season with salt.
6. Place equal portions of crispy tortillas on plates. Serve with green mango and tomato salsa on the side.

Nutrition:
Calories: 128

Carbohydrates: 8.6g
Fat: 3.6g
Sodium: 117mg
Protein: 2.7g
Fiber: 5.7g

669. SKINNY PUMPKIN CHIPS

Preparation Time: 20 minutes
Cooking Time: 10 minutes
Servings: 2
Ingredients:
- 1 pound pumpkin, cut into sticks
- 1 tablespoon coconut oil
- ½ teaspoon rosemary
- ½ teaspoon basil
- Salt and ground black pepper, to taste

Directions:
1. Start by preheating the air fryer to 395°F. Brush the pumpkin sticks with coconut oil; add the spices and toss to combine.
2. Cook for 13 minutes, shaking the basket halfway through the cooking time.
3. Serve with mayonnaise. Bon appétit!

Nutrition:
Calories: 100
Fat: 6.9g
Carbohydrates: 10g
Protein: 1.56g
Sugars: 4.13g
Sodium: 389.23mg

670. GARLIC BREAD WITH CHEESE DIP

Preparation Time: 10 minutes
Cooking Time: 10 minutes
Servings: 8
Ingredients:
Fried garlic bread
- 1 medium baguette, halved lengthwise, cut sides toasted
- 2 garlic cloves, whole
- 4 tablespoons of extra-virgin olive oil
- 2 tablespoons of fresh parsley, minced

For the Blue Cheese Dip:
- 1 tablespoon of fresh parsley, minced
- ¼ cup of fresh chives, minced
- ¼ teaspoon of Tabasco sauce
- 1 tablespoon of lemon juice, freshly squeezed
- ½ cup of Greek yogurt, low-fat
- ¼ cup of bleu cheese, reduced-fat
- 1/16 teaspoon of salt

- 1/16 teaspoon of white pepper

Directions:
1. Preheat machine to 400°F.
2. Mix oil and parsley in a small bowl.
3. Vigorously rub garlic cloves on cut/toasted sides of the baguette. Dispose of garlic nubs.
4. Using a pastry brush, spread parsley-infused oil on the cut side of the bread.
5. Place the bread cut side down on a chopping board. Slice into inch-thick half-moons.
6. Place bread slices in an air fryer basket. Fry for 3-5 minutes or until bread browns a little. Shake contents of the basket once midway through. Place cooked pieces on a serving platter. Repeat the step for the remaining bread.
7. To prepare blue cheese dip: mix all the ingredients in a bowl.
8. Place equal portions of fried bread on plates. On the side, serve bleu cheese dip.

Nutrition:
Calories: 174
Carbohydrates: 17.4g
Fat: 9g
Protein: 5.38g
Fiber: 1.12g
Sodium: 237mg

671. FRIED MIXED VEGGIES WITH AVOCADO DIP

Preparation Time: 10 minutes
Cooking Time: 10 minutes
Servings: 4
Ingredients:
- Cooking spray

Avocado-feta dip:
- 1 avocado, pitted, peeled, flesh scooped out
- 4 oz. of feta cheese, reduced fat
- 2 leeks, minced
- 1 lime, freshly squeezed
- ¼ cup of fresh parsley, chopped roughly
- 1/16 teaspoon of black pepper
- 1/16 teaspoon of salt

Vegetables:
- 1 zucchini, sliced into matchsticks
- 1 carrot, sliced into matchsticks
- 1 cup of panko breadcrumbs. Add more if needed
- 1 parsnip, sliced into matchsticks

- 1 large egg, whisked, add more if needed
- 1 cup of almond flour, add more if needed
- ⅛ teaspoon flaky sea salt

Directions:
1. Preheat the Air Fryer to 400°F.
2. Season carrots, parsnips, and zucchini with salt.
3. Dredge carrots with flour first, then dip them into the whisked egg, and finally into breadcrumbs. Place breaded pieces on a baking sheet lined with parchment paper. Repeat the step for all carrots. Then do the same for parsnips and zucchini.
4. Lightly spray vegetables with oil. Place a generous handful of carrots in the air fryer basket. Fry for 10 minutes or until breading turns golden brown, shaking contents of the basket once midway. Place cooked pieces on a plate. Repeat the step for the remaining carrots.
5. Do the previous step for parsnips and then zucchini.
6. For the dip, except for salt, place the remaining ingredients in a food processor. Pulse a couple of times, and then process to desired consistency scraping down sides of the machine often. Taste. Add salt only if needed. Place in an airtight container. Chill until needed.
7. Place equal portions of cooked vegetables on plates. Serve with a small amount of avocado-feta dip on the side.

Nutrition:
Calories: 375
Carbohydrates: 30g
Fat: 22.6g
Protein: 16g
Fiber: 9g
Sodium: 562mg

672. AIR-FRIED PLANTAINS IN COCONUT SAUCE

Preparation Time: 10 minutes
Cooking Time: 10 minutes
Servings: 8
Ingredients:
- 6 ripe plantains, peeled, quartered lengthwise
- 1 can of coconut cream
- 1 tablespoon of Splenda

Directions:
1. Preheat the air fryer to 330°F.

2. Pour coconut cream in a thick-bottomed saucepan set over high heat; bring to boil. Reduce heat to lowest setting; simmer uncovered until the cream is reduced by half and darkens in color. Turn off heat.
3. Whisk in honey until smooth. Cool completely before using. Lightly grease a non-stick skillet with coconut oil.
4. Layer plantains in the air fryer basket and fry until golden on both sides; drain on paper towels. Place plantain into plates.
5. Drizzle in a small amount of coconut sauce. Serve.

Nutrition:
Calories: 348
Fat: 8.65g
Protein: 2.3g
Fiber: 3.19g
Carbs: 70.8g
Sodium: 23.37mg

673. KALE CHIPS WITH LEMON YOGURT SAUCE

Preparation Time: 10 minutes
Cooking Time: 5 minutes
Servings: 4
Ingredients:
- 1 cup of plain Greek yogurt
- 3 tablespoons of freshly squeezed lemon juice
- 2 tablespoons of honey mustard
- ½ teaspoon of dried oregano
- 1 bunch of curly kale
- 2 tablespoons of olive oil
- ½ teaspoon of salt
- ⅛ teaspoon of pepper

Directions:
1. In a small bowl, mix the yogurt, lemon juice, honey mustard, and oregano, and set aside.
2. Remove the stems and ribs from the kale with a sharp knife. Cut the leaves into 2- to 3-inch pieces.
3. Toss the kale with olive oil, salt, and pepper. Rub the oil into the leaves with your hands.
4. Air fry the kale in batches at 390°F (199°C) until crisp, about 5 minutes, shaking the basket once during cooking time. Serve with the yogurt sauce.

Nutrition:

Calories: 155
Fat: 8g
Protein: 8g
Carbohydrates: 13g
Fiber: 1g
Sugar: 3g
Sodium: 378mg

674. CINNAMON PEAR CHIPS

Preparation Time: 15 minutes
Cooking Time: 9-13 minutes
Servings: 4
Ingredients:
- 2 firm Bosc pears, cut crosswise into ⅛ inch-thick slices
- 1 tablespoon of freshly squeezed lemon juice
- ½ teaspoon of ground cinnamon
- ⅛ teaspoon of ground cardamom or ground nutmeg

Directions:
1. Separate the smaller stem-end pear rounds from the bigger seeded rounds. Take the core and seeds out of the bigger chunks. Sprinkle lemon juice, cinnamon, and cardamom over all slices.
2. Place the smaller chips in the basket of the air fryer. Air fry at 380ºF (193ºC) for 3 to 5 minutes, until light golden brown, shaking the basket once during cooking. Remove from the air fryer.
3. Repeat with the bigger pieces, air frying for 6 to 8 minutes each time., until light golden brown, shaking the basket once during cooking.
4. Remove the chips from the air fryer. Cool completely before serving, or keep in an airtight jar at room temperature for up to 2 days.

Nutrition:
Calories: 47.4
Protein: 0.28g
Carbohydrates: 11.51g
Fiber: 2g
Sugar: 5g
Sodium: 0.76mg

675. PHYLLO VEGETABLE TRIANGLES

Preparation Time: 15 minutes
Cooking Time: 6 to 11 minutes
Servings: 6
Ingredients:
- 3 tablespoons of minced onion
- 2 garlic cloves, minced

- 2 tablespoons of grated carrot
- 1 teaspoon of olive oil
- 3 tablespoons of frozen baby peas, thawed
- 2 tablespoons of nonfat cream cheese, at room temperature
- 6 sheets of frozen phyllo dough, thawed
- Olive oil spray, for coating the dough

Directions:
1. In a baking pan, combine the onion, garlic, carrot, and olive oil. Air fry at 390ºF (199ºC) for 2 to 4 minutes, or until the vegetables are crisp-tender. Transfer to a bowl.
2. Stir in the peas and cream cheese to the vegetable mixture. Let it cool while you prepare the dough.
3. Lay one sheet of phyllo on a work surface and lightly spray with olive oil spray. Top with another sheet of phyllo. Repeat with the remaining 4 phyllo sheets; you'll have 3 stacks with 2 layers each. Cut each stack lengthwise into 4 strips (12 strips total).
4. Place a scant 2 teaspoons of the filling near the bottom of each strip. Bring one corner up over the filling to make a triangle; continue folding the triangles over, as you would fold a flag. Seal the edge with a bit of water. Repeat with the remaining strips and filling.
5. Air fry the triangles, in 2 batches, for 4 to 7 minutes, or until golden brown. Serve.

Nutrition:
Calories: 67
Fat: 2g
Protein: 2g
Carbohydrates: 11g
Fiber: 1g
Sugar: 1g
Sodium: 121mg

676. RED CABBAGE AND MUSHROOM POT STICKERS

Preparation Time: 12 minutes
Cooking Time: 11-18 minutes
Servings: 4
Ingredients:
- 1 cup of shredded red cabbage
- ¼ cup of chopped button mushrooms
- ¼ cup of grated carrot
- 2 tablespoons of minced onion
- 2 garlic cloves, minced

- 2 teaspoons of grated fresh ginger
- 12 gyoza/pot sticker wrappers
- 2½ teaspoons of olive oil, divided

Directions:
1. In a baking pan, combine the red cabbage, mushrooms, carrot, onion, garlic, and ginger. Add 1 tablespoon of water. Place in the air fryer and bake at 370ºF (188ºC) for 3 to 6 minutes, until the vegetables are crisp-tender. Drain and set aside.
2. Working one at a time, place the pot sticker wrappers on a work surface. Top each wrapper with a scant 1 tablespoon of the filling. Fold half of the wrapper over the other half to form a half-circle. Dab one edge with water and press both edges together.
3. To the baking pan, add 1¼ teaspoons of olive oil. Put half of the pot stickers, seam-side up, in the pan. Air fry for 5 minutes, or until the bottoms are light golden brown. Add 1 tablespoon of water and return the pan to the air fryer.
4. Air fry for 4 to 6 minutes more, or until hot. Repeat with the remaining pot stickers, remaining 1¼ teaspoons of oil, and another tablespoon of water. Serve immediately.

Nutrition:
Calories: 88
Fat: 3g
Protein: 2g
Carbohydrates: 14g
Fiber: 1g
Sugar: 1g
Sodium: 58mg

677. GARLIC ROASTED MUSHROOMS

Preparation Time: 3 minutes
Cooking Time: 22-27 minutes
Servings: 4
Ingredients:
- 16 garlic cloves, peeled
- 2 teaspoons of olive oil, divided
- 16 button mushrooms
- ½ teaspoon of dried marjoram
- ⅛ teaspoon of freshly ground black pepper
- 1 tablespoon of white wine or low-sodium vegetable broth

Directions:

1. In a baking pan, mix the garlic with 1 teaspoon of olive oil. Roast in the air fryer at 350ºF (177ºC) for 12 minutes.
2. Add the mushrooms, marjoram, and pepper. Stir to coat. Drizzle with the remaining 1 teaspoon of olive oil and white wine.
3. Return to the air fryer and roast for 10 to 15 minutes more, or until the mushrooms and garlic cloves are tender. Serve.

Nutrition:
Calories: 128
Fat: 4g
Protein: 13g
Carbohydrates: 17g
Fiber: 4g
Sugar: 8g
Sodium: 20mg

678. BAKED SPICY CHICKEN MEATBALLS

Preparation Time: 10 minutes
Cooking Time: 11-14 minutes
Servings: 24 meatballs
Ingredients:
- 1 medium red onion, minced
- 2 garlic cloves, minced
- 1 jalapeño pepper, minced
- 2 teaspoons of olive oil
- 3 tablespoons of ground almonds
- 1 egg
- 1 teaspoon of dried thyme
- 1 pound (454 g) of ground chicken breast

Directions:
1. In a baking pan, combine the red onion, garlic, jalapeño, and olive oil. Bake at 400ºF (204ºC) for 3 to 4 minutes, or until the vegetables are crisp-tender. Transfer to a medium bowl.
2. Mix in the almonds, egg, and thyme to the vegetable mixture. Add the chicken and mix until just combined.
3. Form the chicken mixture into about 24 1-inch balls. Bake the meatballs, in batches, for 8 to 10 minutes, until the chicken reaches an internal temperature of 165ºF (74ºC) on a meat thermometer.

Nutrition:
Calories: 186
Fat: 7g
Protein: 29g
Carbohydrates: 5g
Fiber: 1g
Sugar: 3g

Sodium: 55mg

679. MINI ONION BITES

Preparation Time: 10 minutes
Cooking Time: 16-20 minutes
Servings: 20 onion bites
Ingredients:

- 20 white boiler onions
- 1 cup of buttermilk
- 2 eggs
- 1 cup of wheat flour
- 1 cup of whole wheat breadcrumbs
- 1 tablespoon of smoked paprika
- 1 teaspoon of salt
- 1 teaspoon of ground black pepper
- 1 teaspoon of granulated garlic
- ¾ teaspoon of chili powder
- Olive oil spray

Directions:

1. Place a parchment liner in the air fryer basket.
2. Slice off the root end of the onions, taking off as little as possible.
3. Peel off the papery skin and make cuts halfway through the tops of the onions. Don't cut too far down; you want the onion to hold together still.
4. In a large bowl, beat the buttermilk and eggs.
5. In a medium bowl, mix the flour, breadcrumbs, paprika, salt, pepper, garlic, and chili powder.
6. Add the prepared onions to the buttermilk mixture and allow to soak for at least 10 minutes.
7. Working in batches, remove the onions from the batter and dredge them with the bread crumb mixture.
8. Place the prepared onions in the air fryer basket in a single layer.
9. Spray lightly with the olive oil and air fry at 360ºF (182ºC) for 8 to 10 minutes, until golden and crispy. Repeat with any remaining onions and serve.

Nutrition:
Calories: 166
Fat: 2g
Protein: 6g
Carbohydrates: 31g
Fiber: 4g
Sugar: 7g
Sodium: 372mg

680. CRISPY PARMESAN CAULIFLOWER

Preparation Time: 12 minutes
Cooking Time: 14 to 17 minutes
Servings: 20 cauliflower bites
Ingredients:

- 4 cups of cauliflower florets
- 1 cup of whole wheat breadcrumbs
- ¼ cup of grated Parmesan cheese
- 1 teaspoon of coarse sea salt or kosher salt
- ¼ cup of unsalted butter
- ¼ cup of mild hot sauce
- Olive oil spray

Directions:

1. Place a parchment liner in the air fryer basket.
2. Cut the cauliflower florets in half and set them aside.
3. In a small bowl, mix the breadcrumbs, salt, and Parmesan; set aside.
4. In a small microwave-safe bowl, combine the butter and hot sauce. Heat in the microwave until the butter is melted, about 15 seconds. Whisk.
5. Holding the stems of the cauliflower florets, dip them in the butter mixture to coat. Shake off any excess mixture.
6. Dredge the dipped florets with the bread crumb mixture, then put them in the Air Fryer basket. There's no need for a single layer; just toss them all in there.
7. Spray the cauliflower lightly with olive oil and air fry at 350ºF (177ºC) for 14 to 17 minutes, shaking the basket a few times throughout the cooking process. The florets are done when they are lightly browned and crispy. Serve warm.

Nutrition:
Calories: 106
Fat: 6g
Protein: 3g
Carbohydrates: 10g
Fiber: 1g
Sugar: 1g
Sodium: 416mg

681. CREAM CHEESE STUFFED JALAPEÑOS

Preparation Time: 12 minutes
Cooking Time: 6-8 minutes
Servings: 10 poppers
Ingredients:

- 8 ounces (227 g) of cream cheese, at room temperature
- 1 cup of whole wheat breadcrumbs, divided
- 2 tablespoons of fresh parsley, minced
- 1 teaspoon of chili powder
- 10 jalapeño peppers, halved and seeded

Directions:

1. In a small bowl, combine the cream cheese, ½ cup of breadcrumbs, the parsley, and the chili powder. Whisk to combine.
2. Stuff the cheese mixture into the jalapeños.
3. Sprinkle the tops of the stuffed jalapeños with the remaining ½ cup of breadcrumbs.
4. Place in the air fryer basket and air fry at 360ºF (182ºC) for 6 to 8 minutes, until the peppers are softened, and the cheese is melted. Serve warm.

Nutrition:
Calories: 126
Fat: 8g
Protein: 3g
Carbohydrates: 9.95g
Fiber: 0.9g
Sugar: 2g
Sodium: 158mg

682. HONEYDEW & GINGER SMOOTHIES

Preparation Time: 10 minutes
Cooking Time: 3 Minutes
Servings: 3
Ingredients:

- 1½ cup honeydew melon, cubed
- ½ cup banana
- ½ cup non-fat vanilla yogurt
- ¼ teaspoon fresh ginger, grated
- ½ cup ice cubes

Directions:

1. Place all ingredients in a blender and pulse until smooth. Pour into glasses and serve immediately.

Nutrition:
Calories: 83
Total Carbohydrates: 16g
Net Carbohydrates: 15g
Protein: 2g
Sugar: 12g
Sodium: 40.4mg
Fiber: 1g

683. BROILED STONE FRUIT

Preparation Time: 10 minutes
Cooking Time: 5 Minutes

Servings: 2

Ingredients:

- 1 peach
- 1 nectarine
- 2 tablespoon sugar-free whipped topping
- 1 tablespoon Splenda brown sugar
- Non-stick cooking spray

Directions:

2. Heat oven to broil. Line a shallow baking dish with foil and spray with cooking spray.
3. Cut the peach and nectarine in half and remove pits. Place cut side down in prepared dish. Broil 3 minutes.
4. Turn fruit over and sprinkle with Splenda brown sugar. Broil another 2-3 minutes.
5. Transfer 1 of each fruit to a dessert bowl and top with 1 tablespoon of whipped topping. Serve.

Nutrition:

Calories: 101
Total Carbohydrates: 22g
Net Carbohydrates: 20g
Protein: 1g
Sodium: 3.6mg
Fat: 1g
Sugar: 19g
Fiber: 2g

DESSERT

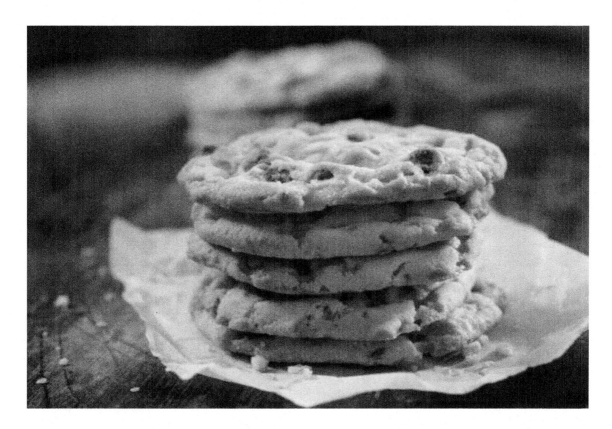

684. "OREO" COOKIES WITH CREAM CHEESE FILLING

Preparation Time: 15 minutes
Cooking Time: 12 minutes
Servings: 25
Ingredients:
- 3 tablespoons of coconut flour
- 2¼ cups hazelnut or almond flour
- 4 tablespoons of cocoa powder
- 1 teaspoon of baking powder
- ½ teaspoon of xanthan gum
- ¼ teaspoon of salt
- ½ cup of softened unsalted butter
- 1 large egg
- ½ cup of Stevia
- 1 teaspoon vanilla extract

For the Cream Filling:
- 2 tablespoons of almond butter
- 4 oz of softened cream cheese
- ½ cup of powdered Swerve
- ½ teaspoon of pure vanilla extract

Directions:
1. Preheat your oven to 350°F.
2. In a large mixing bowl, thoroughly combine the hazelnut or almond flour, baking powder, cocoa powder, xanthan gum, Stevia, salt, egg, and vanilla extract.
3. Add the almond butter and mix again.
4. In a separate medium bowl, cream all with the Swerve and the butter until it becomes light and extremely fluffy for 2 to 3 minutes.
5. Mix in the vanilla extract and egg until everything is well mixed.
6. Mix in the previously prepared dry ingredients until thoroughly blended.
7. Roll out the dough between 2 rectangular waxed paper sheets; make sure the thickness is about ⅛".
8. Place the dough on a cookie sheet that has been lined with parchment paper.
9. Continue rolling the cookie dough until it reaches the finish.
10. Bake the cookies for about 12 minutes; then let cool completely before starting to fill.

To Make the Filling:
1. Whip the cream cheese and the butter together, then add the vanilla extract.
2. Gradually add in the powdered Swerve.
3. Fill the cookies with the cream.
4. Serve and enjoy your delicious cookies!

Nutrition:
Calories: 120.5
Fat: 11.69 g
Protein: 2.6 g
Carbs: 9.33 g

Sodium: 65.38mg

685. WHIPPED CREAM ICING CAKE

Preparation Time: 20 minutes
Cooking Time: 25 minutes
Servings: 7
Ingredients:
- ¾ cup coconut flour
- ¾ cup of Swerve sweetener
- ½ cup of cocoa powder
- 2 teaspoons of baking powder
- 6 large eggs
- ⅔ cup of heavy whipping cream
- ½ cup of melted almond butter

For the Whipped Cream Icing:
- 1 cup of heavy whipping cream
- ¼ cup of Swerve sweetener
- 1 teaspoon of vanilla extract
- ⅓ cup of sifted cocoa powder

Directions:
1. Pre-heat your oven to 350°F.
2. Cooking spray should be used to grease an 8x8 cake tray.
3. Combine the coconut flour, Swerve sweetener, cocoa powder, baking powder, eggs, and melted butter in a large mixing bowl using an electric or manual mixer.
4. Bake for 25 minutes after pouring the batter into the cake pan.
5. Pull the cake pan from the oven and set aside for 5 minutes to cool.

For the Icing:
6. Whip the cream until creamy, then fold in the Swerve, vanilla, and cocoa powder.
7. Mix in the Swerve, vanilla, and cocoa powder until all of the ingredients are thoroughly incorporated.
8. Frost your baked cake with the frosting, then slice it, serve, and enjoy your delectable cake!

Nutrition:
Calories: 530
Fat: 37g
Protein: 14.3g
Carbs: 42.89g
Sodium: 266.55mg

686. FRUIT CAKE WITH WALNUTS

Preparation Time: 15 minutes
Cooking Time: 20 minutes
Servings: 6
Ingredients:
- ½ cup of almond butter (softened)
- ¼ cup of granulated erythritol
- 1 tablespoon of ground cinnamon
- ½ teaspoon of ground nutmeg
- ¼ Teaspoon of ground cloves
- 4 large eggs
- 1 teaspoon of vanilla extract
- ½ teaspoon of almond extract
- 2 cups of almond flour
- ½ cup of chopped walnuts
- ¼ cup of dried unsweetened cranberries
- ¼ cup of seedless raisins

Directions:
1. First pre-heat oven to 350°F and grease an 8-inch round baking tin with coconut oil.
2. Beat the granulated erythritol at a high speed until it becomes fluffy.
3. Blend in the cinnamon, nutmeg, and cloves until the mixture is smooth.
4. Batter in the eggs and beat them in well, one at a time, along with the almond extract and vanilla extract.
5. Whisk in the almond flour until the batter is smooth, then fold in the nuts and fruit.
6. Spread the mixture into the prepared baking sheet and bake for 20 minutes.
7. Take the cake from the oven and set aside for 5 minutes to cool.
8. Dust the cake with powdered erythritol.
9. Serve and enjoy your cake!

Nutrition:
Calories: 469.48
Fat: 37.7g
Protein: 17.45g
Carbs: 30.53g
Sodium: 95.35mg

687. CINNAMON AND GINGER CAKE

Preparation Time: 15 minutes
Cooking Time: 20 minutes
Servings: 9
Ingredients:
- 4 large eggs
- ½ tablespoon almond butter, unsalted to grease the pan
- ¼ cup coconut milk
- 2 tablespoons of unsalted almond butter
- 1½ teaspoons of Stevia
- 1 tablespoon of natural cocoa powder
- 1 tablespoon of ground cinnamon
- 1 tablespoon of fresh ground ginger
- ½ teaspoon of kosher salt
- 1½ cups of blanched almond flour
- ½ teaspoon of baking soda

Directions:
1. Preheat your oven to 325°F.
2. Grease an 8X8" glass baking tray thoroughly with almond butter.
3. In a large bowl, whisk all together with the coconut milk, the eggs, the melted almond butter, the Stevia, the cinnamon, the cocoa powder, the ginger, and the kosher salt.
4. Whisk in the almond flour, followed by the baking soda, and thoroughly combine.
5. Bake for 20 to 25 minutes, depending on the size of the pan.
6. Allow the cake to cool for 5 minutes before slicing, serving, and enjoying your delectable cake.

Nutrition:
Calories: 175
Fat: 15g
Protein: 7.4g
Carbs: 6.6g
Sodium: 138.57mg

688. KETO DONUTS

Preparation Time: 5 minutes
Cooking Time: 0 minutes
Servings: 4
Ingredients:
For the Donut:
- ½ cup of sifted almond flour
- 3 to 4 tablespoons of coconut milk
- 2 large eggs
- 2 to 3 tablespoons granulated of stevia
- 1 teaspoon of Keto-friendly baking powder
- 1 heaping teaspoon of apple cider vinegar
- 1 pinch of salt
- 1½ tablespoons of sifted cacao powder
- 3 teaspoons of Ceylon cinnamon
- 1 teaspoon of powdered vanilla beans
- 1 tablespoon of grass-fed ghee
- 2 tablespoons of coconut oil for greasing

For the Icing:

- Blend 1 to 2 teaspoons of coconut oil with 4 tablespoons of melted coconut butter

Optional Garnish:
- Edible rose petals, or shredded cacao

Directions:
1. Preheat the oven to 350F.
2. Grease a donut tray with coconut oil.
3. Stir all together with the sifted almond flour the coconut milk, eggs, the granulated Stevia, the Keto-friendly baking powder, the apple cider vinegar, the salt, the sifted cocoa powder, the Ceylon cinnamon, the powdered vanilla bean, and the grass-fed ghee.
4. Mix all of the doughnut ingredients together until they are uniformly distributed.
5. Divide the batter into the donut molds making sure to fill each to ¾ full.
6. Bake for 8 minutes, then gently remove the tray from the oven and place it on a wire rack to cool.
7. Serve and enjoy your doughnut, or top it with your favourite frosting and garnish.
8. Serve and enjoy your delicious treat!

Nutrition:
Calories: 357.36
Fat: 32.46g
Protein: 7.7g
Carbs: 16.25g
Sodium: 204.81mg

689. COCONUT MILK PEAR SHAKE

Preparation Time: 2 minutes
Cooking Time: 0 minutes
Servings: 4
Ingredients:
- 4 ripe chopped pears
- 4 lettuce leaves finely torn into pieces
- ¼ cup of unsweetened coconut milk
- 5 dried and toasted almonds
- 4 leaves of mint
- 2 tablespoons of unsweetened orange juice
- ½ tablespoon of apple sauce
- 5 ice cubes

Directions:
1. Place the chopped pears in the blender.
2. Add the lettuce leaves.

3. Pour in the almond milk and the remaining ingredients, including the ice cubes.
4. For around 3 minutes, combine all of the ingredients in a blender.
5. Serve and enjoy!

Nutrition:
Calories: 166.43
Fat: 3.9g
Protein: 5.45g
Carbs: 32g
Sodium: 108.9mg

690. CHOCOLATE PUDDING

Preparation Time: 5 minutes
Cooking Time: 0 minutes
Servings: 3
Ingredients:
- 1 avocado
- ¼ cup of apple sauce
- ¼ cup of organic raw unsweetened cacao powder
- 2 organic Medjool dates
- 1 tablespoon of organic coconut oil
- 1 tablespoon of homemade almond milk

For the Crust:
- 1 cup of organic walnuts
- 2 organic Medjool dates
- 2 tablespoons of organic raw cacao powder
- 1 tablespoon of coconut oil

Directions
1. Start by preparing the crust.
2. In a food processor, mix all the ingredients and process until you get a sticky consistency.
3. Divide the mixture in half, then press it into the bottoms of two tart molds cavities and put aside.
4. To make your pudding, combine all of your ingredients in a blender and blend until you have a creamy concoction.
5. Transfer your smooth mixture to the mound you have prepared on the crust and make sure to spread it evenly.
6. Pistachios, walnuts, raw cacao nibs, or hemp seeds can be sprinkled on top.
7. Serve and enjoy!

Nutrition:
Calories: 589
Fat: 51g
Protein: 12.5g
Carbs: 29g
Sodium: 27.4mg

691. RASPBERRY SMOOTHIE

Preparation Time: 5 minutes
Cooking Time: 0 minutes
Servings: 3
Ingredients:
- 1 cup of water
- 2 cups of chopped lettuce
- 1 cup of fresh or frozen raspberries
- 1 tablespoon of flax seeds
- 1 teaspoon of chia seeds
- A little bit of unsweetened apple sauce
- 1 teaspoon of coconut oil

Directions:
1. Place your ingredients into your blender.
2. Blend your components for around 1 minute on high speed.
3. Make sure the smoothie is creamy and smooth before serving.

Nutrition:
Calories: 63
Fat: 3.34g
Protein: 1.5g
Carbs: 8.07g
Sodium: 9.9mg

692. COCOA MOUSSE

Preparation Time: 3 minutes
Cooking Time: 0 minutes
Servings: 2
Ingredients:
- 1 cup of heavy whipping coconut cream
- ¼ cup of sifted, unsweetened cocoa powder
- ¼ cup of Swerve
- 1 teaspoon of vanilla extract
- ¼ teaspoon of kosher salt

Directions:
1. Begin by whisking the cream until it stiffens.
2. Whisk in the Stevia, vanilla extract, and salt until thoroughly combined.
3. Add the cocoa powder to the ingredients and mix once more.
4. Serve and enjoy your cocoa mousse!

Nutrition:
Calories: 458
Fat: 20.9g
Protein: 3g
Carbs: 94g
Sodium: 277.9mg

693. COCONUT ICE CREAM

Preparation Time: 3 minutes
Cooking Time: 0 minutes

Servings: 2

Ingredients:

- 2 cups of canned coconut milk
- 1½ teaspoons of pure vanilla bean paste or pure vanilla extract
- ⅓ cup of stevia
- ⅛ Teaspoon of salt
- optional ingredients for the desired flavor

Directions:

1. Use only full-fat canned coconut milk.
2. Instead of extract, you can use the seeds of a vanilla bean.
3. To prepare the ice cream, combine the milk, Swerve, salt, and vanilla extract in a mixing bowl.
4. You can use a cream machine. If you have one, simply churn as per the manufacturer's directions.
5. Freeze the resulting mixture in ice cube trays, then combine at high speed in a blender.
6. For around 30 minutes, place the ice cream in the freezer.
7. Serve and enjoy your ice cream!

Nutrition:

Calories: 436
Fat: 46g
Protein: 4.3g
Carbs: 36.5g
Sodium: 173.4mg

694. CHOCO-NUT MILKSHAKE

Preparation Time: 10 minutes
Cooking Time: 0 minute
Servings: 2
Ingredients:

- 2 cups unsweetened coconut and almonds
- 1 banana, sliced and frozen
- ¼ cup unsweetened coconut flakes
- 1 cup ice cubes
- ¼ cup macadamia nuts, chopped
- 3 tablespoons sugar-free sweetener
- 2 tablespoons raw unsweetened cocoa powder
- Whipped coconut cream

Directions:

1. Put all ingredients into a blender and blend on high until smooth and creamy.
2. Divide evenly between 4 "mocktail" glasses and top with whipped coconut cream, if desired.

3. Add a cocktail umbrella and toasted coconut for added flair.
4. Enjoy your delicious choco-nut smoothie!

Nutrition:

Carbohydrates: 12g
Protein: 3g
Calories: 199
Sodium: 115.7mg

695. PINEAPPLE & STRAWBERRY SMOOTHIE

Preparation Time: 7 minutes
Cooking Time: 0 minute
Servings: 2
Ingredients:

- 1 cup strawberries
- 1 cup pineapple, chopped
- ¾ cup almond milk
- 1 tablespoon almond butter

Directions:

1. Add all ingredients to a blender.
2. Blend until smooth.
3. Add additional almond milk as needed to get the desired consistency.
4. Chill before serving.

Nutrition:

Calories: 155
Carbohydrates: 24.68g
Protein: 3.6g
Sodium: 81.25mg

696. CANTALOUPE SMOOTHIE

Preparation Time: 11 minutes
Cooking Time: 0 minute
Servings: 2
Ingredients:

- ¾ cup carrot juice
- 4 cups cantaloupe, sliced into cubes
- Pinch of salt
- Frozen melon balls
- Fresh basil

Directions:

1. Add the carrot juice and cantaloupe cubes to a blender. Sprinkle with salt.
2. Process until smooth.
3. Transfer to a bowl.
4. Chill in the refrigerator for at least 30 minutes.
5. Top with the frozen melon balls and basil before serving.

Nutrition:

Calories: 172
Carbohydrates: 41.3g
Protein:3.4g
Sodium: 196mg

697. BERRY SMOOTHIE WITH MINT

Preparation Time: 7 minutes
Cooking Time: 0 minute
Servings: 2
Ingredients:

- ¼ cup orange juice
- ½ cup blueberries
- ½ cup blackberries
- 1 cup reduced-fat plain kefir
- 1 tablespoon honey
- 2 tablespoons fresh mint leaves

Directions:

1. Add all the ingredients to a blender.
2. Blend until smooth.

Nutrition:

Calories: 137
Carbohydrates: 27g
Protein: 6g
Sodium: 50.44mg

698. GREEN SMOOTHIE

Preparation Time: 12 minutes
Cooking Time: 0 minute
Servings: 2
Ingredients:

- 1 cup vanilla almond milk (unsweetened)
- ¼ ripe avocado, chopped
- 1 cup kale, chopped
- 1 banana
- 2 teaspoons honey
- 1 tablespoon chia seeds
- 1 cup ice cubes

Directions:

1. Combine all the ingredients in a blender.
2. Process until creamy.

Nutrition:

Calories: 155.21
Carbohydrates: 26.25g
Protein: 3.8g
Sodium: 100mg

699. BANANA, CAULIFLOWER & BERRY SMOOTHIE

Preparation Time: 9 minutes
Cooking Time: 0 minute
Servings: 2
Ingredients:

- 2 cups almond milk (unsweetened)
- 1 cup banana, sliced
- ½ cup blueberries
- ½ cup blackberries
- 1 cup cauliflower rice
- 2 teaspoons maple syrup

Directions:

1. Pour almond milk into a blender.

2. Stir in the rest of the ingredients.
3. Process until smooth.
4. Chill before serving.

Nutrition:
Calories: 172
Carbohydrates: 34.35g
Protein:4.1g
Sodium: 203mg

700. BERRY & SPINACH SMOOTHIE

Preparation Time: 11 minutes
Cooking Time: 0 minute
Servings: 2
Ingredients:
- 2 cups strawberries
- 1 cup raspberries
- 1 cup blueberries
- 1 cup fresh baby spinach leaves
- 1 cup pomegranate juice
- 3 tablespoons milk powder (unsweetened)

Directions:
1. Mix all the ingredients in a blender.
2. Blend until smooth.
3. Chill before serving.

Nutrition:
Calories: 270
Carbohydrates: 54g
Protein:4.6g
Sodium: 126mg

701. PUMPKIN & BANANA ICE CREAM

Preparation Time: 5 minutes
Cooking Time: 10 minutes
Servings: 4
Ingredients:
- 15 oz. pumpkin puree
- 4 bananas, sliced and frozen
- 1 teaspoon pumpkin pie spice
- Chopped pecans

Directions:
1. Add pumpkin puree, bananas, and pumpkin pie spice in a food processor.
2. Pulse until smooth.
3. Chill in the refrigerator.
4. Garnish with pecans.

Nutrition:
Calories: 185
Carbohydrates: 36g
Protein: 2.77g
Sodium: 5.6mg

702. BRULEE ORANGES

Preparation Time: 5 minutes
Cooking Time: 10 minutes
Servings: 4

Ingredients:
- 4 oranges, sliced into segments
- 1 teaspoon ground cardamom
- 6 teaspoons brown sugar
- 1 cup non-fat Greek yogurt

Directions:
1. Preheat your broiler.
2. Arrange orange slices in a baking pan.
3. In a bowl, mix the cardamom and sugar.
4. Sprinkle mixture on top of the oranges. Broil for 5 minutes.
5. Serve oranges with yogurt.

Nutrition:
Calories: 94
Carbohydrates: 18g
Protein: 6.8g
Sodium: 20mg

703. FROZEN BLUEBERRY LEMONDAE

Preparation Time: 5 minutes
Cooking Time: 10 minutes
Servings: 4
Ingredients:
- 6 cups fresh blueberries
- 8 sprigs of fresh thyme
- ¾ cup light brown sugar
- 1 teaspoon lemon zest
- ¼ cup lemon juice
- 2 cups water

Directions:
1. Add blueberries, thyme, and sugar to a pan over medium heat.
2. Cook for 6 to 8 minutes.
3. Transfer mixture to a blender.
4. Remove thyme sprigs.
5. Stir in the remaining ingredients.
6. Pulse until smooth.
7. Strain mixture and freeze for 1 hour.

Nutrition:
Calories: 261.56
Carbohydrates: 67.21g
Protein:1.8g
Sodium: 14.5mg

704. PEANUT BUTTER CHOCO CHIP COOKIES

Preparation Time: 5 minutes
Cooking Time: 10 minutes
Servings: 4
Ingredients:
- 1 egg
- ½ cup light brown sugar
- 1 cup natural unsweetened peanut butter
- Pinch salt
- ¼ cup dark chocolate chips

Directions:
1. Preheat your oven to 375°F.
2. Mix egg, sugar, peanut butter, salt, and chocolate chips in a bowl.
3. Form into cookies and place in a baking pan.
4. Bake the cookie for 10 minutes.
5. Let cool before serving.

Nutrition:
Calories: 542
Carbohydrates: 42g
Protein:16.22g
Sodium: 70.26mg

705. WATERMELON SHERBET

Preparation Time: 5 minutes
Cooking Time: 3 minutes
Servings: 4
Ingredients:
- 6 cups watermelon, sliced into cubes
- 14 oz. almond milk
- 1 tablespoon honey
- ¼ cup lime juice
- Salt to taste

Directions:
1. Freeze watermelon for 4 hours.
2. Add frozen watermelon and other ingredients to a blender.
3. Blend until smooth.
4. Transfer to a container with a seal.
5. Seal and freeze for 4 hours.

Nutrition:
Calories: 126
Carbohydrates: 29.45g
Protein: 1.89g
Sodium: 259.11mg

706. STRAWBERRY & MANGO ICE CREAM

Preparation Time: 5 minutes
Cooking Time: 10 minutes
Servings: 4
Ingredients:
- 8 oz. strawberries, sliced
- 12 oz. mango, sliced into cubes
- 1 tablespoon lime juice

Directions:
1. Add all ingredients to a food processor.
2. Pulse for 2 minutes.
3. Chill before serving.

Nutrition:
Calories: 54
Carbohydrates: 13.3g
Protein:0.86g
Sodium: 1.21mg

707. SPARKLING FRUIT DRINK

Preparation Time: 5 minutes
Cooking Time: 10 minutes
Servings: 4
Ingredients:

- 8 oz. unsweetened grape juice
- 8 oz. unsweetened apple juice
- 8 oz. unsweetened orange juice
- 1 qt. homemade ginger ale
- Ice

Directions:

1. Makes 7 servings. Mix the first 4 ingredients together in a pitcher. Stir in ice cubes and 9 ounces of the beverage to each glass. Serve immediately.

Nutrition:
Calories: 178
Protein:0.65g
Carbs: 44.67g
Sodium: 26.46mg

708. TIRAMISU SHOTS

Preparation Time: 5 minutes
Cooking Time: 10 minutes
Servings: 4
Ingredients:

- 1 pack silken tofu
- 1 oz. dark chocolate, finely chopped
- ¼ cup sugar substitute
- 1 teaspoon lemon juice
- ¼ cup brewed espresso
- Pinch salt
- 24 slices angel food cake
- Cocoa powder (unsweetened)

Directions:

1. Add tofu, chocolate, sugar substitute, lemon juice, espresso, and salt in a food processor.
2. Pulse until smooth.
3. Add angel food cake pieces into shot glasses.
4. Sprinkle with the cocoa powder.
5. Pour the tofu mixture on top.
6. Top with the remaining angel food cake pieces.
7. Chill for 30 minutes and serve.

Nutrition:
Calories: 727
Carbohydrates: 150g
Protein:18.8g
Sodium: 1823mg

709. ICE CREAM BROWNIE CAKE

Preparation Time: 5 minutes
Cooking Time: 10 minutes
Servings: 4
Ingredients:

- Cooking spray
- 12 oz. no-sugar brownie mix
- ¼ cup oil
- 2 egg whites
- 3 tablespoons water
- 2 cups sugar-free ice cream

Directions:

1. Preheat your oven to 325°F.
2. Spray your baking pan with oil.
3. Mix brownie mix, oil, egg whites, and water in a bowl.
4. Pour into the baking pan.
5. Bake for 25 minutes.
6. Let cool.
7. Freeze brownie for 2 hours.
8. Spread ice cream over the brownie.
9. Freeze for 8 hours.

Nutrition:
Calories: 518
Carbohydrates: 88g
Protein:3g
Sodium: 223mg

710. PEANUT BUTTER CUPS

Preparation Time: 5 minutes
Cooking Time: 10 minutes
Servings: 4
Ingredients:

- 1 packet plain gelatin
- ¼ cup sugar substitute
- 2 cups nonfat cream
- ½ teaspoon vanilla
- ¼ cup low-fat peanut butter
- 2 tablespoons unsalted peanuts, chopped

Directions:

1. Mix gelatin, sugar substitute, and cream in a pan.
2. Let sit for 5 minutes.
3. Place over medium heat and cook until gelatin has been dissolved.
4. Stir in vanilla and peanut butter.
5. Pour into custard cups. Chill for 3 hours.
6. Top with the peanuts and serve.

Nutrition:
Calories: 533
Carbohydrates: 21g
Protein:6.8g
Sodium: 223mg

711. FRUIT PIZZA

Preparation Time: 5 minutes
Cooking Time: 10 minutes
Servings: 4
Ingredients:

- 1 teaspoon maple syrup
- ¼ teaspoon vanilla extract
- ½ cup coconut milk yogurt

- 2 round slices of watermelon
- ½ cup blackberries, sliced
- ½ cup strawberries, sliced
- 2 tablespoons coconut flakes (unsweetened)

Directions:

1. Mix maple syrup, vanilla, and yogurt in a bowl.
2. Spread the mixture on top of the watermelon slice.
3. Top with the berries and coconut flakes.

Nutrition:
Calories: 127.25
Carbohydrates: 19g
Protein:2.35g
Sodium: 14.63mg

712. CHOCO PEPPERMINT CAKE

Preparation Time: 5 minutes
Cooking Time: 10 minutes
Servings: 4
Ingredients:

- Cooking spray
- ⅓ cup oil
- 15 oz. package chocolate cake mix
- 3 eggs, beaten
- 1 cup water
- ¼ teaspoon peppermint extract

Directions:

1. Spray slow cooker with oil.
2. Mix all the ingredients in a bowl.
3. Use an electric mixer on a medium-speed setting to mix ingredients for 2 minutes.
4. Pour the mixture into the slow cooker.
5. Cover the pot and cook on low for 3 hours.
6. Let cool before slicing and serving.

Nutrition:
Calories: 642
Carbohydrates: 85g
Protein: 9.04g
Sodium: 864mg

713. ROASTED MANGO

Preparation Time: 5 minutes
Cooking Time: 10 minutes
Servings: 4
Ingredients:

- 2 mangoes, sliced
- 2 teaspoons crystallized ginger, chopped
- 2 teaspoons orange zest
- 2 tablespoons coconut flakes (unsweetened)

Directions:

1. Preheat your oven to 350°F.
2. Add mango slices in custard cups.
3. Top with ginger, orange zest, and coconut flakes.
4. Bake in the oven for 10 minutes.

Nutrition:
Calories: 104
Carbohydrates: 20g
Protein:1.22g
Sodium: 3.33mg

714. ROASTED PLUMS

Preparation Time: 5 minutes
Cooking Time: 10 minutes
Servings: 4

Ingredients:
- Cooking spray
- 6 plums, sliced
- ½ cup pineapple juice (unsweetened)
- 1 tablespoon brown sugar
- 2 tablespoons brown sugar
- ¼ teaspoon ground cardamom
- ½ teaspoon ground cinnamon
- ⅛ teaspoon ground cumin

Directions:
1. Mix all the ingredients in a baking pan.
2. Roast in the oven at 450°F for 20 minutes.

Nutrition:
Calories: 104
Carbohydrates: 22.9g
Protein:0.8g
Sodium: 4mg

715. FIGS WITH HONEY & YOGURT

Preparation Time: 5 minutes
Cooking Time: 10 minutes
Servings: 4
Ingredients:
- ½ teaspoon vanilla
- 8 oz. nonfat yogurt
- 2 figs, sliced
- 1 tablespoon walnuts, chopped and toasted
- 2 teaspoons honey

Directions:
1. Stir vanilla into yogurt.
2. Mix well.
3. Top with the figs and sprinkle with walnuts.
4. Drizzle with honey and serve.

Nutrition:
Calories: 77.95
Carbohydrates: 9.5g
Protein:6.6g
Sodium: 30.68mg

716. FLOURLESS CHOCOLATE CAKE

Preparation Time: 10 minutes
Cooking Time: 45 minutes
Servings: 6
Ingredients:
- ½ cup of Stevia
- 12 ounces of unsweetened baking chocolate
- ⅔ cup of ghee
- ⅓ cup of warm water
- ¼ teaspoon of salt
- 4 large eggs
- 2 cups of boiling water

Directions:
1. With parchment paper, line the bottom of a 9-inch springform pan.
2. In a small pot, heat the water; then sprinkle the salt and stevia over the water and wait until the combination is completely dissolved.
3. Melt the baking chocolate over a double boiler or in the microwave for 30 seconds.
4. In a large mixing bowl, mix the melted chocolate and the butter using an electric mixer.
5. After adding each egg, beat in your heated mixture, then break in the egg and stir.
6. Fill the prepared springform tray halfway with the prepared mixture.
7. Wrap the springform tray with foil.
8. Place the springform tray in a large cake tray and fill it halfway with boiling water; the depth should not exceed 1 inch.
9. Now bake the cake for 45 minutes at 350°F in a water bath.
10. Take the tray from the boiling water and place it on a cooling rack to cool.
11. Let the cake chill overnight in the refrigerator.

Nutrition:
Calories: 609
Carbohydrates: 30.35g
Fiber: 9.41g
Sodium: 160mg

717. RASPBERRY CAKE WITH WHITE CHOCOLATE SAUCE

Preparation Time: 15 minutes
Cooking Time: 60 minutes
Servings: 5
Ingredients:
- 5 ounces of melted cacao butter
- 2 ounces of grass-fed ghee
- ½ cup of coconut cream
- 1 cup of green banana flour
- 3 teaspoons of pure vanilla
- 4 large eggs
- ½ cup of Lakanto's powdered monk fruit
- 1 teaspoon of baking powder
- 2 teaspoons of apple cider vinegar
- 2 cups of raspberries

For White Chocolate Sauce:
- 3½ ounces of cacao butter
- ½ cup of coconut cream
- 2 teaspoons of pure vanilla extract
- 1 pinch of salt

Directions:
1. Preheat your oven to 280°F.
2. Mix the green banana flour, pure vanilla extract, baking powder, coconut cream, eggs, cider vinegar, and monk fruit in a large mixing bowl and well combine.
3. Set aside the raspberries and line a cake loaf pan with parchment paper.
4. Spread the raspberries over the top of the cake after pouring the mixture into the baking tray.
5. Place the tray in the oven for about 60 minutes; in the meantime, make the sauce.

Directions for sauce:
1. In a saucepan over low heat, combine the cacao cream, vanilla extract, cacao butter, and salt.
2. With a fork, mix all of the ingredients, making sure the cacao butter is properly combined with the cream.
3. Remove from the fire and set aside to cool slightly but not solidify.
4. Drizzle with the chocolate sauce.
5. Scatter the cake with more raspberries.
6. Slice your cake; serve and enjoy it!

Nutrition:
Calories: 773
Carbohydrates: 49g
Fiber: 5.2g
Sodium: 194mg

718. LAVA CAKE

Preparation Time: 10 minutes
Cooking Time: 10 minutes
Servings: 2
Ingredients:

- 1 tablespoon of super-fine almond flour
- 2 oz of dark chocolate; use chocolate of 85% cocoa solids
- 2 oz of unsalted almond butter
- 2 large eggs

Directions:
1. Heat your oven to 350°F
2. Grease 2 heat-proof ramekins with almond butter.
3. Now, combine the chocolate and almond butter in a mixing bowl and well combine.
4. Using a mixer, thoroughly combine the eggs.
5. Add the eggs to the chocolate and butter mixture and thoroughly combine with the almond flour and swerve; then whisk.
6. Pour the dough into 2 ramekins.
7. Bake for about 9 to 10 minutes.
8. Serve the cakes on plates topped with pomegranate seeds!

Nutrition:
Calories: 427
Carbohydrates: 21.2g
Fiber: 5.57g
Sodium: 75.82mg

719. CHEESECAKE

Preparation Time: 15 minutes
Cooking Time: 50 minutes
Servings: 6
Ingredients:
For Almond Flour Cheesecake Crust:
- 2 cups of blanched almond flour
- ⅓ cup of almond butter
- 3 tablespoons of erythritol (powdered or granular)
- 1 teaspoon of vanilla extract

For Keto Cheesecake Filling:
- 32 oz of softened cream cheese
- 1¼ cups of powdered erythritol
- 3 large eggs
- 1 tablespoon of lemon juice
- 1 teaspoon of vanilla extract

Directions:
1. Preheat your oven to 350°F.
2. Grease a 9" springform pan with cooking spray or just line its bottom with parchment paper.
3. In order to make the cheesecake crust, stir in the melted butter, the almond flour, the vanilla extract, and the erythritol in a large bowl.
4. Because the dough will be crumbly, press it into the bottom of your prepared tray.

5. Bake for 12 minutes, then set aside for 10 minutes to cool.
6. Meanwhile, mix the softened cream cheese and powdered sweetener together on low speed until smooth.
7. Crack in the eggs and beat on low to medium speed until the mixture is frothy. Make a point of adding one at a time.
8. Mix in the lemon juice and vanilla essence with a mixer on low to medium speed.
9. Filling should be poured directly on top of the crust in your pan. Smooth the top of the cake with a spatula.
10. Bake for about 45 to 50 minutes.
11. Remove the cooked cheesecake from the oven and carefully run a knife around the edge.
12. Allow the cake to chill in the refrigerator for about 4 hours.
13. Serve and enjoy your delicious cheesecake!

Nutrition:
Calories: 839
Carbohydrates: 54g
Fiber: 5.47g
Sodium: 541.89mg

720. CAKE WITH WHIPPED CREAM ICING

Preparation Time: 20 minutes
Cooking Time: 25 minutes
Servings: 7
Ingredients:
- ¾ cup coconut flour
- ¾ cup of Swerve sweetener
- ½ cup of cocoa powder
- 2 teaspoons of baking powder
- 6 large eggs
- ⅔ cup of heavy whipping cream
- ½ cup of melted almond butter

For Whipped Cream Icing:
- 1 cup of heavy whipping cream
- ¼ cup of Swerve sweetener
- 1 teaspoon of vanilla extract
- ⅓ cup of sifted cocoa powder

Directions:
1. Pre-heat your oven to 350°F.
2. Cooking spray should be used to grease an 8x8 cake pan.
3. Combine the coconut flour, Swerve sweetener, cocoa powder, baking powder, eggs, and melted butter in a large mixing bowl using an electric or manual mixer.

4. Bake for 25 minutes after pouring the batter into the cake pan.
5. Take the cake pan from the oven and set aside for 5 minutes to cool.

For the Icing:
1. Whip the cream until creamy, then fold in the Swerve, vanilla, and cocoa powder.
2. Mix in the Swerve, vanilla, and cocoa powder until all of the ingredients are thoroughly incorporated.
3. Frost your baked cake with the icing!

Nutrition:
Calories: 530
Carbohydrates: 42g
Fiber: 10g
Sodium: 266.55mg

721. GINGER CAKE

Preparation Time: 15 minutes
Cooking Time: 20 minutes
Servings: 9
Ingredients:
- 4 large eggs
- ½ tablespoon of unsalted almond butter to grease the pan
- ¼ cup coconut milk
- 1½ teaspoons of Stevia
- 2 tablespoons of unsalted almond butter
- 1 tablespoon of ground cinnamon
- 1 tablespoon of natural cocoa powder
- 1 tablespoon of fresh ground ginger
- ½ teaspoon of kosher salt
- 1½ cups of blanched almond flour
- ½ teaspoon of baking soda

Directions:
1. Preheat your oven to 325°F.
2. Grease an 8x8" glass baking tray thoroughly with almond butter.
3. In a large bowl, whisk all together with the coconut milk, the eggs, the melted almond butter, the Stevia, the cinnamon, the cocoa powder, the ginger, and the kosher salt.
4. Whisk in the almond flour, followed by the baking soda, and thoroughly combine.
5. Bake for 20 to 25 minutes, depending on the size of the pan.
6. Allow the cake to cool for 5 minutes.

Nutrition:
Calories:175
Carbohydrates: 5g
Fiber: 1.9g
Sodium: 137mg

722. ORANGE CAKE

Preparation Time: 10 minutes
Cooking Time: 50minutes
Servings: 8
Ingredients:
- 2 Unwaxed washed oranges
- 2 and ½ cups of almond flour
- 5 Large separated eggs
- 2 Teaspoons of orange extract
- 1 teaspoon of baking powder
- 1 teaspoon of vanilla bean powder
- 16 drops liquid stevia; about 3 teaspoons
- 6 Seeds of cardamom pods crushed
- 1 Handful of flaked almonds to decorate

Directions:
1. Preheat your oven to 350 Fahrenheit.
2. Line a rectangular bread baking tray with parchment paper.
3. Put the oranges in a pan with cold water and cover with a lid.
4. Bring the pot to a boil, then reduce to a low heat for about 1 hour, making sure the oranges are well immersed.
5. To eliminate any bitterness from the oranges, keep them immersed at all times.
6. Cut the oranges in halves and remove any seeds before draining the water and setting the oranges aside to cool.
7. Cut the oranges in halves and remove the seeds before pureeing them in a blender or food processor.
8. Separate the eggs and whisk the egg whites until firm peaks form.
9. Mix all of the ingredients except the egg whites to the orange mixture, then add the egg whites.
10. Pour the batter into the prepared cake pan and top with the flaked almonds.
11. Bake your cake for about 50 minutes.
12. Take the cake from the oven and set it aside to cool for 5 minutes.

Nutrition:

Calories:164
Carbohydrates:7.1g
Fiber: 2.7g
Sodium: 110mg

723. LEMON CAKE

Preparation Time: 20 minutes
Cooking Time: 20minutes
Servings: 9
Ingredients:
- 2 medium lemons grated zest
- 4 large eggs
- 2 tablespoons of almond butter
- 4-5 tablespoons of honey (or sweetener of your choice)
- 2 tablespoons of avocado oil
- ⅓ cup of coconut flour
- ½ tablespoon baking soda

Directions:
1. Preheat your oven to 350°F.
2. In a large mixing bowl, crack the eggs and put aside 2 egg whites.
3. Whisk together the two egg whites, the egg yolks, the honey, the oil, the almond butter, the lemon zest, and the juice.
4. Mix the baking soda and coconut flour together, then gradually add this dry combination to the wet ingredients while stirring for a few minutes.
5. Beat the 2 eggs with a hand mixer and beat the egg into foam.
6. Using a silicone spatula, gradually incorporate the white egg foam into the mixture.
7. Transfer your batter to a tray covered with baking paper.
8. Bake the cake for 20-22 minutes.
9. Allow the cake to cool for 5 minutes before slicing.

Nutrition:
Calories: 127
Carbohydrates: 11.32g
Fiber: 7.6g
Sodium: 44mg

724. CINNAMON CAKE

Preparation Time: 15 minutes
Cooking Time: 35minutes
Servings: 8
Ingredients:
For Cinnamon Filling:
- 3 tablespoons of Swerve sweetener
- 2 teaspoons of ground cinnamon

For the Cake:
- 3 cups of almond flour
- ¾ cup of Swerve sweetener
- ¼ cup of unflavored whey protein powder
- 2 teaspoons of baking powder
- ½ teaspoon of salt
- 3 large eggs
- ½ cup of melted coconut oil
- ½ teaspoon of vanilla extract
- ½ cup of almond milk
- 1 tablespoon of melted coconut oil

For Cream Cheese Frosting:
- 3 tablespoons of softened cream cheese
- 2 tablespoons of powdered Swerve sweetener
- 1 tablespoon of coconut heavy whipping cream
- ½ teaspoon of vanilla extract

Directions:
1. Preheat oven to 325°F and grease a 8x8" baking tray.
2. To make the filling, combine the Swerve and cinnamon in a mixing bowl and combine; put aside.
3. For the preparation of the cake, whisk it all together with the almond flour, the sweetener, the protein powder, the baking powder, and the salt in a mixing bowl.
4. Mix in the eggs, melted coconut oil, and vanilla extract well.
5. Stir in the almond milk until all of the ingredients are fully blended.
6. Spread half of the batter in the prepared pan, followed with two-thirds of the filling mixture.
7. Spread the remaining batter mixture over the filling and level it out with a spatula.
8. Bake for 35 minutes at 350°F.
9. Brush the remaining cinnamon filling with the melted coconut oil and sprinkle with the remaining cinnamon filling.
10. To make the frosting, combine the cream cheese, powdered erythritol, cream, and vanilla extract in a mixing dish and beat until smooth.
11. Drizzle frost over the cooled cake.

Nutrition:
Calories: 491
Carbohydrates: 34.8g
Fiber: 4.9g
Sodium: 333.58mg

725. MADELEINE

Preparation Time: 10 minutes
Cooking Time: 15 minutes
Servings: 12
Ingredients:
- 2 large eggs
- ¾ cup of almond flour
- 1½ tablespoons of Swerve
- ¼ cup of cooled, melted coconut oil
- 1 teaspoon of vanilla extract
- 1 teaspoon of almond extract
- 1 teaspoon of lemon zest
- ¼ teaspoon of salt

Directions:
1. Preheat your oven to 350°F.
2. Whisk the eggs with the salt for roughly 5 minutes on high speed.
3. Slowly add the Swerve and continue to mix on high for 2 minutes.
4. Stir in the almond flour until well combined, then add the vanilla and almond extracts.
5. Stir in the melted coconut oil until all of the ingredients are combined.
6. Pour the batter onto a greased Madeleine tray in equal halves.
7. Bake your ketogenic Madeleine for 13 minutes, or when the edges begin to brown.
8. Remove the Madeleine from the baking tray.

Nutrition:
Calories: 87
Carbohydrates: 3g
Fiber: 3g
Sodium: 60.36mg

726. WAFFLES

Preparation Time: 20 minutes
Cooking Time: 30 minutes
Servings: 3
Ingredients:
For Ketogenic Waffles:
- 8 oz of cream cheese
- 5 large eggs
- ⅓ cup of coconut flour
- ½ teaspoon of xanthan gum
- 1 pinch of salt
- ½ teaspoon of vanilla extract
- 2 tablespoons of Swerve
- ¼ teaspoon of baking soda
- ⅓ cup of almond milk

Optional Ingredients:
- ½ teaspoon of cinnamon pie spice
- ¼ teaspoon of almond extract

For Low-Carb Maple Syrup:
- 1 cup of water

- 1 tablespoon of maple flavor
- ¾ cup of powdered Swerve
- 1 tablespoon of almond butter
- ½ teaspoon of xanthan gum

Directions:
For the Waffles:
1. Check that all of your components are at room temperature.
2. Using a food processor, combine all of the ingredients for the waffles, except the almond milk, including the cream cheese, pastured eggs, coconut flour, xanthan gum, salt, vanilla extract, Swerve, baking soda, and almond milk.
3. Blend the ingredients together until smooth and creamy, then transfer the batter to a bowl.
4. With a spatula, combine the almond milk and the remaining ingredients.
5. Preheat a waffle maker to a high setting.
6. Spray waffle maker with coconut oil and spoon approximately 1/4 of the batter into it equally with a spatula.
7. Close your waffle maker and cook until the desired colour is achieved.
8. Carefully remove the waffles to a platter.

For the Ketogenic Maple Syrup:
1. In a small saucepan, bring 1 and 1/4 cups of water, the Swerve, and the maple to a boil over low heat, then reduce to a simmer for approximately 10 minutes.
2. Add the coconut oil.
3. Sprinkle the xanthan gum on top of the waffle and combine with an immersion blender until smooth.
4. Serve and enjoy your delicious waffles!

Nutrition:
Calories: 484
Carbohydrates: 59g
Fiber: 6.45g
Sodium: 457mg

727. PRETZELS

Preparation Time: 10 minutes
Cooking Time: 20 minutes
Servings: 8
Ingredients:
- 1½ cups of pre-shredded mozzarella

- ¾ cup of almond flour + 2 tablespoons of ground almonds or almond meal
- 2 tablespoons of full-fat cream cheese
- 1 large egg
- 1 pinch of coarse sea salt
- ½ teaspoon of baking powder

Directions:
1. Heat your oven to 355°F.
2. Melt the cream cheese and mozzarella cheese together in a small saucepan over low heat, stirring constantly until the cheeses are completely melted.
3. If you want to microwave the cheese, do it for no more than 1 minute, and if you want to do it on the stove, turn off the heat as soon as the cheese is completely melted.
4. Stir the egg into the prepared heated cheese dough until everything is completely blended. You will need to gently warm the egg if it is cold.
5. Stir in the ground almonds or almond flour and the baking powder until everything is thoroughly blended.
6. Toll or stretch one pinch of cheese dough between your hands until it is about 18 to 20 cm in length; if your dough is sticky, you may oil your hands to avoid this.
7. Form pretzels from the cheese dough and shape them properly before placing them on a baking sheet.
8. Bake for about 17 minutes, sprinkled with a pinch of salt.

Nutrition:
Calories: 149
Carbohydrates: 2.8g
Fiber: 1.2g
Sodium: 169.92mg

728. SEED AND NUT SQUARES

Preparation Time: 30 minutes
Cooking Time: 10 minutes
Servings: 10
Ingredients:
- ½ cup of desiccated coconut
- 2 cups of almonds, sunflower seeds, pumpkin seeds, and walnuts
- 1 tablespoon of chia seeds
- 2 tablespoons of coconut oil
- ¼ teaspoon of salt
- 1 teaspoon of vanilla extract
- 3 tablespoons of almond or peanut butter

- ⅓ cup of Sukrin gold fiber syrup

Directions:
1. Line a square baking pan using parchment paper and gently oil it with cooking spray.
2. All of the nuts should be roughly chopped and gently oiled; you may alternatively leave them whole.
3. In a large mixing bowl, combine the nuts; then blend them with the coconut, chia seeds, and salt.
4. In a microwave-safe bowl, combine the coconut oil, vanilla, coconut butter or oil, almond butter, and fibre syrup, and microwave for about 30 seconds.
5. Stir your ingredients thoroughly, then pour the melted mixture directly on top of the nuts.
6. With the back of a measuring cup, press the mixture into the prepared baking tin and push down firmly.
7. Before cutting your dessert, place it in the freezer for about 1 hour.
8. Cut the frozen nut batter into equal-sized chunks or squares.

Nutrition:
Calories: 320.67
Carbohydrates: 17g
Fiber: 11.2g
Sodium: 73.8mg

729. COCONUT SNACK BARS

Preparation Time: 30 minutes
Cooking Time: 0 minutes
Servings: 13
Ingredients:
- 2 cups of coconut flakes
- ¾ cup of melted coconut oil
- 1½ cups of macadamia nuts
- 1 large scoop of vanilla protein powder
- ¼ cup of unsweetened dark chocolate chips

Directions:
1. In a large mixing bowl, mix the coconut flakes, melted coconut oil, macadamia nuts, vanilla protein powder, and dark chocolate chips.
2. Using parchment paper, line an 8x8 baking pan.
3. In a food processor, combine the macadamia nuts and coconut oil until smooth.

4. Pour the batter into a pan and place it in the freezer for about 30 minutes.
5. Cut the frozen batter into bars using a sharp knife.

Nutrition:
Calories: 306.5
Fat: 29g
Protein: 3.2g
Carbs: 11.38g
Sodium: 47.59mg

730. FLAX SEED CRACKERS

Preparation Time: 8 minutes
Cooking Time: 10 minutes
Servings: 25
Ingredients:
- 2½ cups of almond flour
- ½ cup of coconut flour
- 1 teaspoon of ground flaxseed meal
- ½ teaspoon of dried rosemary, chopped
- ½ teaspoon of onion powder
- ¼ teaspoon of kosher salt
- 3 large organic eggs
- 1 tablespoon of extra-virgin olive oil

Directions:
1. Preheat your oven to 325°F.
2. Line a baking sheet with parchment paper.
3. In a large mixing bowl, add the flours, rosemary, flax meal, salt, and onion powder.
4. Crack in the eggs and add the oil; then thoroughly combine your ingredients.
5. Continue mixing for about 1 minute, or until you get the shape of a huge ball.
6. Put the dough between two sheets of parchment paper and roll it out to a 14-inch thickness.
7. Cut the dough into squares and place it on the baking sheet that has been prepared.
8. Bake your dough for 13 to 15 minutes, then set aside to cool for 15 minutes.
9. Serve and enjoy your crackers or store them in a container.

Nutrition:
Calories: 80
Fat: 6.34g
Protein: 3.7g
Carbs: 3.47g
Sodium: 29mg

731. KETO SUGAR-FREE CANDIES

Preparation Time: 30 minutes
Cooking Time: 0 minutes

Servings: 12
Ingredients:
- 4 oz of coconut oil, melted
- 4.5 oz of shredded unsweetened coconut
- 1 teaspoon of Stevia
- 3 oz of erythritol
- 1 large egg white
- 1 teaspoon of vanilla extract
- 3 drops of red food coloring
- ½ teaspoon of strawberry extract

Directions:
1. In a large bowl, mix all together with the erythritol the shredded coconut, the Stevia, and the vanilla with a hand blender on low speed.
2. In a small saucepan over low heat, melt the coconut oil.
3. Mix the oil into the shredded coconut mixture well.
4. Mix in the egg white, then divide half of the mixture into an 8x8 square dish and leave aside.
5. Add the strawberry extract and the food coloring to the mixture and mix very well.
6. Press the mixture right on top of the white mixture into the square dish and set it aside in the fridge for about 1 hour.
7. Cut into 16 pieces after it has completely set.
8. Serve and enjoy!

Nutrition:
Calories: 163.95
Fat: 16.5g
Protein: 1g
Carbs: 10.29g
Sodium: 8.17mg

732. COCONUT FAT BOMBS

Preparation Time: 15 minutes
Cooking Time: 0 minutes
Servings: 14
Ingredients:
- ½ cup of shredded coconut
- 1½ cups of walnuts or any type of nuts of your choice
- ¼ cup of coconut butter + 1 tablespoon of extra coconut butter
- 2 tablespoons of chia seeds
- 2 tablespoons of almond butter
- 2 tablespoons of flax meal
- 2 tablespoons of hemp seeds
- ½ teaspoon of vanilla bean powder
- 1 teaspoon of cinnamon
- ¼ teaspoon of kosher salt

- 2 tablespoons of cacao nibs

For the Chocolate Drizzle:

- 1 oz of unsweetened chocolate, chopped
- ½ teaspoon of coconut oil

Directions:

1. Mix the walnuts with the coconut butter; the chia seeds, the almond butter, the flax meal, the cinnamon, the hemp seeds, the vanilla bean powder, the shredded coconut, and the chopped; then drizzle with the coconut oil in the mixing bowl of your food processor.
2. Pulse your ingredients for 1-2 minutes, or until the mixture begins to break down.
3. Continue to process the mixture until it begins to stay together, but be cautious not to overmix.
4. Add the cacao nibs and pulse until the ingredients are combined.
5. Divide the mixture into equal-sized pieces using a tiny cookie scoop or a tablespoon.
6. With your hands to roll the mixture into balls; then arrange it over a platter.
7. Put the balls in an airtight container or freeze them for about 15 minutes.

Nutrition:
Calories: 230
Fat: 22g
Protein: 5.1g
Carbs: 7.71g
Sodium: 43.28mg

733. NUT AND RASPBERRY BALLS

Preparation Time: 15 minutes
Cooking Time: 0 minutes
Servings: 14
Ingredients:

- ¼ cup of cashew or almond butter
- 1⅓ cups of raw cashews or almonds
- 2 tablespoons of coconut oil
- ½ teaspoon of vanilla extract
- 2 pitted Medjool dates, pre-soaked in hot water for about 10 minutes
- ¼ teaspoon of kosher salt
- ⅓ cup of chopped dark chocolate
- ½ cup of freeze-dried and lightly crushed raspberries

Directions:

1. In a high-powered blender or Vitamix, add the cashews or almonds, butter, coconut oil, Medjool dates, vanilla extract, and salt and process for 1 to 2 minutes, or until the batter begins to stick together.
2. Pulse in the dried raspberries and dark chocolate until you get a thick mixture.
3. Divide the mixture into equal-sized balls using a tablespoon or a tiny cookie scoop.
4. Refrigerate the balls in a jar or zip-top bag for around 2 weeks, or just serve and enjoy your wonderful cashew balls!

Nutrition:
Calories: 155.5
Fat: 11.89g
Protein: 3.17g
Carbs: 11g
Sodium: 36.5mg

734. COCOA AND COCONUT BALLS

Preparation Time: 90 minutes
Cooking Time: 0 minutes
Servings: 9
Ingredients:

- 1 Cup coconut oil, at room temperature
- 1 Cup of almond butter
- ½ Cup of unsweetened cocoa powder
- ⅓ Cup of coconut flour
- ¼ Teaspoon of powdered stevia
- 1/16 teaspoon of pink Himalayan salt

Directions:

1. In a small pot and over medium-high heat, melt the almond butter and combine it with the coconut oil.
2. After adding stir in the coconut flour, cocoa powder, and Himalayan salt.
3. Mix in the stevia again, then set aside to chill.
4. Pour the mixture into a large bowl and transfer it to the freezer to solidify for about 60 to 90 minutes.
5. When the bowl has set, take it from the freezer and roll it into balls.
6. Form the batter into balls and place them on a pan lined with parchment paper.
7. Refrigerate the balls for about 15 minutes.
8. Serve and enjoy your delicious Ketogenic bombs!

Nutrition:

Calories: 411
Fat: 41g
Protein: 7.28g
Carbs: 10.48g
Sodium: 83mg

735. PINE NUT COOKIES

Preparation Time: 10 minutes
Cooking Time: 12 minutes
Servings: 20
Ingredients:

- 1 large egg
- 1 teaspoon of almond extract
- 1 pinch of salt
- 1 cup of Stevia
- 2 cups of super-fine blanched almond flour
- ⅓ cup of pine nuts

Directions:

1. Preheat your oven to 325°F.
2. In a medium mixing bowl, combine the eggs, almond extract, salt, and sweetener.
3. Mix the ingredients in a mixing bowl for about 2 minutes, or until the mixture turns glossy.
4. Add the almond flour and continue to beat until the mixture is frothy.
5. If the dough becomes too dry, add roughly a tablespoon of water until it holds together properly.
6. Arrange the nuts on a small plate.
7. Take a pinch of the dough and roll it into a 1-inch-diameter round.
8. With the side up, press the top of the spherical dough into the nut.
9. Place the cookie on a cookie sheet that has been lined with parchment paper.
10. Repeat with the remaining dough; you should be able to make around 20 cookies.
11. Bake your cookies for 12 minutes at 350°F.
12. Pull the cookies from the oven and set aside for 6 minutes to cool.
13. Serve and enjoy your cookies.

Nutrition:
Calories: 74.28
Fat: 6.44g
Protein: 2.65g
Carbs: 10.95g
Sodium: 13mg

736. PEANUT BUTTER SMOOTHIE WITH BLUEBERRIES

Preparation Time: 12 minutes
Cooking Time: 0 minutes
Servings: 2
Ingredients:

- 2 tablespoons creamy peanut butter
- 1 cup vanilla almond milk (unsweetened)
- 6 oz. soft silken tofu
- ½ cup grape juice
- 1 cup blueberries
- Crushed ice

Directions:

1. Mix all the ingredients in a blender.
2. Process until smooth.

Nutrition:
Calories: 239
Carbohydrates: 26g
Protein: 10.7g
Sodium: 151mg

737. PEACH & APRICOT SMOOTHIE

Preparation Time: 11 minutes
Cooking Time: 0 minutes
Servings: 2
Ingredients:

- 1 cup almond milk (unsweetened)
- 1 teaspoon honey
- ½ cup apricots, sliced
- ½ cup peaches, sliced
- ½ cup carrot, chopped
- 1 teaspoon vanilla extract

Directions:

1. Mix milk and honey.
2. Pour into a blender.
3. Add the apricots, peaches, and carrots.
4. Stir in the vanilla.
5. Blend until smooth.

Nutrition:
Calories: 83
Carbohydrates: 15g
Protein:1.98g
Sodium: 115mg

738. TROPICAL SMOOTHIE

Preparation Time: 8 minutes
Cooking Time: 0 minutes
Servings: 2
Ingredients:

- 1 banana, sliced
- 1 cup mango, sliced
- 1 cup pineapple, sliced
- 1 cup peaches, sliced
- 6 oz. non-fat coconut yogurt

- Pineapple wedges

Directions:

1. Freeze the fruit slices for 1 hour.
2. Transfer to a blender.
3. Stir in the rest of the ingredients except pineapple wedges.
4. Process until smooth.
5. Garnish with pineapple wedges.

Nutrition:
Calories: 299
Carbohydrates: 56g
Protein:5g
Sodium: 37mg

739. BANANA & STRAWBERRY SMOOTHIE

Preparation Time: 7 minutes
Cooking Time: 0 minutes
Servings: 2
Ingredients:

- 1 banana, sliced
- 4 cups fresh strawberries, sliced
- 1 cup ice cubes
- 6 oz. yogurt
- 1 kiwi fruit, sliced

Directions:

1. Add banana, strawberries, ice cubes, and yogurt in a blender.
2. Blend until smooth.
3. Garnish with kiwi fruit slices and serve.

Nutrition:
Calories: 222.39
Carbohydrates: 45.77g
Protein: 6g
Sodium: 44mg

740. CANTALOUPE & PAPAYA SMOOTHIE

Preparation Time: 9 minutes
Cooking Time: 0 minutes
Servings: 2
Ingredients:

- ¾ cup low-fat milk
- ½ cup papaya, chopped
- ½ cup cantaloupe, chopped
- ½ cup mango, cubed
- 4 ice cubes
- Lime zest

Directions:

1. Pour milk into a blender.
2. Add the chopped fruits and ice cubes.
3. Blend until smooth.
4. Garnish with lime zest and serve.

Nutrition:

Calories: 100.4
Carbohydrates: 18.4g
Protein: 3.9g
Sodium: 45.6mg

741. WATERMELON & CANTALOUPE SMOOTHIE

Preparation Time: 10 minutes
Cooking Time: 0 minutes
Servings: 2
Ingredients:

- 2 cups watermelon, sliced
- 1 cup cantaloupe, sliced
- ½ cup nonfat yogurt
- ¼ cup orange juice

Directions:

1. Add all the ingredients to a blender.
2. Blend until creamy and smooth.
3. Chill before serving.

Nutrition:
Calories: 114
Carbohydrates: 23.4g
Sodium: 42mg
Protein:8g

742. RASPBERRY AND PEANUT BUTTER SMOOTHIE

Preparation Time: 10 minutes
Cooking Time: 0 minute
Servings: 2
Ingredients:

- 2 tablespoon peanut butter, smooth and natural
- 2 tablespoon skim milk
- 1 or 1½ cups raspberries, fresh
- 1 cup ice cubes
- 2 teaspoons Stevia

Directions:

1. Combine all the ingredients in your blender. Set the mixer to puree. Serve.

Nutrition:
Calories: 133
Fat: 8.6g
Carbohydrates: 15.12g
Sodium: 75.19mg

743. STRAWBERRY, KALE, AND GINGER SMOOTHIE

Preparation Time: 13 minutes
Cooking Time: 0 minutes
Servings: 2
Ingredients:

- 6 pieces curly kale leaves, fresh and large with stems removed

- 2 teaspoon grated ginger, raw and peeled
- ½ cup cold water
- 3 tablespoons lime juice
- 2 teaspoons honey
- 1 or 1½ cups strawberries, fresh and trimmed
- 1 cup ice cubes

Directions:
1. Combine all the ingredients in your blender. Set to puree. Serve.

Nutrition:
Calories: 205
Fat: 2.9g
Carbohydrates: 42.4g
Sodium: 256mg

744. GREEN DETOX SMOOTHIE

Preparation Time: 10 minutes
Cooking Time: 0 minutes
Servings: 4
Ingredients:
- 2 cups baby spinach
- 2 cups baby kale
- 2 ribs celery, chopped
- 1 medium green apple, chopped
- 1 cup frozen sliced banana
- 1 cup almond milk
- 1 tablespoon grated fresh ginger
- 1 tablespoon chia seeds
- 1 tablespoon honey

Directions:
1. In a blender, combine all of the ingredients and mix until smooth.
2. Serve.

Nutrition:
Calories:136
Fat:2.02g
Carbs:28.9g
Sodium: 75.6mg
Protein:2.48g

745. CUCUMBER GINGER DETOX

Preparation Time: 5 minutes
Cooking Time: 0 minutes
Servings: 2
Ingredients:
- 1½ oz. Spinach
- 1 orange, peeled
- ½ inch ginger, peeled
- 1 cup water
- 1 cucumber, chopped
- ½ avocado, chopped
- 1 cup ice
- 1 teaspoon rosehips

Directions:

1. In a blender, combine all of the ingredients and mix until smooth.
2. Serve.

Nutrition:
Calories: 92
Fat: 4.3g
Carbs: 12.23g
Sodium: 25mg
Protein: 3g

746. GREEN PROTEIN SMOOTHIE

Preparation Time: 5 minutes
Cooking Time: 0 minutes
Servings: 2
Ingredients:
- 1 oz. kale
- 4 oz. pineapple
- 1 tablespoon pea protein
- 1 cup water
- 1 tangerine, peeled
- ½ avocado
- 3 tablespoons almonds
- 1 cup ice

Directions:
1. Except for the almonds, blend everything in the blender.
2. Top with almonds and serve.

Nutrition:
Calories:185
Fat: 12.35g
Protein: 7.38g
Carbs: 15.07g
Sodium: 44.13mg

747. GINGER DETOX TWIST

Preparation Time: 5 minutes
Cooking Time: 0 minutes
Servings: 2
Ingredients:
- 1½ oz. collard greens
- 1 apple, chopped
- ½ inch ginger
- 1 cup water
- 2 Persian cucumbers, chopped
- 1 Meyer lemon, peeled
- ½ teaspoon chlorella
- 1 cup ice

Directions:
1. Blend everything in a blender and serve.

Nutrition:
Calories: 59.46
Fat: 0.24g
Protein: 1.4g
Carbs: 15.55g
Sodium: 10.09mg

748. CLASSIC APPLE DETOX SMOOTHIE

Preparation Time: 5 minutes
Cooking Time: 0 minute
Servings: 2
Ingredients:
- 1½ oz. baby spinach
- 2 oz. celery, chopped
- 1 lemon, juiced
- 1 cup water
- 1 apple, chopped
- 1 mini cucumber, chopped
- ½ inch ginger, peeled and chopped
- 1 cup ice

Directions:
1. Blend everything in a blender and enjoy.

Nutrition:
Calories: 66
Fat: 0.32g
Protein: 1..26g
Carbs: 14.6g
Sodium: 39.39mg

749. ENERGY-BOOSTING GREEN SMOOTHIE

Preparation Time: 15 minutes
Cooking Time: 0 minutes
Servings: 4
Ingredients:
- 2 handfuls of greens
- ½ seeded cucumber
- 1 apple
- 1 burro banana
- ½ teaspoon Bromide Plus Powder
- 1 tablespoon walnuts
- ½ lb. soft jelly coconut milk

Directions:
1. To prepare your green smoothie, mix all the ingredients in a food processor. Pour into a glass and enjoy.

Nutrition:
Calories: 222
Fat: 16.5g
Carbs: 16.66g
Sodium: 9.33mg
Protein: 2.9g

750. ZUCCHINI RELAXING SMOOTHIE

Preparation Time: 15 minutes
Cooking Time: 10 minutes
Servings: 4
Ingredients:
- 1 zucchini, chopped
- 0.2 lb. herbal tea
- ½ lb. soft jelly coconut water

Directions:

1. To make your smoothie, first, brew the tea according to the instructions and let it cool.
2. Combine all ingredients in a blender. Blend well.
3. Pour into serving glasses and enjoy!

Nutrition:
Calories: 18.9
Fat: 0.26g
Carbs: 3.55g
Sodium: 63.48mg
Protein: 1.1g

751. MAGNESIUM-BOOSTING SMOOTHIE

Preparation Time: 10 minutes
Cooking Time: 0 minutes
Servings: 2
Ingredients:
- ½ lb. fresh spring water
- 0.7 lb. Brazil nuts
- ½ burro banana
- 2 strawberries
- ½ lb. figs

Directions:
1. Mix all the ingredients using a high-speed mixer. Enjoy.

Nutrition:
Calories: 182
Fat: 3g
Sodium: 8.37mg
Carbs: 34g
Protein: 2.8g

752. DETOX SMOOTHIE

Preparation Time: 20 minutes
Cooking Time: 0 minutes
Servings: 4
Ingredients:
- ½ avocado
- ½ lb. homemade soft jelly coconut milk
- 1 handful of approved greens, such as callaloo, watercress, or dandelion greens
- 1 squeeze of key lime
- 1 teaspoon of Dr. Sebi's Bromide Plus Powder

Directions:
1. Mix all the ingredients in a high-speed mixer. Fill in more water if the mixture is too concentrated. Enjoy.

Nutrition:
Calories: 155.43
Fat: 15.6g
Protein: 1.7g
Carbs: 4.91g
Sodium: 9.45mg

753. IMMUNITY-BOOSTING SMOOTHIE

Preparation Time: 35 minutes
Cooking Time: 20 minutes
Servings: 2
Ingredients:
- 1 mango
- 1 Seville orange
- ½ lb. brewed Dr. Sebi's Immune Support Herbal Tea
- 1 tablespoon coconut oil
- 1 tablespoon date sugar or agave syrup
- 1 lime, juiced

Directions:
1. Boil distilled water and pour 1 ½ teaspoon of Dr. Sebi's Immune Support Herbal Tea. Cook for about 15 minutes. Let cool, strain. Add Seville orange peel and mango cut into pieces.
2. Mix all ingredients in a high-speed mixer. Add to serving glasses and enjoy!

Nutrition:
Calories:97
Fat: 3.7g
Protein: 9g
Sodium: 3.09mg
Carbs: 30.79g

754. BLUEBERRY AND STRAWBERRY SMOOTHIE

Preparation Time: 5 minutes
Cooking Time: 0 minutes
Servings: 2
Ingredients:
- 6-7 strawberries, sliced
- ½ lb. blueberries
- ½ pint of almond milk

Directions:
1. Add all ingredients to a blender jar. Blend until smooth. Add to serving glasses.
2. Serve and enjoy.

Nutrition:
Calories: 135
Fat: 2.09g
Protein: 1.7g
Carbs: 29g
Sodium: 99.21mg

755. BLUEBERRY AND APPLE SMOOTHIE

Preparation Time: 25 minutes
Cooking Time: 15 minutes
Servings: 4
Ingredients:
- Brae burn apple, or another kind of organic apple
- ½-1 lb. of Brazil nuts

- ½ lb. homemade walnut milk
- ½ lb. blueberries
- ½ lb. of approved greens (dandelion greens, turnip greens, watercress, etc.)
- ½ tablespoon of date sugar or agave syrup

Directions:
1. Combine all the ingredients in a high-speed mixer. Stir more water if the mixture is too concentrated.

Nutrition:
Calories: 466
Fat: 40g
Protein: 10.3g
Carbs: 24.6g
Sodium: 8.56mg

756. BLUEBERRY PIE SMOOTHIE

Preparation Time: 20 minutes
Cooking Time: 0 minutes
Servings: 2
Ingredients:
- 1 oz. fresh blueberries
- 1 burro banana
- 1 glass coconut milk
- ½ lb. cooked amaranth
- 1 teaspoon Bromide Plus Powder
- 1 tablespoon homemade walnut butter
- 1 tablespoon date sugar

Directions:
1. Combine all the ingredients in a high-speed mixer. Fill in more water if too concentrated.

Nutrition:
Calories: 543
Fat: 37.22g
Protein: 9.4g
Carbs: 51.44g
Sodium: 26.9mg

757. CUCUMBER AND CARLEY GREEN SMOOTHIE

Preparation Time: 10 minutes
Cooking Time: 0 minutes
Servings: 4
Ingredients:
- 1 lb. soft jelly coconut water
- 4 seeded cucumbers
- 2-3 key limes
- 1 bunch basil or sweet basil leaves
- ½ teaspoon Bromide Plus Powder

Directions:
1. Mix cucumbers, basil, and lime. If you don't have a juicer,

combine them in a grinder with sweet coconut jelly.

2. Transfer to a tall glass and stir in coconut water to make it smooth and add powdered bromide. Mix well and enjoy.

Nutrition:
Calories: 62.7
Fat:0.6g
Protein: 2.8g
Carbs: 14.6g
Sodium: 124mg

758. FRUITY AND GREEN SMOOTHIE

Preparation Time: 10 minutes
Cooking Time: 0 minute
Servings: 2
Ingredients:
- ½ cup of lettuce
- 1 cup of water
- 3 medium-size bananas
- 2 teaspoons of lime juice
- ½ cup of raspberries
- ¼ teaspoon of ginger

Directions:
1. Mash the banana and blend all ingredients for 30 seconds at a time.
2. Serve in a cup and add some ice cubes or place in a refrigerator.

Nutrition:
Calories: 176.38
Protein: 2.45g
Fiber: 6.7g
Carbs:44.8g
Sodium: 7.19mg

759. BLUEBERRY CRISP

Preparation Time: 10 minutes
Cooking Time: 3-4 hours
Servings: 10
Ingredients:
- ¼ cup unsalted butter, melted
- 24 oz. blueberries, frozen
- ¾ teaspoon salt
- 1 ½ cups rolled oats, coarsely ground
- ¾ cup almond flour, blanched
- ¼ cup coconut oil, melted
- 6 tablespoons Stevia sweetener
- 1 cup pecans or walnuts, coarsely chopped

Directions:
1. Using a non-stick cooking spray, spray the slow cooker pot well.
2. Into a bowl, add ground oats and chopped nuts along with salt, blanched almond flour, brown sugar, Stevia granulated

sweetener, and then stir in the coconut/butter mixture. Stir well to combine.
3. When done, spread crisp topping over blueberries. Cook for 3-4 hours, until the mixture has become bubbling hot, and you can smell the blueberries.
4. Serve while still hot with whipped cream or ice cream if desired. Enjoy!

Nutrition:
Calories: 316
Fat: 22.36g
Total Carbohydrates: 27.92g
Protein: 4 g
Sodium: 176.6mg

760. MAPLE CUSTARD

Preparation Time: 10 minutes
Cooking Time: 2 hours
Servings: 6
Ingredients:
- 1 teaspoon maple extract
- 2 egg yolks
- 1 cup heavy cream
- 2 eggs
- ½ cup whole milk
- ¼ teaspoon salt
- ¼ cup sugar-free brown sugar substitute
- ½ teaspoon cinnamon

Directions:
1. Combine all ingredients together in a blender, process well.
2. Grease 6 ramekins and then pour the batter evenly into each ramekin.
3. To the bottom of the slow cooker, add 4 ramekins and then arrange the remaining 2 against the side of a slow cooker, and not at the top of the bottom ramekins.
4. Close the lid and cook on high for 2 hours, until the center is cooked through, but the middle is still jiggly.
5. Let cool at room temperature for an hour after removing from the slow cooker, and then chill in the fridge for at least 2 hours.
6. Serve and enjoy with a sprinkle of cinnamon and little sugar-free whipped cream.

Nutrition:
Calories: 217
Fat: 17.69g
Total Carbohydrates: 10.5g
Protein: 4g
Sodium: 138mg

761. RASPBERRY CREAM CHEESE COFFEE CAKE

Preparation Time: 10 minutes
Cooking Time: 4 hours
Servings: 12
Ingredients:
- 1¼ cups almond flour
- ⅔ cup water
- ½ cup Swerve
- 3 eggs
- ¼ cup coconut flour
- ¼ cup protein powder
- ¼ teaspoon salt
- ½ teaspoon vanilla extract
- 1½ teaspoons baking powder
- 6 tablespoons unsalted butter, melted

For the Filling:
- 1½ cup fresh raspberries
- 8 oz. cream cheese
- 1 large egg
- ⅓ cup powdered Swerve
- 2 tablespoon whipping cream

Directions:
1. Grease the slow cooker pot. Prepare the cake batter. In a bowl, combine almond flour together with coconut flour, sweetener, baking powder, protein powder, and salt, and then stir in the melted butter along with eggs and water until well combined. Set aside.
2. Prepare the filling. Beat cream cheese thoroughly with the sweetener until have smoothened, and then beat in whipping cream along with the egg and vanilla extract until well combined.
3. Assemble the cake. Spread around ⅔ of batter in the slow cooker as you smoothen the top using a spatula or knife.
4. Pour cream cheese mixture over the batter in the pan, evenly spread it, and then sprinkle with raspberries. Add the rest of the batter over filling.
5. Cook for 3-4 hours on low. Let cool completely.
6. Serve and enjoy!

Nutrition:
Calories: 239
Fat: 19.18 g
Total Carbohydrates: 18.86 g
Protein: 7.5 g
Sodium: 197mg

762. PUMPKIN PIE BARS

Preparation Time: 10 minutes
Cooking Time: 3 hours
Servings: 16
Ingredients:
For the Crust:
- ¾ cup coconut, shredded
- 4 tablespoons butter, unsalted, softened
- ¼ cup cocoa powder, unsweetened
- ¼ teaspoon salt
- ½ cup of raw sunflower seeds or sunflower seed flour
- ¼ cup confectioners Swerve

For the Filling:
- 2 teaspoons cinnamon liquid Stevia
- 1 cup heavy cream
- 1 can pumpkin puree
- 6 eggs
- 1 tablespoon pumpkin pie spice
- ½ teaspoon salt
- 1 tablespoon vanilla extract
- ½ cup sugar-free chocolate chips, optional

Directions:
1. Add all the crust ingredients to a food processor. Then process until fine crumbs are formed.
2. Grease the slow cooker pan well. When done, press crust mixture onto the greased bottom.
3. In a stand mixer, combine all the ingredients for the filling, and then blend well until combined.
4. Top the filling with chocolate chips if using, and then pour the mixture onto the prepared crust.
5. Close the lid and cook for 3 hours on low. Open the lid and let cool for at least 30 minutes, and then place the slow cooker into the refrigerator for at least 3 hours.
6. Slice the pumpkin pie bar and serve it with sugar-free whipped cream. Enjoy!

Nutrition:
Calories: 169
Fat: 15 g
Total Carbohydrates: 6 g
Sodium: 140mg
Protein: 4 g

763. LEMON CUSTARD

Preparation Time: 10 minutes
Cooking Time: 3 hours
Servings: 4
Ingredients:
- 2 cups whipping cream or coconut cream
- 5 egg yolks
- 1 tablespoon lemon zest
- 1 teaspoon vanilla extract
- ¼ cup fresh lemon juice, squeezed
- ½ teaspoon liquid Stevia
- Lightly sweetened whipped cream

Directions:
1. Whisk egg yolks together with lemon zest, liquid Stevia, lemon zest, and vanilla in a bowl, and then whisk in heavy cream.
2. Divide the mixture among 4 small jars or ramekins.
3. To the bottom of a slow cooker add a rack, and then add ramekins on top of the rack and add enough water to cover half of the ramekins.
4. Close the lid and cook for 3 hours on low. Remove ramekins.
5. Let cool to room temperature, and then place into the refrigerator to cool completely for about 3 hours.
6. When through, top with the whipped cream and serve. Enjoy!

Nutrition:
Calories: 497
Fat: 50g
Total Carbohydrates: 6.4g
Protein: 7g
Sodium: 43.8mg

764. BAKED STUFFED PEARS

Preparation Time: 15 minutes
Cooking Time: 35 minutes
Servings: 04
Ingredients:
- 4 tablespoons agave syrup
- ¼ teaspoon cloves
- 4 tablespoon chopped walnuts
- 1 cup currants
- 4 pears

Directions:
1. Make sure your oven has been warmed to 375°F.
2. Slice the pears in 2 lengthwise and remove the core. To get the pear to lay flat, you can slice a small piece off the backside.
3. Place the agave syrup, currants, walnuts, and cloves in a small bowl and mix well. Set this to the side to be used later.
4. Put the pears on a cookie sheet that has parchment paper on it. Make sure the cored sides are facing up. Sprinkle each pear half with about ½ tablespoon of the chopped walnut mixture.
5. Place into the oven and cook for 25 to 30 minutes. Pears should be tender.

Nutrition:
Calories: 210.29
Fiber: 4.8g
Carbohydrates: 41.87g
Sodium: 3.24mg

765. BUTTERNUT SQUASH PIE

Preparation Time: 25 minutes
Cooking Time: 35 minutes
Servings: 4
Ingredients:
For the Crust:
- Cold water
- Agave, splash
- Sea salt, pinch
- 1/4 cup grapeseed oil
- 1 cup coconut flour
- 1 cup spelt flour

For the Filling:
- Butternut squash, peeled, chopped
- Water
- Allspice, to taste
- Agave syrup, to taste
- 1 cup hemp milk
- 4 tablespoons sea moss

Directions:
1. You will need to warm your oven to 350°F.
2. For the Crust: Place the grapeseed oil and water into the refrigerator to get it cold. This will take about one hour.
3. Place all ingredients into a large bowl. Now you need to add in the cold water a little bit in small amounts until a dough forms. Place this onto a surface that has been sprinkled with some coconut flour. Knead for a few minutes and roll the dough as thin as you can get it. Carefully, pick it up and place it inside a pie plate.
4. Place the butternut squash into a Dutch oven and pour in enough water to cover. Bring

this to a full rolling boil. Let this cook until the squash has become soft.

5. Completely drain and place in a bowl. Using a potato masher, mash the squash. Add in some allspice and agave to taste. Add in the sea moss and hemp milk. Using a hand mixer, blend well. Pour into the pie crust.

6. Place into an oven and bake for about one hour.

Nutrition:
Calories: 441.21
Carbohydrates: 55g
Fat: 20g
Sodium: 88.71mg

766. COCONUT CHIA CREAM POT

Preparation Time: 5 minutes
Cooking Time: 5 minutes
Servings: 4
Ingredients:
- 1 date
- 1 cup coconut milk (organic)
- 1 cup coconut yogurt
- ½ teaspoon vanilla extract
- ¼ cup chia seeds
- 1 teaspoon sesame seeds
- 1 tablespoon flaxseed (ground) or flax meal

Toppings:
- 1 fig
- 1 handful blueberries
- Mixed nuts (Brazil nuts, almonds, pistachios, macadamia, etc.)
- 1 teaspoon cinnamon (ground)

Directions:
1. First, blend the date with coconut milk (the idea is to sweeten the coconut milk).
2. Get a mixing bowl and add the coconut milk with the vanilla, sesame seeds, chia seeds, and flax meal.
3. Refrigerate for between twenty to thirty minutes or wait till the chia expands.
4. To serve, pour a layer of coconut yogurt in a small glass, then add the chia mix, followed by pouring another layer of coconut yogurt.
5. It's alkaline, creamy, and delicious.

Nutrition:
Calories: 364
Carbohydrates: 25.9g
Protein: 7.11g
Sodium: 59mg
Fiber: 8.1g

767. CHOCOLATE AVOCADO MOUSSE

Preparation Time: 10 minutes
Cooking Time: 5 minutes
Servings: 04
Ingredients:
- ⅔ cup coconut water
- ½ Hass avocado
- 2 teaspoon raw cacao
- 1 teaspoon vanilla
- 3 dates
- 1 teaspoon sea salt
- Dark chocolate shavings

Directions:
1. Blend all ingredients.
2. Blast until it becomes thick and smooth, as you wish.
3. Put in a fridge and allow it to get firm.

Nutrition:
Calories: 109.1
Fat: 3.9g
Protein: 1.4g
Carbs: 18.6g
Sodium: 518.68mg

768. CHIA VANILLA COCONUT PUDDING

Preparation Time: 5 minutes
Cooking Time: 5 minutes
Servings: 2
Ingredients:
- 2 tablespoon coconut oil
- ½ cup raw cashews
- ½ cup coconut water
- 1 teaspoon cinnamon
- 3 dates (pitted)
- 2 teaspoon vanilla
- 1 teaspoon coconut flakes (unsweetened)
- Salt (Himalayan or Celtic grey)
- 6 tablespoon chia seeds
- Cinnamon or pomegranate seeds for garnish (optional)

Directions:
1. Get a blender, add all the ingredients (minus the pomegranate and chia seeds), and blend for about forty to sixty seconds.
2. Reduce the blender speed to the lowest and add the chia seeds.
3. Pour the content into an airtight container and put it in a refrigerator for five to six hours.
4. To serve, you can garnish with the cinnamon powder of pomegranate seeds.

Nutrition:
Calories: 622
Fat: 41.42g
Sodium: 462mg
Carbs: 58.1g

769. SWEET TAHINI DIP WITH GINGER CINNAMON FRUIT

Preparation Time: 10 minutes
Cooking Time: 5 minutes
Servings: 2
Ingredients:
- 1 teaspoon cinnamon
- 1 green apple
- 1 pear
- 2-3 fresh ginger root
- 1 teaspoon Celtic sea salt

Ingredients for sweet tahini:
- 3 teaspoons almond butter (raw)
- 3 teaspoons tahini (one big scoop)
- 2 teaspoons coconut oil
- ¼ teaspoon cayenne (optional)
- 2 teaspoons wheat-free tamari
- 1 teaspoon liquid coconut nectar

Directions:
1. Get a clean mixing bowl.
2. Grate the ginger, add cinnamon, sea salt and mix together in the bowl.
3. Dice apple and pear into little cubes, turn into the bowl, and mix.
4. Get a mixing bowl and mix all the ingredients.
5. Sprinkle the sweet tahini dip all over the ginger cinnamon fruit.
6. Serve.

Nutrition:
Calories: 313.37
Fat: 15g
Sodium: 1314mg
Carbs: 42.8g

770. COCONUT BUTTER AND CHOPPED BERRIES WITH MINT

Preparation Time: 5 minutes
Cooking Time: 5 minutes
Servings: 4
Ingredients:
- 1 tablespoon chopped mint
- 2 tablespoon coconut butter (melted)
- Mixed berries (strawberries, blueberries, and raspberries)

Directions:
1. Get a small bowl and add the berries.
2. Drizzle the melted coconut butter and sprinkle the mint.
3. Serve.

Nutrition:
Calories: 58.82
Fat: 5g
Carbohydrates: 2.59g

Sodium: 2.63mg

771. ALKALINE RAW PUMPKIN PIE

Preparation Time: 5 minutes
Cooking Time: 5 minutes
Servings: 4
Ingredients:
For the Pie Crust:
- 1 teaspoon cinnamon
- 1 cup dates/Turkish apricots
- 1 cup raw almonds
- 1 cup coconut flakes (unsweetened)

For the Pie Filling:
- 6 dates
- ½ teaspoon cinnamon
- ½ teaspoon nutmeg
- 1 cup pecans (soaked overnight)
- 1¼ cup organic pumpkin blends (12 oz.)
- ½ teaspoon nutmeg
- ¼ teaspoon of sea salt (Himalayan or Celtic sea salt)
- 1 teaspoon vanilla
- Gluten-free tamari

Directions:
For the Pie Crust:
1. Get a food processor and blend all the pie crust Ingredients at the same time.
2. Make sure the mixture turns oily and sticky before you stop mixing.
3. Put the mixture in a pie pan and mold it against the sides and floor, to make it stick properly.

For the Pie Filling:
1. Mix ingredients together in a blender.
2. Add the mixture to fill in the pie crust.
3. Pour some cinnamon on top.
4. Then refrigerate till it's cold.
5. Then mold.

Nutrition:
Calories: 865
TotalFat: 59.97
Carbs: 79.26g
Cholesterol: 0mg
Sodium: 381.34mg

772. STRAWBERRY SORBET

Preparation Time: 5 minutes
Cooking Time: 4 hours
Servings: 4
Ingredients:
- 2 cups of strawberries
- 1½ teaspoon of spelt flour
- ½ cup of date sugar
- 2 cups of spring water

Directions:
1. Add date sugar, spring water, and spelt flour to a medium pot and boil on low heat for about ten minutes. The mixture should thicken, like syrup.
2. Allow the pot to cool after removing it from the heat.
3. After cooling, add strawberries and mix gently.
4. Put the mixture in a container and freeze.
5. Cut it into pieces, put the sorbet into a processor, and blend until smooth.
6. Put everything back in the container and leave it in the refrigerator for at least 4 hours.
7. Serve and enjoy your Strawberry Sorbet!

Nutrition:
Calories: 117.87
Carbohydrates: 30.58g
Fat: 0.25g
Sodium: 3.17mg

773. BLUEBERRY MUFFINS

Preparation Time: 5 minutes
Cooking Time: 1 hour
Servings: 3
Ingredients:
- ½ cup of blueberries
- ¾ cup of teff flour
- ¾ cup of spelt flour
- ⅓ cup of agave syrup
- ½ teaspoon of pure sea salt
- 1 cup of coconut milk
- ¼ cup of sea moss gel (optional)
- Grapeseed oil

Directions:
1. Preheat your oven to 365°F.
2. Grease or line 6 standard muffin cups.
3. Add teff, spelt flour, pure sea salt, coconut milk, sea moss gel, and agave syrup to a large bowl. Mix them together.
4. Add blueberries to the mixture and mix well.
5. Divide muffin batter among the 6 muffin cups.
6. Bake for 30 minutes until golden brown.
7. Serve and enjoy your blueberry muffins!

Nutrition:
Calories: 565
Fat: 25g
Carbohydrates: 78g
Protein: 10.44g
Fiber: 9.8g
Sodium: 337mg

774. BANANA STRAWBERRY ICE CREAM

Preparation Time: 5 minutes
Cooking Time: 4 Hours
Servings: 5
Ingredients:
- 1 cup of strawberries
- 5 quartered baby bananas
- ½ avocado, chopped
- 1 tablespoon of agave syrup
- ¼ cup of homemade walnut milk

Directions:
1. Mix ingredients into the blender and blend them well.
2. Taste. If it is too thick, add extra milk or agave syrup if you want it sweeter.
3. Put in a container with a lid and allow to freeze for at least 5 to 6 hours.
4. Serve it and enjoy your banana strawberry ice cream!

Nutrition:
Calories: 85
Fat: 2.23g
Carbohydrates: 17.24g
Sodium: 3mg

775. HOMEMADE WHIPPED CREAM

Preparation Time: 5 minutes
Cooking Time: 10 minutes
Servings: 1 cup
Ingredients:
- 1 cup of aquafaba
- ¼ cup of agave syrup

Directions:
1. Add agave syrup and aquafaba into a bowl.
2. Mix at high speed around 5 minutes with a stand mixer or 10 to 15 minutes with a hand mixer.
3. Serve and enjoy your homemade whipped cream!

Nutrition:
Calories: 299
Sodium: 10.51g
Carbohydrates: 5.3g
Sugar: 4.7g

776. CHOCOLATE CRUNCH BARS

Preparation Time: 5 minutes
Cooking Time: 5 minutes
Servings: 4
Ingredients:
- 1½ cups sugar-free chocolate chips
- 1 cup almond butter
- Stevia to taste
- ¼ cup coconut oil

- 3 cups pecans, chopped

Directions:
1. Layer an 8-inch baking pan with parchment paper.
2. Mix chocolate chips with butter, coconut oil, and sweetener in a bowl.
3. Melt it by heating in a microwave for 2 to 3 minutes until well mixed.
4. Stir in nuts and seeds. Mix gently.
5. Pour this batter carefully into the baking pan and spread evenly.
6. Refrigerate for 2 to 3 hours.
7. Slice and serve.

Nutrition:
Calories: 316
Total Fat: 30.9g
Saturated Fat: 8.1g
Total Carbohydrates: 8.3g
Sugar 1.8g
Fiber: 3.8g
Sodium: 8mg
Protein: 6.4g

777. HOMEMADE PROTEIN BAR

Preparation Time: 5 minutes
Cooking Time: 10 minutes
Servings: 4
Ingredients:
- 1 cup nut butter
- 4 tablespoons coconut oil
- 2 scoops vanilla protein
- Stevia, to taste
- ½ teaspoon sea salt

Optional Ingredient:
- 1 teaspoon cinnamon

Directions:
1. Mix coconut oil with butter, protein, stevia, and salt in a dish.
2. Stir in cinnamon and chocolate chip.
3. Press the mixture firmly and freeze until firm.
4. Cut the crust into small bars.
5. Serve and enjoy.

Nutrition:
Calories: 179
Total Fat: 15.7g
Saturated Fat: 8g
Total Carbohydrates: 4.8g
Sugar 3.6g
Fiber: 0.8g
Sodium: 43mg
Protein: 5.6g

778. SHORTBREAD COOKIES

Preparation Time: 10 minutes
Cooking Time: 70 minutes

Servings: 6
Ingredients:
- 2½ cups almond flour
- 6 tablespoons nut butter
- ½ cup erythritol
- 1 teaspoon vanilla extract

Directions:
1. Preheat your oven to 350°F.
2. Layer a cookie sheet with parchment paper.
3. Beat butter with erythritol until fluffy.
4. Stir in vanilla extract and almond flour. Mix well until becomes crumbly.
5. Spoon out a tablespoon of cookie dough onto the cookie sheet.
6. Add more dough to make as many cookies as possible.
7. Bake for 15 minutes until brown.
8. Serve.

Nutrition:
Calories: 288
Total Fat: 25.3g
Saturated Fat: 6.7g
Cholesterol: 23mg
Total Carbohydrates: 9.6g
Sugar 0.1g
Fiber: 3.8g
Sodium: 74mg
Potassium: 3mg
Protein: 7.6g

779. COCONUT CHIP COOKIES

Preparation Time: 10 minutes
Cooking Time: 15 minutes
Servings: 4
Ingredients:
- 1 cup almond flour
- ½ cup cacao nibs
- ½ cup coconut flakes, unsweetened
- ⅓ cup erythritol
- ½ cup almond butter
- ¼ cup nut butter, melted
- ¼ cup almond milk
- Stevia, to taste
- ¼ teaspoon sea salt

Directions:
1. Preheat your oven to 350°F.
2. Layer a cookie sheet with parchment paper.
3. Add and then combine all the dry ingredients in a glass bowl.
4. Whisk in butter, almond milk, vanilla essence, stevia, and almond butter.
5. Beat well then stir in dry mixture. Mix well.

6. Spoon out a tablespoon of cookie dough on the cookie sheet.
7. Add more dough to make as many as 16 cookies.
8. Flatten each cookie using your fingers.
9. Bake for 25 minutes until golden brown.
10. Let them sit for 15 minutes.
11. Serve.

Nutrition:
Calories: 192
Total Fat: 17.44g
Saturated Fat: 11.5g
Cholesterol: 125mg
Total Carbohydrates: 2.2g
Sugar 1.4g
Fiber: 2.1g
Sodium: 135mg
Protein: 4.7g

780. PEANUT BUTTER BARS

Preparation Time: 10 minutes
Cooking Time: 10 minutes
Servings: 6
Ingredients:
- ¾ cup almond flour
- 2 oz. almond butter
- ¼ cup Swerve
- ½ cup peanut butter
- ½ teaspoon vanilla

Directions:
1. Combine all the ingredients for bars.
2. Transfer this mixture to a 6-inch small pan. Press it firmly.
3. Refrigerate for 30 minutes.
4. Slice and serve.

Nutrition:
Calories: 214
Total Fat: 19g
Saturated Fat: 5.8g
Cholesterol: 15mg
Total Carbohydrates: 6.5g
Sugar 1.9g
Fiber: 2.1g
Sodium: 123mg
Protein: 6.5g

781. ZUCCHINI BREAD PANCAKES

Preparation Time: 15 minutes
Cooking Time: 35 minutes
Servings: 12
Ingredients:
- 1 tablespoon grapeseed oil
- 5 cups chopped walnuts
- 2 cups walnut milk
- 1 cup shredded zucchini
- ¼ cups mashed burro banana
- 2 tablespoon date sugar
- 2 cups kamut flour or spelt

Directions:

1. Place the date sugar and flour into a bowl. Whisk together.
2. Add in the mashed banana and walnut milk. Stir until combined. Remember to scrape the bowl to get all the dry mixture. Add in walnuts and zucchini. Stir well until combined.
3. Place the grapeseed oil onto a griddle and warm.
4. Pour ¼ cup batter on the hot griddle. Leave it along until bubbles begin forming on to surface. Carefully turn over the pancake and cook another 4 minutes until cooked through.
5. Place the pancakes onto a serving plate and enjoy with some agave syrup.

Nutrition:
Calories: 440
Carbohydrates: 25g
Fiber: 4.6g
Protein: 7.8g

782. BANANA NUT MUFFINS

Preparation Time: 5 minutes
Cooking Time: 1 hour
Servings: 6
Ingredients:
Dry Ingredients:

- 1½ cups of spelt or teff flour
- ½ teaspoon of pure sea salt
- ¾ cup of date syrup

Wet Ingredients:

- 2 medium-blend burro bananas
- ¼ cup of grapeseed oil
- ¾ cup of walnut milk
- 1 tablespoon of key lime juice

For the Filling:

- ½ cup of chopped walnuts (plus extra for decorating)
- 1 chopped burro banana

Directions:

1. Preheat your oven to 400°F.
2. Take a muffin tray and grease 12 cups or line with cupcake liners.
3. Put all dry ingredients in a large bowl and mix them thoroughly.
4. Add all wet ingredients to a separate, smaller bowl and mix well with bananas.
5. Mix ingredients from the 2 bowls in one large container. Be careful not to over mix.
6. Add the filling ingredients and fold in gently.
7. Pour muffin batter into the 12 prepared muffin cups and

garnish with a couple of Walnuts.

8. Bake it for 22 to 26 minutes until golden brown.
9. Allow to cool for 10 minutes.
10. Serve and enjoy your banana nut muffins!

Nutrition:
Calories: 429.8
Fat: 17.59g
Carbohydrates: 64.29g
Protein: 7.1g
Fiber: 5.81g
Sodium: 181.74mg

783. MANGO NUT CHEESECAKE

Cooking Time: 4 hours 30 minutes
Servings: 8
Ingredients:
For the Filling:

- 2 cups of Brazil nuts
- 5 to 6 dates
- 1 tablespoon of sea moss gel
- ¼ cup of agave syrup
- ¼ teaspoon of pure sea salt
- 2 tablespoons of lime juice
- 1½ cups of walnut milk

For the Crust:

- 1½ cups of quartered dates
- ¼ cup of agave syrup
- 1½ cups of coconut flakes
- ¼ teaspoon of pure sea salt

For the Toppings:

- Sliced mango
- Sliced strawberries

Directions:

1. Put all crust ingredients, in a food processor and blend for 30 seconds.
2. With parchment paper, cover a baking form and spread out the blended crust Ingredients.
3. Put sliced mango across the crust and freeze for 10 minutes.
4. Mix all filling ingredients, using a blender until it becomes smooth
5. Pour the filling above the crust, cover with foil or parchment paper and let it stand for about 3 to 4 hours in the refrigerator.
6. Take out from the baking form and garnish with toppings.
7. Serve and enjoy your mango nut cheesecake!

Nutrition:
Calories: 463.24
Fat: 27.9g
Carbohydrates: 54.6g
Protein: 6.4g
Fiber: 7.16g
Sodium: 111.47mg

784. BLACKBERRY JAM

Preparation Time: 5 minutes
Cooking Time: 4 hours 30 minutes
Servings: 1 cup
Ingredients:

- ¾ cup of blackberries
- 1 tablespoon of key lime juice
- 3 tablespoons of agave syrup
- ¼ cup of sea moss gel + extra 2 tablespoons

Directions:

1. Put rinsed blackberries into a medium pot and cook on medium heat.
2. Stir blackberries until liquid appears.
3. Once berries soften, use your immersion blender to chop up any large pieces. If you don't have a blender, put the mixture in a food processor, mix it well, then return to the pot.
4. Add sea moss gel, key lime juice, and agave syrup to the blended mixture. Boil on medium heat and stir well until it becomes thick.
5. Remove from the heat and leave it to cool for 10 minutes.
6. Serve it with bread pieces or flatbread.
7. Enjoy your blackberry jam!

Nutrition:
Calories: 240
Fat: 0.8g
Carbohydrates: 58g
Sodium: 3.7mg

785. BLACKBERRY BARS

Preparation Time: 5 minutes
Cooking Time: 1 hour 20 minutes
Servings: 6
Ingredients:

- 3 burro bananas or 4 baby bananas
- 1 cup of spelt flour
- 2 cups of quinoa flakes
- ¼ cup of agave \syrup
- ¼ teaspoon of pure sea salt
- ½ cup of grapeseed oil
- 1 cup of prepared blackberry jam

Directions:

1. Preheat your oven to 350°F.
2. Remove the skin of bananas and mash with a fork in a large bowl.
3. Combine agave syrup and grapeseed oil with the blend and mix well.

4. Add spelt flour and quinoa flakes. Knead the dough until it becomes sticky to your fingers.
5. Cover a 9x9-inch baking pan with parchment paper.
6. Take ⅔ of the dough and smooth it out over the parchment pan with your fingers.
7. Spread blackberry jam over the dough.
8. Crumble the remaining dough and sprinkle on the top.
9. Bake for 20 minutes.
10. Remove from the oven and let it cool for 10 to 15 minutes.
11. Cut into small pieces.
12. Serve and enjoy your Blackberry Bars!

Nutrition:
Calories: 611
Fat: 21.3g
Carbohydrates: 98g
Protein: 8.4g
Fiber: 7.14g
Sodium: 99mg

786. DETOX BERRY SMOOTHIE

Preparation Time: 15 minutes
Cooking Time: 0
Servings: 1
Ingredients:
- 1 Cup of Spring water
- ¼ avocado pitted
- One medium burro banana
- One Seville orange
- 2 cups of fresh lettuce
- 1 tablespoon of hemp seeds
- 1 cup of berries (blueberries or an aggregate of blueberries, strawberries, and raspberries)

Directions:
1. Add the spring water to your blender.
2. Put the fruits and veggies right inside the blender.
3. Blend all ingredients till smooth.

Nutrition:
Calories: 294.29
Fat: 9.88g
Carbohydrates: 52.9g
Protein: 7.3g
Sodium: 30.91mg

787. RASPBERRY CAKE WITH WHITE CHOCOLATE SAUCE

Preparation Time: 15 minutes

Cooking Time: 60 minutes
Servings: 5-6
Ingredients:
- 5 ounces of melted cacao butter
- 2 ounces of grass-fed ghee
- ½ cup of coconut cream
- 1 cup of green banana flour
- 3 teaspoons of pure vanilla
- 4 large eggs
- ½ cup of Lakanto monk fruit
- 1 teaspoon of baking powder
- 2 teaspoons of apple cider vinegar
- 2 cups of raspberries

For the White Chocolate Sauce:
- 3½ ounces of cacao butter
- ½ cup of coconut cream
- 2 teaspoons of pure vanilla extract
- 1 pinch of salt

Directions:
1. Preheat your oven to 280°F.
2. Mix together the green banana flour, pure vanilla extract, baking powder, coconut cream, eggs, cider vinegar, and monk fruit until thoroughly combined.
3. Set aside the raspberries and line a cake loaf pan with parchment paper.
4. Spread the raspberries over the top of the cake after pouring the mixture into the baking tray.
5. Place the tray in the oven for about 60 minutes; in the meantime, make the sauce.

For the Sauce:
6. In a saucepan over low heat, combine the coconut cream, vanilla extract, cacao butter, and salt.
7. With a fork, combine all of the ingredients, making sure the cacao butter is properly combined with the cream.
8. Remove from the fire and set aside to cool slightly but not solidify.
9. Drizzle with the chocolate sauce.
10. Scatter the cake with more raspberries.
11. Serve and enjoy your cake once it has been sliced.

Nutrition:
Calories: 644
Fat: 56g
Carbohydrates: 47g
Fiber: 4.34g
Protein: 5.56g

Sodium: 161.57mg

788. WALNUT-FRUIT CAKE

Preparation Time: 15 minutes
Cooking Time: 20 minutes
Servings: 6
Ingredients:
- ½ cup of almond butter (softened)
- ¼ cup of granulated erythritol
- 1 tablespoon of ground cinnamon
- ½ teaspoon of ground nutmeg
- ¼ teaspoon of ground cloves
- 4 large eggs
- 1 teaspoon of vanilla extract
- ½ teaspoon of almond extract
- 2 cups of almond flour
- ½ cup of chopped walnuts
- ¼ cup of dried unsweetened cranberries
- ¼ cup of seedless raisins

Directions:
1. Preheat the oven to 350°F and grease an 8-inch circular baking pan with coconut oil.
2. Beat the granulated erythritol at a high speed until it becomes fluffy.
3. Blend in the cinnamon, nutmeg, and cloves until the mixture is smooth.
4. Crack in the eggs and beat them in well, one at a time, along with the almond extract and vanilla extract.
5. Whisk in the almond flour until the batter is smooth, then fold in the nuts and fruit.
6. Spread the mixture into the prepared baking sheet and bake for 20 minutes.
7. Remove the cake from the oven and set aside for 5 minutes to cool.
8. Dust the cake with powdered erythritol.
9. Serve and enjoy your cake!

Nutrition:
Calories: 469
Fat: 137.74g
Carbohydrates: 30g
Fiber: 8.79g
Protein: 17.45g
Sodium: 95.35mg

6 WEEK MEAL PLAN

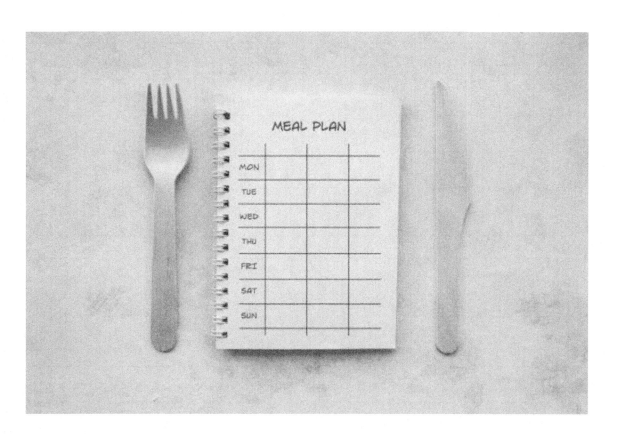

WEEK 1

Day	Breakfast	Lunch	Dinner	Dessert
1	Blueberry Breakfast Cake	Vegetarian Club Salad	Beef Steak Fajitas	Pine Nut Cookies
2	Berry-Oat Breakfast Bars	Pita Pizza	Chickpeas & Veggie Stew	Nut and Raspberry Balls
3	Turkey Meatballs	Lemon Garlic Shrimp Pasta	Spicy Turkey Tacos	Keto Sugar-Free Candies
4	Breakfast Bowl of Yogurt	Egg Salad Stuffed Avocado	Quick and Easy Shrimp Stir-Fry	Cheesy Taco Bites
5	Yogurt and Kale Smoothie	Smoky Carrot & Black Bean Stew	Nori Burritos	Coconut Fat Bombs
6	Basil and Tomato Baked Eggs	Corn Tortillas & Spinach Salad	Rosemary Chicken	Seed and Nut Squares
7	Crispy Pita With Canadian Bacon	Chicken Thighs	Air Fryer Meatloaf	Cinnamon Cake

WEEK 2

Day	Breakfast	Lunch	Dinner	Dessert
1	Coconut and Berry Smoothie	Fettuccine Chicken Alfredo	Dijon Salmon	Waffles
2	Buckwheat Crêpes	Beef Pizza	Zucchini Herb	""Oreo"" Cookies with Cream Cheese Filling
3	Banana Barley Porridge	Bell Pepper Basil Pizza	Veggie Burgers	Cinnamon and Ginger Cake
4	Tomato Waffles	Nacho Steak in the Skillet	Spinach Curry	Keto Donuts
5	Healthy Baked Eggs	Portobello Bun Cheeseburgers	Pork Rind Nachos	Ketogenic Cheesecake
6	Greek Yogurt and Oat Pancakes	Balsamic Beef Pot Roast	Air Fryer Hamburgers	Lemon Cake
7	Spinach And Cheese Quiche	Cumin Spiced Beef Wraps	Air-Fried Beef Schnitzel	Walnut-Fruit Cake

WEEK 3

Day	Breakfast	Lunch	Dinner	Dessert
1	Keto Salad	Barbecue Brisket	Homestyle Herb Meatballs	Madeleine
2	Niçoise Salad Tuna	Roasted Carrot and Leek Soup	Orange-Marinated Pork Tenderloin	Fruit Cake with Walnuts
3	Greek-Style Yogurt	Lemon-Tarragon Soup	Chipotle Chili Pork Chops	Tropical Smoothie
4	Shrimp and Grits Cajun-Style	Beef Goulash	Pork Chop Diane	Ginger Detox Twist
5	Blackberry-Mango Shake	Chicken Cordon Bleu	Mediterranean Steak Sandwiches	Cantaloupe & Papaya Smoothie
6	Whole Grain Breakfast Cookies	Cajun Beef & Rice Skillet	Chicken with Creamy Thyme Sauce	Raspberry Smoothie
7	Buckwheat Grouts Breakfast Bowl	Thai Pork Salad	Almond-Crusted Salmon	Peanut Butter Smoothie with Blueberries

WEEK 4

Day	Breakfast	Lunch	Dinner	Dessert
1	Bulgur Porridge Breakfast	Pasta Salad	Beef & Asparagus	Butternut Squash Pie
2	Cheesy Low-Carb Omelet	Courgettes In Cider Sauce	Roasted Pork & Apples	Chocolate Crunch Bars
3	Coconut and Berry Oatmeal	Zucchini Noodles with Portabella Mushrooms	Coffee-and-Herb-Marinated Steak	Shortbread Cookies
4	Avocado Lemon Toast	Lemony Salmon Burgers	Rosemary Lamb	Coconut Chip Cookies
5	Tofu and Vegetable Scramble	Grilled Tempeh with Pineapple	Stuffed Mushrooms	Homemade Whipped Cream
6	Chia and Coconut Pudding	Lighter Shrimp Scampi	Easy Egg Salad	Baked Stuffed Pears
7	Mushroom Frittata	Lighter Eggplant Parmesan	Greek Broccoli Salad	Homemade Protein Bar

WEEK 5

Day	Breakfast	Lunch	Dinner	Dessert
1		Brunswick Stew	Spicy Chicken Cacciatore	Keto Orange Cake
2	Banana Crêpe Cakes	Chicken Vera Cruz	Veggies Casserole	Cocoa Mousse
3	Tacos with Pico De Gallo	Roasted Pork & Apples	Sweet & Spicy Chickpeas	Green Smoothie
4	Spicy Jalapeño Popper Deviled Eggs	Tomato and Guaca Salad	Italian Pork Chops	Banana & Strawberry Smoothie
5	Salty Macadamia Chocolate Smoothie	Chicken Tortilla Soup	Mushrooms with Bell Peppers	Crackers
6	Whole-Grain Dutch Baby Pancake	Gazpacho	Ginger Citrus Chicken Thighs	Pretzels
7	Banana Smoothie for Breakfast	Carnitas Tacos	Coffee-and-Herb-Marinated Steak	Cake with Whipped Cream Icing

WEEK 6

Day	Breakfast	Lunch	Dinner	Dessert
1	Instant Pot Chicken Chili	Spiced Okra	Baked Chicken Legs	Chocolate Avocado Mousse
2	Cheese Yogurt	Millet Pilaf	Barbecue Beef Brisket	Lemon Custard
3	Muffins of Savory Egg	Coconut-Lentil Curry	Sesame Pork with Mustard Sauce	Blueberry Muffins
4	Peach and Pancakes with Blueberry	Sweet and Sour Onions	Pork with Cranberry Relish	Peanut Butter Bars
5	Lox, Eggs, and Onion Scramble	Maple-Mustard Salmon	Chicken and Roasted Vegetable Wraps	Blackberry Bars
6	Tex-Mex Migas	Cauliflower Rice with Chicken	Chipotle Chili Pork Chops	Detox Berry Smoothie
7	Rolls with Spinach	Spinach Curry	Pork Chop Diane	Walnut-Fruit Cake

CONCLUSION

A healthy diet may be the best medicine for diabetes. In fact, a diabetic diet, which is really just a healthy diet with good portion control, can help you achieve more than just blood sugar control. Among the advantages are reduced risks of serious health conditions such as heart disease and cancer.

Eating a well-balanced diet is essential for overall health and lowering your risk of other health problems. Other advantages of a diabetic diet include maintaining a normal blood sugar level in your body, reducing the amount of medication your body requires, preventing blood sugar levels from becoming too low or too high, assisting you in controlling weight, and increasing your metabolism to better manage food processing.

Putting together the perfect diabetic diet meal isn't difficult, but it can be challenging at first. While you may have to get used to cooking for yourself and your loved ones and not always relying on fast-food chains, you will reap the benefits of living a healthy lifestyle in the end.

This cookbook includes comprehensive step-by-step methods for preparing a variety of meals. We truly have it all: breakfast, lunch, dinner, sides, salads, soups and stews, seafood, vegetarian meals, snacks, and desserts. This book is perfect for beginners who want to try out a diabetic diet and learn how to cook at home. With this cookbook, we are sure you will be able to enjoy a healthy lifestyle. It includes simple recipes for all meal types that are described in a way that is easy to understand. Any beginner can easily prepare the recipes without any challenges.

As we near the end of this cookbook, we hope you've come to appreciate the beauty that comes with healthy living. We included 800+ recipes in this cookbook to demonstrate that having diabetes does not require you to eat only boring, healthy foods. While you may be hesitant to try this diet at first, I am confident that you will grow accustomed to it and come to appreciate it along the way. We hope that you and your family enjoy all of the recipes within this cookbook.

Diabetes is not something that should limit your life, especially the food you eat. Food is such an important aspect of life, and we should not be limited to bland flavors just because of something we cannot control. There are many delicious meals available to you; all you need to do is learn how to put them together.

To take it a step further, we highly recommend that you try out the included meal plan as well, as it can be really helpful in your journey. Learning a new way to eat might be difficult, but it is feasible. To put the diet into action, all you need is motivation and willpower. Not only your body will thank you for taking care of it, but it will also reward you by making you feel more energized and prepared throughout the day.

INDEX OF RECIPES

Printed in Great Britain
by Amazon